ADVANCES IN SURGICAL PATHOLOGY

# COLORECTAL CARCINOMA AND TUMORS OF THE VERMIFORM APPENDIX

## ADVANCES IN SURGICAL PATHOLOGY SERIES

**Series Editors: Philip T. Cagle, MD, and Timothy C. Allen, MD, JD**

**Advances in Surgical Pathology: Lung Cancer**
Philip T. Cagle and Timothy C. Allen, 2010

**Advances in Surgical Pathology: Gastric Cancer**
Dongfeng Tan and Gregory Y. Lauwers, 2010

**Advances in Surgical Pathology: Endometrial Cancer**
Anna Sienko, 2012

**Advances in Surgical Pathology: Prostate Cancer**
Jae Y. Ro, Steven S. Shen, and Alberto G. Ayala, 2012

**Advances in Surgical Pathology: Mesothelioma**
Richard Attanoos and Timothy C. Allen 2013

**Advances in Surgical Pathology: Colorectal Carcinoma and Tumors of the Vermiform Appendix**
Rhonda K. Yantiss, 2013

**Advances in Surgical Pathology: Breast Cancer**
Omar Hameed, 2014

**Advances in Surgical Pathology: Thyroid Cancer**
Mojgan Amrikachi and Rose Anton, 2015

**Advances in Surgical Pathology: Brain Cancer**
Andreana Rivera and Hidehiro Takei, 2015

# ADVANCES IN SURGICAL PATHOLOGY

# COLORECTAL CARCINOMA AND TUMORS OF THE VERMIFORM APPENDIX


**Rhonda K. Yantiss, MD**
Associate Professor of Pathology and Laboratory Medicine
Department of Pathology and Laboratory Medicine
Weill Cornell Medical College of Cornell University
New York–Presbyterian Hospital
New York, New York

SERIES EDITORS

**Philip T. Cagle, MD**
Professor of Pathology and Laboratory Medicine
Weill Cornell Medical College of Cornell University
New York, New York
Director, Pulmonary Pathology
The Methodist Hospital
Houston, Texas

**Timothy C. Allen, MD, JD**
Professor of Pathology
Chairman, Department of Pathology
The University of Texas Health Science Center at Tyler
Tyler, Texas



Wolters Kluwer | Lippincott Williams & Wilkins
Health
Philadelphia • Baltimore • New York • London
Buenos Aires • Hong Kong • Sydney • Tokyo

*Acquisitions Editor:* Ryan Shaw
*Product Manager:* Kate Marshall
*Vendor Manager:* Alicia Jackson
*Senior Manufacturing Coordinator:* Beth Welsh
*Marketing Manager:* Alexander Burns
*Designer:* Joan Wendt
*Production Service:* SPi Global


Two Commerce Square
2001 Market Street
Philadelphia, PA 19103 USA
LWW.com



Printed in China

---

**Library of Congress Cataloging-in-Publication Data**

Advances in surgical pathology. Colorectal carcinoma and tumors of the vermiform appendix / [edited by] Rhonda K. Yantiss.

p. ; cm. — (Advances in surgical pathology)

Colorectal carcinoma and tumors of the vermiform appendix

Includes bibliographical references and index.

ISBN 978-1-4511-8277-4

I. Yantiss, Rhonda K., editor of compilation. II. Title: Colorectal carcinoma and tumors of the vermiform appendix. III. Series: Advances in surgical pathology series.

[DNLM: 1. Appendiceal Neoplasms—pathology. 2. Colorectal Neoplasms—pathology. 3. Appendiceal Neoplasms—surgery. 4. Colorectal Neoplasms—surgery. WI 529]

RC280.C6

616.99'4347—dc23

2013017497

---



To purchase additional copies of this book, call our customer service department at (800) 638-3030 or fax orders to (301) 223-2320. International customers should call (301) 223-2300.

Visit Lippincott Williams & Wilkins on the Internet: at LWW.com. Lippincott Williams & Wilkins customer service representatives are available from 8:30 am to 6 pm, EST.

10 9 8 7 6 5 4 3 2 1

CCS0813

# Series Overview

Expectations for the pathologist practicing today exceed those for pathologists in practice only a few years ago. In addition to the rapid growth of knowledge and new technologies in the field of pathology, recent years have seen the emergence of many trends that significantly impact the traditional practice of pathology including the subspecialized multidisciplinary approach to patient care; personalized therapeutics including targeted molecular therapies; and imaging techniques such as endoscopic microscopy, molecular radiology, and imaging multimodality theranostics that compete with conventional light microscopy. In order to remain a viable member of the patient care team, the pathologist must keep up with growing knowledge in traditional subjects as well as in new areas of expertise such as molecular testing. Additionally, the pathologist is subject to an increasing number of credentialing requirements and, for those now completing training, Self-Assessment Modules for Maintenance of Certification, which require the pathologist to be examined on the recent advances in pathology in order to sustain their qualifications to practice.

Each volume in the new series "Advances in Surgical Pathology" focuses on a specific subject in pathology that has undergone recent advancement in terms of knowledge, technical procedures, application, and/or integration as part of current trends in pathology and medicine. This series of books not only updates the pathologist on recently acquired knowledge but also emphasizes the new uses of that knowledge within the context of the changing landscape of pathology practice in the 21st century. Rather than information in a vacuum, the pathologist is educated on how to apply the new knowledge as part of a subspecialized multidisciplinary team and for purposes of personalized patient therapy.

Each volume in the series will be divided into the following sections: (1) Overview—Updates the pathologist on the general topic, including epidemiology, bringing the pathologist generally up-to-date on a topic as a basis for the more specialized sections that follow. (2) Histopathology—Reviews histopathology and specific recent changes that warrant more description and more illustration, for example, recently described entities and recent revisions in classifications. This will also emphasize histopathology figures to illustrate recently described entities and to demonstrate the basis for classification changes so that the pathologist is able to understand and recognize these changes. (3) Imaging—Reviews the impact of imaging techniques on histopathologic diagnosis and on the practice of pathology. An example of the former is the use of increasingly sensitive high-resolution computed tomography scan in the diagnosis of interstitial lung diseases. An example of the latter is the use of multimodality theranostics rather than traditional histopathology for the diagnosis and treatment of lung cancer. Figures linking the radiologic images to the histopathology will be emphasized. (4) Molecular Pathology—A review and update on specific molecular pathology as it applies to specific diseases for the practicing pathologist in regard to molecular diagnostics and molecular therapeutics. An example of the former is the identification of a specific fusion gene to diagnose synovial sarcoma. An example of the latter is the identification of specific epidermal growth factor receptor (EGFR) mutations in pulmonary adenocarcinoma and its relationship to treatment with EGFR antagonists. (5) For those volumes dealing with cancers (Lung Cancer, Breast Cancer, Prostate Cancer, Colon Cancer, etc.), additional sections will include Preneoplastic and Preinvasive Lesions, which will emphasize histopathologic figures and staging, particularly emphasizing the new staging systems and to illustrate specific problems in staging.

These books will assist the pathologist in daily practice in the modern setting and provide a basis for interacting with other physicians in patient care. They will also provide the timely updates in knowledge that are necessary for daily practice, for current credentialing, and for Maintenance of Certification. As such, this series is invaluable to pathologists in practice at all levels of experience who need to keep up with advances for their daily performance and their periodic credentialing and to pathologists in training who will apply this knowledge to their boards and their future practice. In the latter case, this series will serve as a useful library for pathology training programs.

# Contributors

**Debra Beneck, MD**
Professor of Clinical Pathology and Laboratory Medicine
Department of Pathology and Laboratory Medicine
Weill Cornell Medical College of Cornell University
Attending Pathologist
New York–Presbyterian Hospital
New York, New York

**Daniel Cherqui, MD**
Chief, Division of Hepatobiliary Surgery and Liver Transplantation
Department of Surgery
Weill Cornell Medical College of Cornell University
New York–Presbyterian Hospital
New York, New York

**Carl V. Crawford, Jr., MD**
Assistant Professor of Medicine
Division of Gastroenterology and Hepatology
Weill Cornell Medical College of Cornell University
New York–Presbyterian Hospital
New York, New York

**Karen Curtin, PhD**
Research Assistant Professor
Department of Internal Medicine
University of Utah School of Medicine
Salt Lake City, Utah

**Michael D. Kluger, MD, MPH**
Assistant Professor of Surgery
Division of Hepatobiliary Surgery and Liver Transplantation
Department of Surgery
Weill Cornell Medical College of Cornell University
New York–Presbyterian Hospital
New York, New York

**Ser Yee Lee, MBBS, MMed (Surgery), MSc, FRCS, FAMS**
Clinical Fellow, Division of Hepatobiliary Surgery and Liver Transplantation
Weill Cornell Medical College of Cornell University
New York–Presbyterian Hospital
New York, New York
Department of Surgical Oncology
National Cancer Center
Singapore

**Joseph Misdraji, MD**
Associate Pathologist
Department of Pathology
Massachusetts General Hospital
Associate Professor of Pathology
Harvard Medical School
Boston, Massachusetts

**Allyson J. Ocean, MD**
Associate Professor of Clinical Medicine
Weill Cornell Medical College of Cornell University
New York–Presbyterian Hospital
New York, New York

**Romae Palmer**
Data Coordinator
Division of Hematology and Medical Oncology
Weill Cornell Medical College of Cornell University
New York, New York

**Nicole C. Panarelli, MD**
Assistant Professor of Pathology and Laboratory Medicine
Department of Pathology and Laboratory Medicine
Weill Cornell Medical College of Cornell University
New York–Presbyterian Hospital
New York, New York

**Wade S. Samowitz, MD**
Professor of Pathology
Department of Pathology
University of Utah
Salt Lake City, Utah

**Ellen J. Scherl, MD**
Associate Professor of Medicine
Weill Cornell Medical College of Cornell University
New York–Presbyterian Hospital
New York, New York

**Felice Schnoll-Sussman, MD, FACG**
Assistant Professor of Clinical Medicine
Division of Gastroenterology and Hepatology
Weill Cornell Medical College of Cornell University
New York–Presbyterian Hospital
New York, New York

**Manish A. Shah, MD**
Associate Professor of Medicine
Division of Hematology and Medical Oncology
Weill Cornell Medical College of Cornell University
Director, Gastrointestinal Oncology
Director, Gastrointestinal Research
Center for Advanced Digestive Care
New York–Presbyterian Hospital
New York, New York

**Jinru Shia, MD**
Member and Attending Pathologist
Memorial Sloan–Kettering Cancer Center
New York, New York

**Amir Soumekh, MD**
Clinical Fellow, Division of Gastroenterology and Hepatology
Department of Medicine
New York–Presbyterian Hospital
New York, New York

**Rhonda K. Yantiss, MD**
Associate Professor of Pathology and Laboratory Medicine
Department of Pathology and Laboratory Medicine
Weill Cornell Medical College of Cornell University
New York–Presbyterian Hospital
New York, New York

# Preface

Although screening and surveillance practices have impacted its natural history, colorectal carcinoma is still the fourth leading cause of cancer-related death in the United States and remains a global health problem. Several recent advances have enabled investigators to unravel the mechanisms underlying development of these tumors. Emerging endoscopic techniques facilitate detection and complete removal of early cancer precursors, thereby changing the natural history of this disease. The discovery of genetic, epigenetic, and posttranscriptional regulatory mechanisms has allowed us to identify heritable cancer risk factors and elucidate cellular signal transduction pathways that represent potential targets for directed medical therapies. Some of these changes are characteristic of specific tumor types. Their detection improves histologic classification of cancer subtypes and may be prognostically useful. Indeed, evaluation for specific molecular alterations is increasingly essential to the clinical management of colorectal cancer and has become a standard element of pathology reporting.

This book represents a succinct, comprehensive review of issues important to management of patients with colorectal carcinoma. It discusses practical concerns regarding cancer epidemiology and cancer prevention, as well as the pathologic features of cancer precursors. Recent recommendations for pathologic tumor staging and histologic classification are presented in combination with the most relevant molecular features of colorectal carcinoma. These discussions are followed by an introduction to future diagnostic and treatment modalities, including biomarker analysis, chemotherapeutic strategies, targeted molecular therapies, and aggressive multidisciplinary approaches to patients with advanced-stage disease. My intent is that it should provide useful information to practicing surgical pathologists involved in the management of colorectal cancer patients.

*Rhonda K. Yantiss, MD*

ACKNOWLEDGMENT

To Zachary Paul, my new joy

# Contents

ADVANCES IN SURGICAL PATHOLOGY

# COLORECTAL CARCINOMA AND TUMORS OF THE VERMIFORM APPENDIX

SECTION

# I

# Introduction

# Embryology, Anatomy, and Normal Histology of the Colorectum and Appendix

# 1

Debra Beneck

## EMBRYOLOGY

The primordial gut is first recognizable during the 4th week after conception and is formed from the dorsal part of the umbilical vesicle (yolk sac) by embryonic infolding. All three germ cell layers contribute to formation of the gastrointestinal tract. The luminal surface (mucosa) contains cells derived from the endoderm, the wall is composed of mesodermal tissues (splanchnic mesenchyme), and the enteric nervous system originates from the ectoderm.[1] Several genes, including *Hox*, *ParaHox*, *BMP* (bone morphogenetic protein), *CDX1*, *CDX2*, and *Shh* and *Ihh* (Sonic hedgehog and Indian hedgehog), influence patterning along anteroposterior, dorsoventral, left–right and radial axes; cell migration; and interactions between the endodermal and mesodermal components of the gastrointestinal tract.[2–4]

Much of the development of the large intestine is completed during the 4th through the 14th weeks after fertilization (Table 1.1). The proximal large intestine, including the cecum, appendix, ascending colon, and proximal one-half to two-thirds of the transverse colon, is derived from the midgut, which also includes the entire small intestine distal to the ampulla of Vater. The entire midgut receives its vascular supply from the superior mesenteric (midgut) artery. The distal transverse, descending, and sigmoid colon; rectum; and superior two-thirds of the anal canal are derived from the hindgut and are supplied by the inferior mesenteric artery.[1]

The midgut forms a U-shaped loop as it grows. This loop is divided into cranial and caudal limbs by its connection to the omphalomesenteric duct. It herniates into the proximal umbilical cord during the 6th to 10th weeks due to a lack of intra-abdominal space resulting from growth of the liver and kidneys. The loop rotates 90 degrees counterclockwise around the superior mesenteric artery during this time. The cranial limb, which is destined to become the jejunum and ileum, grows more rapidly than does the caudal limb. An elevation on the antimesenteric side of the caudal limb becomes the cecal swelling during the 6th week. Its apex narrows into a diverticulum that develops into the vermiform appendix over the next 4 weeks. The distal limb rotates an additional 180 degrees as the midgut returns to the abdominal cavity during the 10th to 11th weeks. The ascending colon and descending colon become fixed by fusion of their mesenteries to the parietal peritoneum of the posterior body wall, while the transverse colon remains suspended by its mesentery in the peritoneal cavity.[1,2]

The terminal portion of the hindgut expands to form the cloaca, which ends blindly at the cloacal membrane in early development. Ingrowth of the urorectal septum between the 4th and 7th weeks gives rise to the rectum and proximal anal canal dorsally, as well as the urogenital sinus ventrally. The cloacal membrane ruptures at the end of the 8th week and provides communication between the fetal gastrointestinal tract and the amniotic fluid.[1,2]

**Table 1.1 Embryologic and Fetal Development of the Colon and Appendix**

| Developmental Week | Macroscopic Findings | Mucosal Development | Microscopic Findings |
|---|---|---|---|
| 4 | Embryonic infolding to form primordial gut<br>Cloacal septation | Single layer of endodermally derived cells | Neural crest cells begin to migrate into gut wall |
| 5 | | Proliferation of multiple epithelial cell layers | |
| 6 | Midgut herniates into umbilical cord<br>Cecal swelling appears | Gut lumen filled with epithelium | |
| 7 | | | Neural crest cells scattered in mesenchyme |
| 8 | Appendiceal diverticulum<br>Rupture of cloacal membrane to form anal pit | Canalization of gut lumen complete | First identification of circular smooth muscle layer (MP) |
| 9 | | Gut lining is simple columnar epithelium | Interstitial cells of Cajal |
| 10 | Midgut returns to abdomen | Simple villous pattern | Identifiable submucosal and myenteric plexuses |
| 11 | | | Appearance of goblet cells<br>Circular muscle layer complete<br>Longitudinal muscle layer identifiable |
| 12 | Vermiform appendix | | Interstitial cells of Cajal surround myenteric ganglia |
| 14 | | | Muscularis propria complete |

The mucosal epithelial lining of the primitive gut is a uniform single cuboidal layer in early development. The gut lumen fills with a solid growth of epithelium from 6 to 8 weeks and recanalizes *via* apoptosis to form a hollow lumen.[2] The lumen is lined by a simple, polarized columnar epithelium by the 9th week. Goblet cells first appear in gut mucosa during the 11th and 12th weeks.[5] Mesodermal tissues simultaneously grow toward the lumen to form the lamina propria. Subsequent epithelial differentiation is dependent upon cell signaling between endoderm and mesoderm, which continues throughout postnatal life. Proliferation, differentiation, and apoptosis of colonic crypt epithelium are largely controlled by Wnt signaling, but other factors, including homeobox, forkhead, platelet-derived growth factor, and bone morphogenetic protein, have also been identified in developing colonic mucosa. Ephrin-B1 and ephrin-B2 and their receptors, EphB2 and EphB3, regulate intestinal epithelial cell positioning and differentiation and are in turn regulated by β-catenin and *Tcf4* (transcription factor 4) transcriptional activity. A Wnt signaling gradient also regulates intestinal epithelial cell positioning by mediating ephrins.[5–8]

Development of the smooth muscle layers advances from the cranial to caudal end of the gut. The inner circular layer of the muscularis propria forms first, followed by the outer longitudinal layer and, ultimately, the muscularis mucosae. Investment of the large intestine by organized smooth muscle layers is completed by the 14th week of gestation.[1,2]

The neurons and glial cells of the enteric nervous system are derived from ectodermal cells that begin migrating from the neural crest in a craniocaudal fashion as early as the 4th week. Neural crest–derived cells are scattered throughout the mesenchyme of the hindgut by the 8th week and well-formed submucosal and myenteric ganglia are observed by the 14th week. Interstitial cells of Cajal are detectable by the 12th week. These cells are derived from splanchnic mesenchyme and invest the myenteric ganglia to facilitate neuromuscular interactions. Parasympathetic innervation of the large intestine originates in branches of the vagus nerves and nervi erigentes, whereas sympathetic innervation derives from the superior and inferior mesenteric and pelvic ganglia.[9,10]

## ANATOMY AND HISTOLOGY

The cecum, appendix, ascending colon, transverse colon, descending colon, sigmoid colon, and rectum constitute the large intestine, which ranges from 1 to 1.5 m in length. The cecum and appendix, transverse colon, and sigmoid colon are located within the peritoneal cavity, whereas the ascending colon and descending colon are fixed to the posterior body wall by fascial attachments and the rectum lies in the pelvis below the peritoneal reflection.[10] The cecum is a saccular structure with a 3- to 5-cm diameter located at the proximal ascending colon. The fully developed cecum and ascending colon are approximately 15 cm in length. The transverse colon is approximately 50 cm long; the descending colon spans 25 cm in length, and the length of the sigmoid colon varies from 35 to 50 cm, although its redundancy increases with age. The rectum is relatively short, measuring 8 to 15 cm, and is supplied by the inferior mesenteric artery and middle and inferior rectal arteries, which branch from the internal iliac arteries.[11] The average vermiform appendix is 11 cm long, but its length varies depending upon several factors, including height, weight, and body mass index.[12] The appendix usually enters the base of the cecum on its medial aspect, although retrocecal or other locations are relatively common.[1]

The large intestine contains five histologically distinct layers (Figure 1.1). Innermost is the mucosa (Figure 1.2), which consists of the surface and crypt epithelial cells supported by the loose connective tissue of the lamina propria. The epithelial compartment is composed of straight tubular glands (crypts of Lieberkühn) lined by columnar absorptive cells (enterocytes), goblet cells, enteroendocrine cells, and stem cells. Enterocytes and goblet cells are uniformly present in the crypts and surface epithelium, whereas enteroendocrine cells and stem cells are limited to the crypt bases. Paneth cells likely have antimicrobial and host defense functions. They may be found at the crypt base in the appendix, cecum, and ascending and proximal transverse colon but are not normally present in the descending colon, sigmoid colon, or rectum. In fact, their detection in the distal colorectum is considered evidence of chronic mucosal injury.[11] The ratio of enterocytes to goblet cells varies throughout the colorectum, ranging from 4:1 in the cecum and appendix to 1:1 in the rectum. Enterocytes and goblet cells have a lifespan of approximately 6 days, whereas enteroendocrine cells survive for nearly 4 weeks.[6]

All large intestinal epithelial cells are derived from stem cells that are subclassified as long-term quiescent (reserve, label-retaining cells) and actively cycling (primed, crypt base cells).

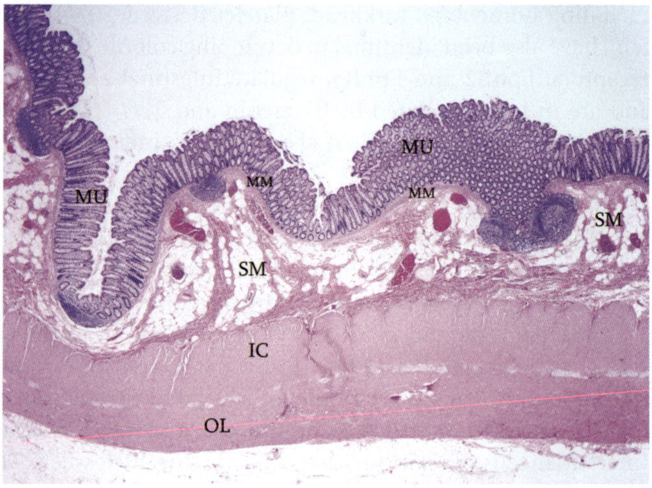


**FIGURE 1.1:** The colonic wall is composed of five layers, including the mucosa, muscularis mucosae, submucosa, muscularis propria, and either subserosa or pericolic soft tissue. (MU, mucosa; MM, muscularis mucosae; SM, submucosa; IC, inner circular layer of muscularis propria; OL, outer longitudinal layer of muscularis propria [H & E; original magnification 200×]).

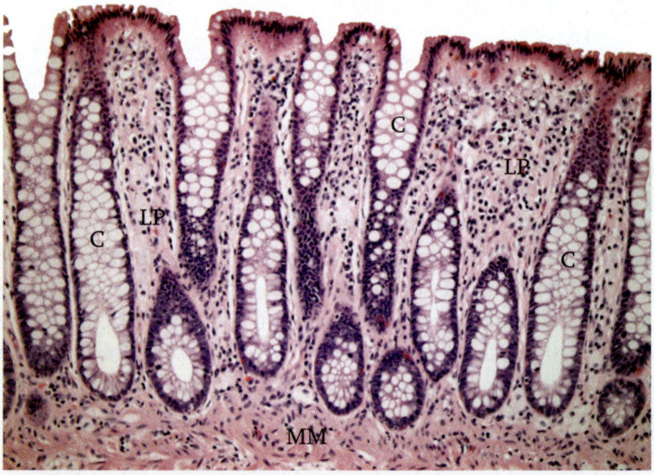


**FIGURE 1.2:** The colonic mucosa contains epithelial cells arranged in crypts, which are supported by areolar tissue of the lamina propria. The surface is flat, and crypt bases rest upon the muscularis mucosae. Most crypt cells are mucin-containing epithelial cells and absorptive cells, although endocrine cells are also present. (C, crypts; LP, lamina propria; MM, muscularis mucosae [H & E; original magnification 200×]).

Each crypt contains four to six stem cells that are limited to the lower third of the deep crypt region. Long-term quiescent stem cells are located above the Paneth cells in the deep lateral region of the crypts. Actively cycling stem cells are located at the crypt bases. Although a universal stem cell marker has yet to be identified, the *Bmi1* gene is exclusively expressed in long-term quiescent stem cells and the Wnt signaling target gene *Lgr5/Gpr49* is exclusively expressed in actively cycling cells.[13–15]

Proliferation, differentiation, and migration of intestinal stem cells depend on epithelial–mesenchymal interactions *via* Wnt and Notch signaling in the lamina propria and continue throughout life. Activation of Wnt signaling is most pronounced near the crypt bases and diffuses toward the luminal surface. Nuclear β-catenin immunolabeling is limited to crypt bases where Tcf4 is expressed in highest concentration. Ephrin-B ligands and their receptors are also differentially expressed along a gradient; EphB receptor expression is highest at the crypt base, whereas ephrin-B expression is highest at the luminal surface.[5,6,13–15]

Each colonic crypt is ensheathed by a cuff of pericryptal myofibroblasts that is most dense at the crypt bases. This layer of cells regulates intestinal stem cells *via* elaboration of growth factors and cytokines. The pericryptal sheath may also harbor stem cells that differentiate into macrophages in the lamina propria.[6] Other components of the lamina propria include capillary endothelial cells, enteric neurons, lymphocytes, and indigenous microbes.[13–15] Lymphocytes, plasma cells, eosinophils, and mast cells occupy the lamina propria in decreasing order of concentration; all are more numerous in the proximal than in the distal colon.[11]

Capillaries are present at all levels of the mucosa, but lymphatic vessels are limited to the deep mucosa near the crypt bases.[6] Lymphoid aggregates are normally present in the lamina propria and may breach the muscularis mucosae, which represents a nearly continuous band of smooth muscle that supports the lamina propria. The muscularis mucosae is discontinuous within large lymphoid aggregates and, in fact, herniations of mucosa through the muscularis mucosae in traumatized polyps usually occur in association with lymphoid aggregates. The submucosa consists of organized connective tissue, large-caliber arteries and veins, and rich lymphatic networks. It also contains the superficial (Meissner) and deep (Henle) plexuses of nerves and ganglion cells. The muscularis propria comprises an inner circular and outer longitudinal layer, between which lies the myenteric (Auerbach) nerve plexus (Figure 1.3). Large-caliber blood vessels and lymphatic channels penetrate the muscularis propria and represent relative weak points in the muscular wall that are prone to herniation of mucosa and submucosa. The outer layer of the muscularis propria is condensed into the three equally spaced longitudinal teniae coli that extend from the cecum to the distal sigmoid colon but exclude the appendix and rectum. Saccular haustra form along the colon between the teniae coli and result from independent contraction of colonic segments.[6] The intraperitoneal colonic segments and appendix are enveloped by serosa composed of fibroelastic tissue and a single layer of mesothelial cells. The ascending colon and descending colon are surfaced anteriorly by serosa, but their retroperitoneal areas are covered by an adventitia. The rectum is surrounded by perirectal soft tissue enveloped by a fascial plane of areolar tissue (mesorectal envelope), but has no serosa except in the upper third, anteriorly.

The large intestine primarily functions to resorb water and inorganic salts from liquid stool delivered by the small intestine. It also secretes lubricating mucus to facilitate stool transport and stores stool in the rectal reservoir prior to excretion.[11] The appendix probably plays a role in gut-mediated immunity, but its precise function is unknown. Although a relationship between appendicitis and/or appendectomy and inflammatory bowel disease has been observed in some series,[16] the nature of this relationship is controversial, and consistent adverse immunologic effects have not been ascribed to appendectomy.

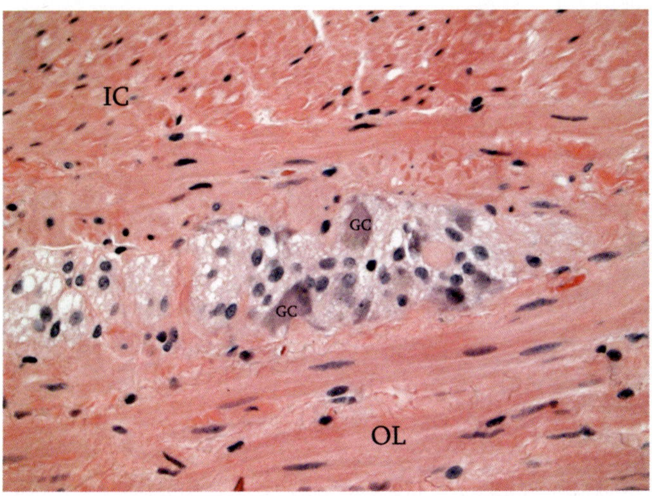


**FIGURE 1.3:** The myenteric plexus lies between the inner circular and outer longitudinal layers of the muscularis propria. It consists of scattered ganglion cells and peripheral nerves and is closely associated with the interstitial cells of Cajal. (GC, ganglion cells; IC, inner circular layer of muscularis propria; OL, outer longitudinal layer of muscularis propria [H & E; original magnification 400×]).

# References


1. Moore KL, Persaud TVN. *The Developing Human: Clinically Oriented Embryology*. 8th ed. Philadelphia, PA: Saunders Elsevier; 2008.
2. Schoenwolf GC, Bleyl SB, Brauer PR, et al. *Larsen's Human Embryology*. 4th ed. Philadelphia, PA: Churchill Livingstone Elsevier; 2009.
3. Rawdon B. Early development of the gut: new light on an old hypothesis. *Cell Biol Int* 2001;25:9–15.
4. Roberts DJ. Molecular mechanisms of development of the gastrointestinal tract. *Dev Dyn* 2000; 219:109–120.
5. Spence JR, Lauf R, Shroyer NF. Vertebrate intestinal endoderm development. *Dev Dyn* 2011;240: 501–520.
6. Ross MH, Pawlina W. *Histology: A Text and Atlas*. 6th ed. Baltimore, MD: Lippincott Williams & Wilkins; 2011.
7. De Santa Barbara P, van den Brink GR, Roberts D. Development and differentiation of the intestinal epithelium. *Cell Mol Life Sci* 2003;60:1322–1332.
8. Gregorieff A, Pinto D, Begthel H, et al. Expression pattern of Wnt signaling components in the adult intestine. *Gastroenterology* 2005;129:626–638.
9. Wallace AS, Burns AJ. Development of the enteric nervous system, smooth muscle and interstitial cells of Cajal in the human gastrointestinal tract. *Cell Tissue Res* 2005;319:367–382.
10. Fu M, Tam PKH, Sham MH, et al. Embryonic development of the ganglion plexuses and the concentric layer structure of the human gut: a topographical study. *Anat Embryol* 2004;208:33–41.
11. Levine DS, Haggit RC. Normal histology of the colon. *Am J Surg Path* 1989;13:966–984.
12. Raschka S, Raschka C. On the relationship between body dimensions and appendix length. *Anthropol Anz* 2008;66:67–72.
13. Scoville DH, Sato T, He XC, et al. Current view: intestinal stem cells and signaling. *Gastroenterology* 2008;134:849–864.
14. Shaker A, Rubin DC. Intestinal stem cells and epithelial-mesenchymal interactions in the crypt and stem cell niche. *Trans Res* 2010;156:180–187.
15. Yen T-H, Wright N. The gastrointestinal tract stem cell niche. *Stem Cell Rev* 2006;2:203–212.
16. Cheluvappa R, Luo AS, Palmer C, et al. Protective pathways against colitis mediated by appendicitis and appendectomy. *Clin Exp Immunol* 2011;165:393–400.

# Epidemiology of Colorectal Adenocarcinoma

2

Karen Curtin

Colorectal cancer is one of the most common cancers worldwide, affecting more individuals in economically developed, affluent nations than in underdeveloped countries. Only a small fraction of colorectal cancers are associated with known genetic syndromes. An estimated 75% to 95% of patients have little or no genetic risk, and most do not have a family history of the disease. Increasing age is strongly associated with colorectal cancer development; evidence suggests that lifestyle and diet may be involved. As the majority of colorectal cancers are sporadic, this chapter focuses on the epidemiology of potentially modifiable factors that have been associated with increasing or decreasing risk of this disease.

Each section of this chapter is based on the most recent information available. Estimates of risk are derived from systematic reviews and meta-analyses of results across dozens of epidemiologic studies published over the past four decades. These cohort-based, case–control, and prospective investigations have been conducted in populations around the globe and thus reflect findings in tens of thousands of individuals collectively. The impact of each factor on colorectal cancer development is portrayed as a percentage of increased or decreased risk at the individual level. Estimates of attributable risk at the population level are also provided.

## INCIDENCE AND MORTALITY OF COLORECTAL CARCINOMA

Colorectal carcinoma is the third most commonly diagnosed cancer worldwide. There were 1.2 million newly diagnosed cases and 608,000 cancer-related deaths in 2008, making it the fourth most common cause of death from cancer.[1,2] Approximately 60% of colorectal cancers are diagnosed in economically developed regions: The highest estimated incidence rates are observed in Australia, New Zealand, and Western Europe. There is less regional variability with respect to colorectal cancer mortality rates. Both incidence and mortality rates are slightly lower in women than in men (Figure 2.1).

Approximately 143,460 individuals (73,420 men and 70,040 women) in the United States have been diagnosed with colorectal cancer, and 51,690 people have died of this malignancy in 2012.[3] The age-adjusted incidence rate is an estimated 46.3 per 100,000 individuals per year, and the age-adjusted annual mortality rate is 16.7 per 100,000. These values are based on 2005 to 2009 data from the Surveillance, Epidemiology and End Results (SEER) Program, National Cancer Institute, U.S. National Institutes of Health (http://seer.cancer.gov), and are based upon findings obtained from specific geographic areas representing 28% of the population.[3] Although incidence rates for colon cancer are similar for men and women, rectal cancers occur more often in men.[4] Recent declines in colorectal cancer incidence in the United States (2.5% annually from 1998 to 2009) reflect the introduction of colonoscopy as a screening tool in the early 1990s and its widespread use beginning in 2001, which coincided with expanded insurance reimbursement.[3,5]

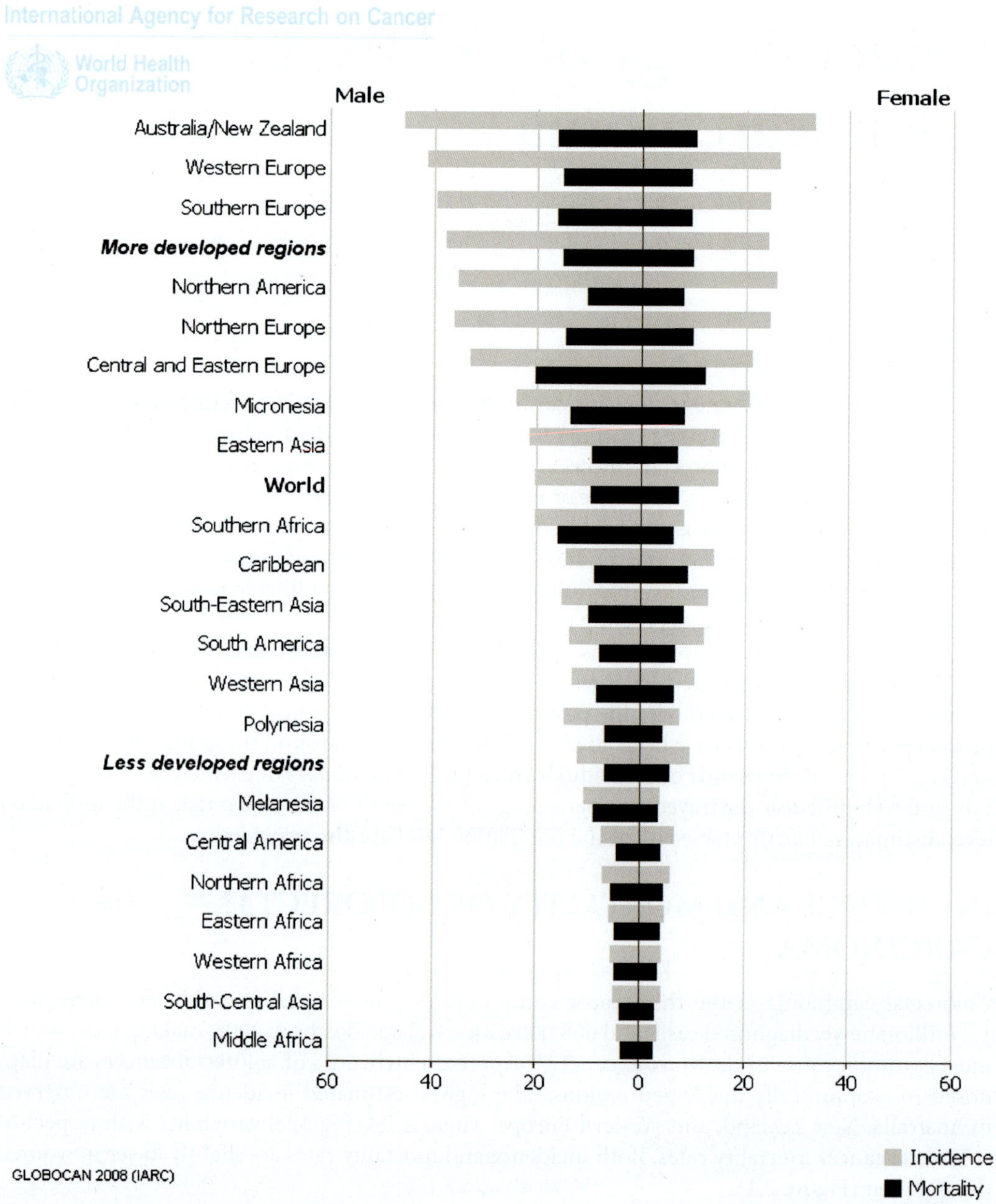


**FIGURE 2.1:** Estimated age-standardized world colorectal cancer rates per 100,000 persons. (Reprinted from Ferlay J, Shin HR, Bray F, et al. GLOBOCAN 2008, cancer incidence and mortality worldwide: IARC CancerBase No. 10 [Internet]. Lyon, France: International Agency for Research on Cancer; 2010. Available from: http://globocan.iarc.fr.)

Five-year survival rates for colorectal cancer range from 90% for localized cancers to 12% for individuals with metastatic disease.[3,6] Stage-independent disparities in survival among regions in the United States and worldwide exist due to differences in access to diagnostic services and treatment. Five-year survival rates have improved significantly over the last few decades in the United States, but death rates continue to be higher among blacks than whites and other racial/ethnic groups (Table 2.1). This disparity in survival has widened in comparison to trends for other cancers.[3,6]

**Table 2.1** Age-Adjusted Colorectal Cancer–Related Death Rates by Race/Ethnicity in the United States, 2005–2009 (per 100,000 Men or Women)

| Race/Ethnicity | Male | Female |
|---|---|---|
| All races | 20.2 | 14.1 |
| White | 19.5 | 13.6 |
| Black | 29.8 | 19.8 |
| Asian/Pacific Islander | 13.1 | 9.6 |
| American Indian/Alaskan Native | 18.8 | 14.6 |
| Hispanic | 15.3 | 10.2 |

Source: SEER Stat Fact Sheets. Colon and rectum, available at http://seer.cancer.gov/statfacts/html/colorect.html

## NONMODIFIABLE RISK FACTORS

Some colorectal cancer risk factors, such as age, history of polyps, and genetic risk, cannot be altered or modified by the individual. Increasing age is strongly associated with increased colorectal cancer incidence: The median age at colorectal cancer diagnosis in the United States is 69 years, and nearly two-thirds of tumors are diagnosed in persons 65 years of age and older, while only 5% are diagnosed before the age of 45 years.[3] Colorectal adenomas are precursor lesions of colorectal cancer.[7] The lifetime risk of developing a colorectal adenoma may be over 18% in the United States, but detection and removal of polyps before malignant transformation reduces the risk of death from colorectal cancer.[8,9] Although hyperplastic polyps have been considered to have little potential for progression to cancer, large nondysplastic serrated polyps (≥1 cm) of the abdominal colon are associated with an increased risk of colon cancer, especially if they are multiple, as discussed in Chapters 4, 11, and 12.[10]

Only 5% to 6% of colorectal cancers develop in association with heritable disease.[11,12] The most common of these inherited disorders are familial adenomatous polyposis, which results from *APC* mutations, and Lynch syndrome, which is caused by mutations in DNA repair genes, as discussed in Chapters 11 and 12. Individuals with familial adenomatous polyposis typically develop hundreds of polyps at a young age, and virtually 100% will develop colorectal cancer unless a prophylactic colectomy is performed.[13] The lifetime risk of colorectal cancer among patients with Lynch syndrome may be as high as 70% to 80%, but cancers are usually diagnosed in the fifth decade of life, which is later than those associated with familial adenomatous polyposis.[4,12]

Approximately 20% to 25% of colorectal cancers occur in patients with a family history of colorectal cancer, unassociated with familial adenomatous polyposis or Lynch syndrome. Such tumors are considered familial cancers and are likely due to inheritance of relatively common, low-penetrance genetic variants that portend low to modest cancer risk.[11] It is unclear whether familial colorectal carcinomas occur due to an inherited predisposition, shared environmental exposure, or a combination of both. Low-penetrance variants affecting *APC, BLM, HRAS1*, and *TGFβR1* have been described, and recent efforts to uncover additional genetic susceptibility variants have revealed a number of genome-wide associations.[11] Genetic variants present in the *SMAD7* gene and regions on chromosomes 8q24 and 18q21, all of which are commonly altered in colorectal cancers, have been identified in many people. These variants are associated with a modest (10% to 30%) increased risk in carriers compared with individuals without the variant.[14–16] Other genetic variants in candidate genes interact with diet and lifestyle factors, such as inflammation or insulin-related pathway, and are associated with very modest effects on colorectal cancer risk. A detailed discussion of the extensive catalog of candidate genetic variants is beyond the scope of this chapter.

## MODIFIABLE RISK FACTORS

Environmental lifestyle and dietary influences are considered to represent modifiable risk factors for colorectal cancer. Epidemiologic studies evaluating associations between the environment and colorectal cancer have shown that colorectal cancer incidence in populations migrating from low-risk to high-risk countries approaches that of the new host nation within a generation or two.[17,18] For example, offspring of Japanese migrants to the United States have a similar colorectal cancer risk to white Americans that is three to four times that of Japanese people in Japan.[18] Colorectal cancer risk is clearly related to a variety of environmental influences, including medications, exposure to cigarette smoke, physical activity, obesity, and alcohol use. Numerous dietary factors have been implicated in colorectal carcinogenesis, although the evidence is generally more inconsistent than that of lifestyle factors. Methods used to measure dietary influences vary widely and include diet records, diet histories and food frequency questionnaires, 24-hour dietary recall, and other forms of self-reporting. Thus, intake is often misreported or imprecise. Only widely studied dietary factors related to colorectal cancer, such as folate and other B vitamins, fiber from grains, fruits and vegetables, calcium and vitamin D, and red and processed meats, are discussed in this chapter.

### Aspirin and Nonsteroidal Anti-inflammatory Drugs

Epidemiologic, clinical, and observational studies have consistently shown that aspirin and other nonsteroidal anti-inflammatory drugs (NSAIDs) protect against colorectal cancer and substantially reduce its incidence. Numerous epidemiologic studies have demonstrated decreased colorectal cancer incidence, prevention of adenoma recurrence, and reduction in colorectal cancer mortality among regular users of these agents.[19,20] The effect of NSAIDs ranges from 20% to 60% reduced risk of colorectal cancer based on relative risk estimates of 0.4 to 0.8.[19] Presumably, inhibition of the cyclooxygenase-2 pathway reduces prostaglandin synthesis and cell growth, although other biologic mechanisms of action unrelated to prostaglandin metabolism may also be important. These agents modulate insulin-mediated metabolism and reduce inflammation, both of which are important to colorectal carcinogenesis, as discussed in subsequent sections.[21]

Despite epidemiologic evidence supporting NSAID use in the prevention of colorectal cancer, the American Cancer Society and other groups have not yet endorsed their routine use in cancer prevention because of concerns regarding toxicity and bleeding risk. However, recent findings suggest that low-dose aspirin (75 mg/day) protects against colorectal cancer in the general population after only 5 years of use and may tip the scale in favor of future recommendations.[22,23]

### Hormone Replacement Therapy

Most colorectal cancer patients are men, especially patients younger than 50 years of age, raising the possibility that hormonal influences play a role in the development of colorectal carcinoma. Estrogens decrease colonic transit time and production of insulin-like growth factor-1, thereby modifying potential cancer risk factors. Some colon cancers express estrogen receptor-β, which could modify the effect of hormone replacement therapy on tumor growth.[24] Epidemiologic studies show that hormone replacement therapy is associated with a decreased risk of colorectal cancer, with few exceptions. Patients who have ever used hormone replacement therapy have a 20% reduced risk of colon or rectal cancer, with the greatest effects seen in those currently using exogenous hormones.[25] These observational results have also been confirmed in a randomized, placebo-controlled trial among nearly 17,000 postmenopausal women that showed a 37% reduced colorectal cancer risk with use of estrogen and progestin combination hormone replacement therapy, but did not show any benefit to estrogen alone.[26] Since hormone replacement therapy may also increase the risk of breast cancer and cardiovascular events, it is not advocated as a strategy in colorectal cancer prevention among postmenopausal women.[24]

## Cigarette Smoking

Tobacco smoke contains several carcinogenic compounds, including polyaromatic hydrocarbons, heterocyclic amines, nitrosamines, and aromatic amines. An estimated 15% to 20% of colorectal cancers in the United States are associated with cigarette smoking. This population-attributable risk may be higher for rectal than for colon cancers.[24] Early studies evaluating the relationship between smoking and colorectal carcinoma did not show a causal association between tobacco smoke and colorectal cancer risk, possibly because the former impacts early carcinogenesis, so a sufficiently long follow-up period is required to demonstrate an association. Several decades of epidemiologic research into cigarette smoking have now amassed abundant evidence supporting a relationship between smoking and increased colorectal cancer risk. Individuals who have smoked at some time have a 20% increased risk of colorectal cancer compared to those who have never smoked. The relationship between cigarette smoking and cancer risk is dose dependent and based upon the number of cigarettes per day after long-term smoking of more than 30 years.[27] Prospective data also provide strong evidence that smoking is associated with increased colorectal cancer risk in former and current smokers, particularly rectal cancer.[28]

Cigarette smoking is strongly associated with certain molecular subtypes of colorectal cancer, which may explain why the overall increase in incidence of colorectal cancer attributable to smoking is modest. Cigarette smoking contributes significantly to colon cancers that exhibit microsatellite instability (MSI): More than 20% of colon cancers with MSI develop in current or ex-smokers, particularly individuals who smoked the equivalent of one pack per day for 20 years or more.[29] Although MSI is not common among rectal tumors, there is a strong association between smoking and rectal cancers with MSI.[30] Other molecular subtypes of colorectal cancer associated with smoking include those with *BRAF* mutations and those with aberrant DNA methylation, or the CpG island methylator phenotype, as described in Chapters 11 and 12.[15,30,31] Each of these molecular changes is more common among tumors with MSI, which may explain the observed association between MSI and smoking.

## Alcohol

The relationship between alcohol and colorectal cancer remains controversial, but most data suggest that high alcohol intake increases cancer risk. Prospective data estimate a 1.2-fold increased risk for colorectal cancer among individuals who consume more than 30 g of alcohol per day compared to those with low or no intake; each increase of 100 g/week results in a 15% increased colorectal cancer risk.[32–34] This association is observed for both rectal and colon cancers, as well as for different types of alcoholic beverage. Thus, the relationship between alcohol and colorectal cancer risk is best established among individuals with the highest intake, but modest alcohol intake (1 to 2 drinks daily) also affects risk. Alcohol may promote colorectal carcinogenesis by reducing folate levels or by antagonizing metabolism of methyl groups, thereby contributing to abnormal DNA methylation. Alcohol may also delay DNA repair, alter bile acid composition, and induce enzymatic activation of hepatic carcinogens.[24]

## Physical Activity

One of the most consistently observed lifestyle associations is that between greater levels of physical activity and decreased colon cancer risk, whereas lack of frequent, vigorous activity may be associated with 12% to 14% of colon cancers.[21] The mechanisms by which physical activity reduces cancer risk probably involve reduced insulin levels, reduced systemic inflammation, and improved gut motility (Figure 2.2). The relationship between physical activity and colon cancer is dose dependent. Risk reductions occur across a wide range of activity frequencies and intensities.[24] Physically active individuals have a 20% to 30% lower risk of colon cancer compared with less active individuals; even moderate levels of physical activity are linked to substantial benefits.[35] High levels of activity substantially reduce cancer risk by 40% to 50% or more.

The relationship between physical activity and rectal cancer risk is less consistent than that with colon cancer, and many studies have failed to detect a significant association. This difference

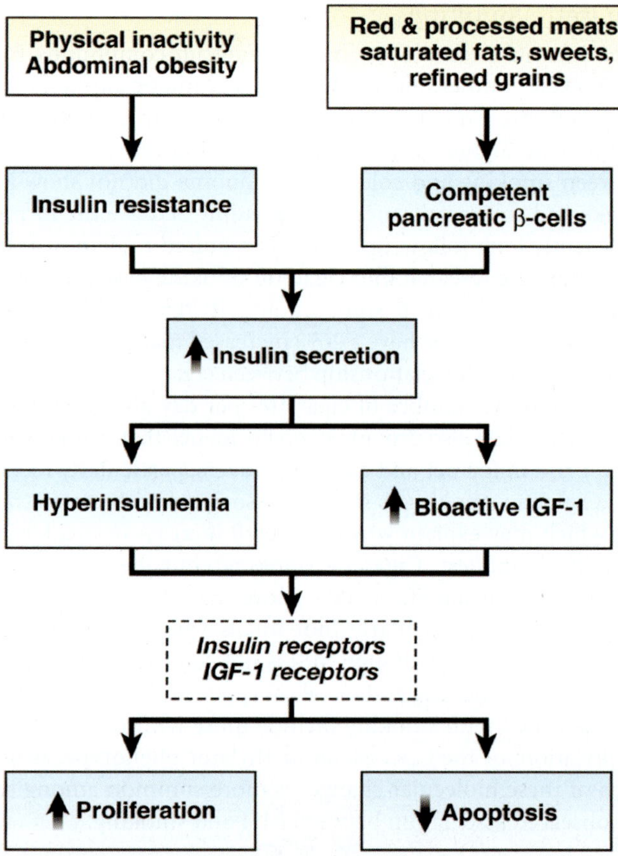


**FIGURE 2.2:** Lack of physical activity, obesity, and some foods common to a Western diet stimulate insulin resulting in repeated cycles of hyperinsulinemia. High insulin levels directly impact susceptible cells through insulin-like growth factor-1 (IGF-1) receptors by decreasing IGF-binding proteins leading to increasing free IGF-1. Activation of insulin and IGF-1 receptors promotes cell proliferation and reduced apoptosis.[24] (Reprinted from Chan AT, Giovannucci EL. Primary prevention of colorectal cancer. *Gastroenterology* 2010;138(6):2029–2043 e10, with permission.)

may reflect different methods used to collect activity data in rectal cancer studies or lack of power to detect significant associations in colorectal cancer studies that include few rectal cancer cases.[36] Moderate and vigorous levels of activity are associated with decreased risk of rectal cancer.[36,37]

## Obesity

Obesity is associated with increased risk of colorectal cancer. The World Health Organization (WHO) defines obesity as an abnormal, or excessive, fat accumulation in adipose tissue to the extent that health is impaired.[38] The classification of obesity for epidemiologic purposes relies on body mass index (BMI) defined by weight in kilograms divided by height in meters squared. *Overweight* is defined as a BMI more than 25 and *obesity* as a BMI more than 30 (Table 2.2). By these definitions, the global prevalence of obesity nearly doubled from 1980 to 2008, and, in the United States, 36% of adults and 17% of children are obese.[39] The WHO estimates that roughly 20% of men and 23% of women in Europe were obese in 2008. These numbers continue to grow.[38]

Increased BMI is associated with increased colorectal cancer risk, especially colon cancer risk.[1] The relative risk for colorectal carcinoma increases by 24% to 59% in obese men and 9% to 22% in obese women compared with individuals of normal weight. There is a clear dose–response relationship between BMI and colorectal cancer risk in populations from North America, Europe, and Asia.[40,41] Body mass indices of 23.0–24.9, 25.0–27.4, 27.5–29.9, and 30.0 or higher are associated with 14%, 19%, 24%, and 41% increased colorectal cancer risk, respectively, compared with a BMI of less than 23.0. The association is stronger for colon than rectal cancer, men more than women, and self-reported BMI compared with directly measured BMI.[41]

Although BMI is used to evaluate adiposity, it has limitations: BMI does not distinguish adipose tissue from lean tissue nor does it reflect either distribution of fat or its metabolic function.

**Table 2.2 Classification of Adiposity by Body Mass Index**

| Classification | BMI ($kg/m^2$) |
|---|---|
| Underweight | ≤18.5 |
| Normal weight | 18.5–25 |
| Overweight | 25–30 |
| Obese class I | 30–35 |
| Obese class II | 35–40 |
| Obese class III | ≥40 |

Central, or visceral, fat is more metabolically active than subcutaneous fat and exerts systemic effects that may promote cancer initiation and progression.[40] Waist circumference and waist-to-hip ratio measurements are widely used as surrogate markers of visceral adiposity. Colon cancer risk increases with waist circumference at a rate of 33% and 10% increased risk per 10 cm increment among men and women, respectively. Increasing waist-to-hip ratio is also associated with an increased cancer risk in men and women, even after controlling for other lifestyle factors.[42]

The mechanisms by which obesity increases colorectal cancer risk are not known. Factors that increase insulin resistance, such as inactivity and obesity, may combine with dietary factors to stimulate insulin secretion and increase colorectal cancer risk (Figure 2.2). Adipose tissue levels affect glucose metabolism and promote insulin resistance.[40] Cytokines produced by adipose tissue, such as interleukin-6 and tumor necrosis factor-α, negatively impact glucose homeostasis and lead to chronic hyperinsulinemia. Obesity also promotes a proinflammatory state by activating cellular pathways involving nuclear factor κB and transcription 3, the latter of which mediates cell proliferation and angiogenesis.[40]

## Dietary Risk Factors

### *Folate*

Many dietary factors may influence colorectal cancer risk. B vitamins, including folates, are important components of one-carbon metabolism that affect DNA synthesis, repair, and methylation (Figure 2.3). Naturally occurring folates are abundant in leafy green vegetables, citrus fruits, and organ meats. Folic acid, the synthetic form of folate, is found in enriched food products and supplements. Both folate and folic acid are hydrolyzed to 5-methyltetrahydrofolate after absorption. Once inside the cell, 5-methyltetrahydrofolate is reduced by dihydrofolate reductase to tetrahydrofolate, which then acts as a methyl donor to regenerate methionine from homocysteine, or it is converted to 5,10-methylenetetrahydrofolate for the production of thymidine or uracil residues used in DNA synthesis. Insufficient folate intake promotes fragility of DNA strands and impairs DNA methylation and repair, thereby promoting cancer development.[43]

The United States, Canada, and several other countries have mandated the fortification of flour, cereals, and other food products with folic acid for primary prevention of neural tube defects since 1998. However, some animal data suggest that heightened folate status and timing of folate exposure may increase colorectal cancer risk. The "dual effect of folate" hypothesis suggests that while adequate folate intake in healthy individuals may decrease colorectal cancer risk, excess folate increases the rate of malignant transformation of colorectal adenomas and other precancerous lesions.[43,44] High total folate intake is associated with no more than a 15% decrease in colorectal cancer risk compared with low total folate intake.[43] Prospective trials have not shown a benefit of daily folic acid supplementation for the prevention of colorectal adenoma

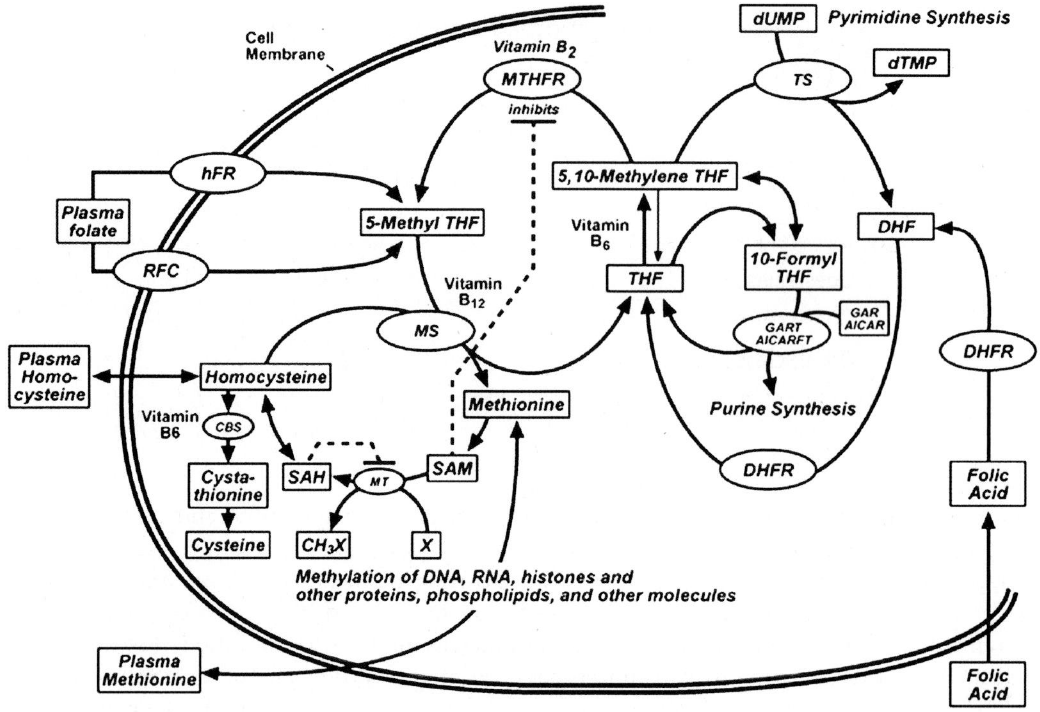


FIGURE 2.3: Overview of folate mediated, one-carbon metabolism.[44] (AICAR, 5-aminoimidazole-4-carboxamide ribonucleotide; AICARFT, 5-aminoimidazole-4-carboxamide ribonucleotide transformylase; CBS, cystathionine-beta-synthase; DHF, dihydrofolate; DHFR, dihydrofolate reductase; dUMP, deoxyuridine monophosphate; GAR, glycinamide ribonucleotide; GART, glycinamide ribonucleotide transformylase; hFR, human folate receptor; MS, methionine synthase; MT, methyltransferases; MTHFR, 5,10-methylenetetrahydrofolate reductase; RFC, reduced folate carrier; SAH (AdoHcy), S-adenosylhomocysteine; SAM (AdoMet), S-adenosylmethionine; THF, tetrahydrofolate; dTMP, deoxythymidine monophosphate; TS, thymidylate synthase; X, a variety of substrates for methylation.) (Reprinted from Ulrich CM, Reed MC, Nijhout FM. Modeling folate, one-carbon metabolism, and DNA methylation. *Nutr Rev* 2008;66(s1):S27–S30, with permission.)

recurrence in patients with a history of adenomas. Few individuals in the United States are folate deficient because of fortification of food, so it remains to be seen whether doses higher than the current recommendations (0.4 mg/day) are beneficial or harmful with respect to colorectal cancer prevention.[24]

### Fiber

The infrequency of colorectal cancer in populations that consume a high-fiber diet led researchers to postulate that diets rich in fruits and vegetables may lower colorectal cancer risk by increasing stool bulk, modulating colonic transit time, absorbing or diluting fecal carcinogens, or altering bile acid metabolism.[24] Data regarding the impact of dietary influences on colorectal cancer risk are conflicting. Older data suggest a 20% to 50% decreased cancer risk in populations that consume high-fiber diets compared with those with low dietary fiber intake.[45] Prospective data show a less substantial association between dietary fiber and colorectal cancer, which likely reflects confounding factors related to lifestyle and dietary practices that also reduce colorectal cancer risk.[46] The most recent information describes an inverse relationship between high intake of dietary fiber from cereal and whole grains; high intake of grain-related fiber is associated with a slight (10%) reduction in colorectal cancer risk.[47]

### Calcium and Vitamin D

Calcium prevents colorectal tumorigenesis by binding ionized fatty acids and toxic secondary bile acids to form insoluble soaps in the colonic lumen, reducing cell proliferation, stimulating differentiation, and inducing apoptosis in the colorectal mucosa.[24] Individuals with high calcium intake have a 22% reduced colorectal cancer risk compared with those with low intake.[48] Randomized, placebo-controlled trials evaluating calcium supplementation in patients with an adenoma history have also demonstrated a modest protective effect of calcium.[24]

Vitamin D reduces colorectal cancer risk by regulating cell proliferation, inhibiting angiogenesis, promoting cell differentiation, and stimulating apoptosis. Data also indicate an anti-inflammatory role for vitamin D supplements; vitamin D deficiency has been associated with inflammatory bowel disease as well as elevated markers of chronic inflammation.[24] Both vitamin D intake and blood levels are inversely related to colorectal cancer risk. High vitamin D intake is associated with a 12% decreased colorectal cancer risk, while highest blood levels of 25-hydroxyvitamin D are associated with a 33% reduction in colorectal cancer risk relative to the lowest levels.[49] A randomized, placebo-controlled trial evaluating daily supplementation of 1,000 mg of calcium and 400 IU of vitamin D per day did not find a difference between the treatment and placebo groups with respect to colorectal cancer risk after 7 years of follow-up.[50]

### *Red Meat*

Consumption of red meat has been implicated as a causal factor in colorectal cancer development for more than 30 years, although evidence supporting this view is limited. Red meat stimulates insulin secretion and serves as a major source of saturated fat, heme iron, and carcinogenic heterocyclic amines.[24] Most data describe a modest (~12%) increase in colorectal cancer risk among individuals with high red meat intake relative to those with low intake. The estimated relative risk is somewhat higher for rectal than colon cancer and stronger in men, who exhibit a 20% increased risk associated with high consumption.[51] Men who eat red meat as a main dish more than five times a week have a threefold increase in colon cancer risk compared with men who eat red meat less than once a month.[24] However, available data are insufficient to support an independent and unequivocal association between red meat intake and increased colorectal cancer risk, because ingestion of large amounts of red meat is often associated with confounding factors, such as diet high in saturated fat, sugar, and alcohol intake.[51] The association between red meat consumption and colorectal cancer may also depend on the cooking method used. Colon cancer is specifically increased among individuals who consume meat with a charred surface or meat exposed to high temperatures for a prolonged time. Grilling and broiling red meat at high temperatures elaborates mutagenic heterocyclic amines and polycyclic aromatic hydrocarbons, both of which are linked to colorectal cancer risk. Individuals with genetic variants in the *N*-acetyltransferase 2 (*NAT2*) gene that mediates metabolism of heterocyclic amines may be more susceptible to colorectal cancer if they consume grilled or broiled red meats. Women in the Nurses' Health Study who had *NAT2* genotypes associated with rapid acetylation of meat-associated carcinogens had a threefold increased risk of colorectal cancer if they also regularly consumed red meat, compared to women with slow acetylation genotypes.[24]

## SUMMARY

Decades of epidemiologic research in human populations have elucidated factors associated with sporadic colorectal cancer and have led to a large body of literature regarding genetic and environmental risk factors for this multifactorial disease. Many are biologically plausible and show consistent associations with colorectal cancer across investigations. Some, such as age, race and ethnicity, and genetic risk, are not modifiable, whereas others represent lifestyle and dietary influences that may be altered. The strength of association, potential for primary prevention, and consistency vary across studies and study designs (Figure 2.4). Regular use of NSAIDs is consistently associated with decreased colorectal cancer incidence and mortality, although concerns for potential negative effects have tempered their utility in primary prevention. Hormone replacement therapy in postmenopausal women is also associated with decreased colorectal cancer risk, but risk of breast cancer and cardiovascular events prevents its widespread advocacy as

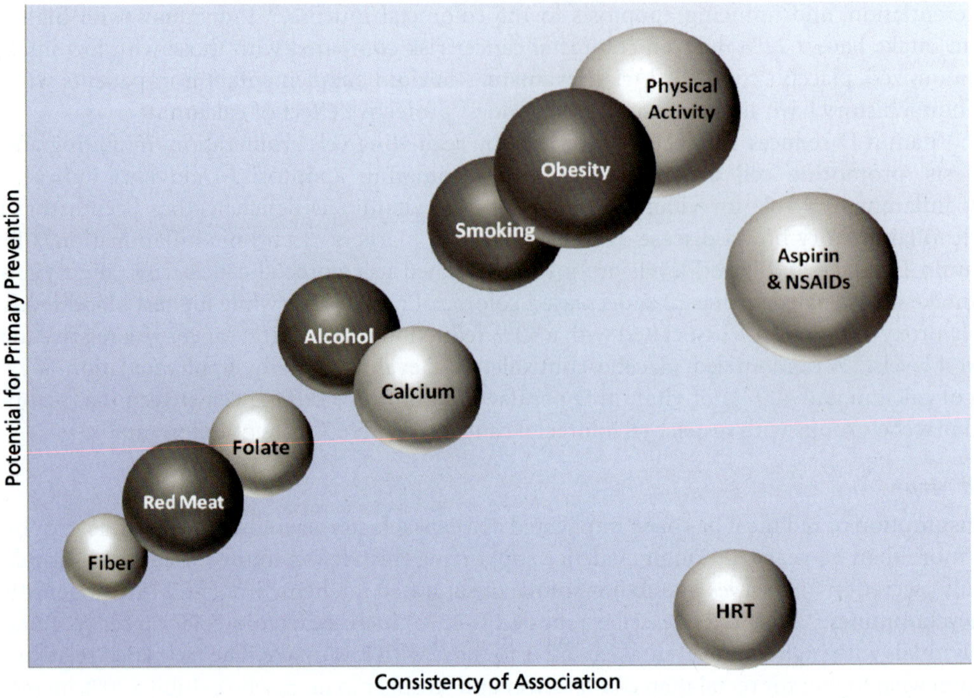


FIGURE 2.4: Evidence for 10 lifestyle and dietary factors associated with colorectal cancer is summarized in the accompanying figure. Each factor has been ranked from 1 through 10 for consistency of associations across multiple studies ($x$-axis) and potential for primary prevention based on summary recommendations and strength of association. *Dark gray spheres* denote factors associated with increased risk, and *light gray spheres* represent factors associated with decreased risk. The size of the *sphere* reflects the average strength of association based on data from prospective cohort and case–control studies.

a preventive tool. Perhaps the greatest potential for reducing the incidence of colorectal cancer lies in efforts that emphasize smoking cessation, moderation of alcohol consumption, and energy balance through increased physical activity and reduction in adipose tissue. Promotion of diets with adequate folate and calcium that are lower in red meat could represent a strategy for modest reductions in colorectal cancer risk.

# References

1. Ferlay J, Shin HR, Bray F, et al. Estimates of worldwide burden of cancer in 2008: GLOBOCAN 2008. *Int J Cancer* 2010;127(12):2893–2917.
2. Ferlay J, Shin HR, Bray F, et al. GLOBOCAN 2008 v 1.2, cancer incidence and mortality worldwide: IARC CancerBase No. 10 [Internet]. Lyon, France: International Agency for Research on Cancer; 2010. Available from http://globocan.iarc.fr, accessed July 20, 2012.
3. Howlander N, Noone AM, Krapcho M, et al. SEER Cancer Statistics Review, 1975–2009 (Vintage 2009 populations), National Cancer Institute. Bethesda, MD, http://seer.cancer.gov/csr/1975_2009_pops09/, based on November 2011 SEER data submission, posted to the SEER Web site 2012.
4. Haggar FA, Boushey RP. Colorectal cancer epidemiology: incidence, mortality, survival, and risk factors. *Clin Colon Rectal Surg* 2009;22(4):191–197.
5. Siegel RL, Jemal A, Thun MJ, et al. Trends in the incidence of colorectal cancer in relation to county-level poverty among blacks and whites. *J Natl Med Assoc* 2008;100(12):1441–1444.
6. American Cancer Society. *Colorectal Cancer Facts & Figures for African Americans 2011–2012*. Atlanta, GA: American Cancer Society; 2011.

7. Schatzkin A, Freedman LS, Dawsey SM, et al. Interpreting precursor studies: what polyp trials tell us about large-bowel cancer. *J Natl Cancer Inst* 1994;86(14):1053–1057.
8. Baxter NN, Warren JL, Barrett MJ, et al. Association between colonoscopy and colorectal cancer mortality in a US cohort according to site of cancer and colonoscopist specialty. *J Clin Oncol* 2012;30(21): 2664–2669.
9. Labianca R, Beretta GD, Mosconi S, et al. Colorectal cancer: screening. *Ann Oncol* 2005;16(suppl 2) :ii127–ii132.
10. Hiraoka S, Kato J, Fujiki S, et al. The presence of large serrated polyps increases risk for colorectal cancer. *Gastroenterology* 2010;139(5):1503–10, 10 e1–e3.
11. de la Chapelle A. Genetic predisposition to colorectal cancer. *Nat Rev Cancer* 2004;4(10):769–780.
12. Jemal A, Bray F, Center MM, et al. Global cancer statistics. *CA Cancer J Clin* 2011;61(2):69–90.
13. Soravia C, Bapat B, Cohen Z. Familial adenomatous polyposis (FAP) and hereditary nonpolyposis colorectal cancer (HNPCC): a review of clinical, genetic and therapeutic aspects. *Schweiz Med Wochenschr* 1997;127(16):682–690.
14. Broderick P, Carvajal-Carmona L, Pittman AM, et al. A genome-wide association study shows that common alleles of SMAD7 influence colorectal cancer risk. *Nat Genet* 2007;39(11):1315–1317.
15. Curtin K, Lin WY, George R, et al. Meta association of colorectal cancer confirms risk alleles at 8q24 and 18q21. *Cancer Epidemiol Biomarkers Prev* 2009;18(2):616–621.
16. Slattery ML, Herrick J, Curtin K, et al. Increased risk of colon cancer associated with a genetic polymorphism of SMAD7. *Cancer Res* 2010;70(4):1479–1485.
17. Flood DM, Weiss NS, Cook LS, et al. Colorectal cancer incidence in Asian migrants to the United States and their descendants. *Cancer Causes Control* 2000;11(5):403–411.
18. Thomas DB, Karagas MR. Cancer in first and second generation Americans. *Cancer Res* 1987;47(21): 5771–5776.
19. Arber N, Levin B. Chemoprevention of colorectal neoplasia: the potential for personalized medicine. *Gastroenterology* 2008;134(4):1224–1237.
20. Kraus S, Arber N. Cancer: do aspirin and other NSAIDs protect against colorectal cancer? *Nat Rev Gastroenterol Hepatol* 2011;8(3):125–126.
21. Slattery ML. Physical activity and colorectal cancer. *Sports Med* 2004;34(4):239–252.
22. Din FV, Theodoratou E, Farrington SM, et al. Effect of aspirin and NSAIDs on risk and survival from colorectal cancer. *Gut* 2010;59(12):1670–1679.
23. Thun MJ, Jacobs EJ, Patrono C. The role of aspirin in cancer prevention. *Nat Rev Clin Oncol* 2012;9(5):259–267.
24. Chan AT, Giovannucci EL. Primary prevention of colorectal cancer. *Gastroenterology* 2010;138(6): 2029–2043 e10.
25. Grodstein F, Newcomb PA, Stampfer MJ. Postmenopausal hormone therapy and the risk of colorectal cancer: a review and meta-analysis. *Am J Med* 1999;106(5):574–582.
26. Rossouw JE, Anderson GL, Prentice RL, et al. Risks and benefits of estrogen plus progestin in healthy postmenopausal women: principal results From the Women's Health Initiative randomized controlled trial. *JAMA* 2002;288(3):321–333.
27. Botteri E, Iodice S, Bagnardi V, et al. Smoking and colorectal cancer: a meta-analysis. *JAMA* 2008;300(23):2765–2778.
28. Liang PS, Chen TY, Giovannucci E. Cigarette smoking and colorectal cancer incidence and mortality: systematic review and meta-analysis. *Int J Cancer* 2009;124(10):2406–2415.
29. Slattery ML, Curtin K, Anderson K, et al. Associations between cigarette smoking, lifestyle factors, and microsatellite instability in colon tumors. *J Natl Cancer Inst* 2000;92(22):1831–1836.
30. Curtin K, Samowitz WS, Wolff RK, et al. Somatic alterations, metabolizing genes and smoking in rectal cancer. *Int J Cancer* 2009;125(1):158–164.
31. Samowitz WS, Albertsen H, Sweeney C, et al. Association of smoking, CpG island methylator phenotype, and V600E BRAF mutations in colon cancer. *J Natl Cancer Inst* [Research Support, N.I.H., Extramural Research Support, Non-U.S. Gov't] 2006;98(23):1731–1738.
32. Cho E, Smith-Warner SA, Ritz J, et al. Alcohol intake and colorectal cancer: a pooled analysis of 8 cohort studies. *Ann Intern Med* 2004;140(8):603–613.
33. Ferrari P, Jenab M, Norat T, et al. Lifetime and baseline alcohol intake and risk of colon and rectal cancers in the European prospective investigation into cancer and nutrition (EPIC). *Int J Cancer* 2007;121(9):2065–2072.

34. Moskal A, Norat T, Ferrari P, et al. Alcohol intake and colorectal cancer risk: a dose-response meta-analysis of published cohort studies. *Int J Cancer* 2007;120(3):664–671.
35. Wolin KY, Yan Y, Colditz GA, et al. Physical activity and colon cancer prevention: a meta-analysis. *Br J Cancer* 2009;100(4):611–616.
36. Slattery ML, Samowitz W, Hoffman M, et al. Aspirin, NSAIDs, and colorectal cancer: possible involvement in an insulin-related pathway. *Cancer Epidemiol Biomarkers Prev* 2004;13(4):538–545.
37. Slattery ML, Edwards S, Curtin K, et al. Physical activity and colorectal cancer. *Am J Epidemiol* 2003;158(3):214–224.
38. World Health Organization. Regional office for Europe. Obesity facts and figures. Available at http://www.euro.who.int/en/what-we-do/health-topics/noncommunicable-diseases/obesity/facts-and-figures, accessed July 25, 2012.
39. Ogden CL, Carroll MD, Kit BK, et al. Prevalence of obesity in the United States, 2009–2010. *NCHS Data Brief* 2012;(82):1–8.
40. Donohoe CL, Pidgeon GP, Lysaght J, et al. Obesity and gastrointestinal cancer. *Br J Surg* 2010;97(5): 628–642.
41. Ning Y, Wang L, Giovannucci EL. A quantitative analysis of body mass index and colorectal cancer: findings from 56 observational studies. *Obes Rev* 2010;11(1):19–30.
42. Larsson SC, Wolk A. Obesity and colon and rectal cancer risk: a meta-analysis of prospective studies. *Am J Clin Nutr* 2007;86(3):556–565.
43. Kennedy DA, Stern SJ, Moretti M, et al. Folate intake and the risk of colorectal cancer: a systematic review and meta-analysis. *Cancer Epidemiol* 2011;35(1):2–10.
44. Ulrich CM, Potter JD. Folate and cancer—timing is everything. *JAMA* 2007;297(21):2408–2409.
45. Howe GR, Benito E, Castelleto R, et al. Dietary intake of fiber and decreased risk of cancers of the colon and rectum: evidence from the combined analysis of 13 case-control studies. *J Natl Cancer Inst* 1992;84(24):1887–1896.
46. Park Y, Hunter DJ, Spiegelman D, et al. Dietary fiber intake and risk of colorectal cancer: a pooled analysis of prospective cohort studies. *JAMA* 2005;294(22):2849–2857.
47. Aune D, Chan DS, Lau R, et al. Dietary fibre, whole grains, and risk of colorectal cancer: systematic review and dose-response meta-analysis of prospective studies. *BMJ* 2011;343:d6617.
48. Cho E, Smith-Warner SA, Spiegelman D, et al. Dairy foods, calcium, and colorectal cancer: a pooled analysis of 10 cohort studies. *J Natl Cancer Inst* 2004;96(13):1015–1022.
49. Ma Y, Zhang P, Wang F, et al. Association between vitamin D and risk of colorectal cancer: a systematic review of prospective studies. *J Clin Oncol* 2011;29(28):3775–3782.
50. Wactawski-Wende J, Kotchen JM, Anderson GL, et al. Calcium plus vitamin D supplementation and the risk of colorectal cancer. *N Engl J Med* 2006;354(7):684–696.
51. Alexander DD, Weed DL, Cushing CA, et al. Meta-analysis of prospective studies of red meat consumption and colorectal cancer. *Eur J Cancer Prev* 2011;20(4):293–307.

# Screening and Surveillance for Prevention of Colorectal Carcinoma

# 3


- Felice Schnoll-Sussman
- Amir Soumekh


Colorectal carcinoma is the most common malignancy of the gastrointestinal tract and the second most common cause of cancer-related death in the United States. Most tumors are preceded by preexisting adenomas, although some develop from nondysplastic serrated polyps, and others arise in the setting of inflammatory bowel disease. Identification and removal of these cancer precursors is a primary goal of gastroenterologists performing screening colonoscopies. Colonic polyps are also routinely encountered during colonoscopies or sigmoidoscopies performed for other indications. Upon identifying and removing a premalignant polyp, clinicians need to provide patients with prognostic information, a plan for colonic surveillance following the initial procedure, and identify patients whose polyps represent a manifestation of a familial cancer syndrome. The purpose of this chapter is to discuss current practice guidelines regarding screening and surveillance of patients with colorectal polyps at risk for cancer development. Surveillance of patients with inflammatory bowel disease is discussed in Chapters 4 and 15.

## ADENOMATOUS POLYPS

The vast majority of colonic cancers arise from adenomatous polyps. Their development is influenced by age, gender, and other risk factors such as body mass index, level of physical activity, and possibly race. Approximately 25% of asymptomatic patients have adenomas at the time of screening colonoscopy, although their prevalence ranges from 2% in patients in their 20s or 30s to 50% by age 70.[1,2] Adenomas occur more commonly among males than females: Men have up to 15% more polyps than women. Adenomas are also associated with abdominal obesity and lack of physical activity.[3–5] Frank adenocarcinoma and larger adenomas are more prevalent among African Americans for unclear reasons; differences between races may reflect variation in location and polyp type or differences in screening rates between Caucasians and African Americans.[6,7]

Adenomatous polyps are endoscopically categorized by size and morphology. Polyps are classified as diminutive (<5 mm diameter), small (5 to 10 mm diameter), or large (>1 cm diameter). Adenoma size increases with age, and larger polyps are seen more frequently in the distal colon.[1] Diminutive polyps are commonly encountered in routine colonoscopic examinations and up to 50% are adenomatous, although less than 5% show high-grade dysplasia or contain villous elements and only 0.1% contain invasive adenocarcinoma.[8,9] It is not clear whether these polyps have potential to grow substantially over time or if endoscopic resection improves outcome.[10–12] Emerging data suggest that diminutive polyps can be resected and discarded without pathologic examination, thereby saving health care costs without significantly impacting clinical care.[13] Nonetheless, current screening guidelines do not distinguish between diminutive adenomatous polyps and those that span 5 to 10 mm. Large polyps are considered to represent advanced adenomas regardless of their pathologic features because they are more likely to have high-risk features, such as a villous architecture, high-grade dysplasia, or even carcinoma, the latter of which may be present in nearly half of these lesions.[14] Thus, current surveillance guidelines require a shorter duration of surveillance for patients with large adenomas.

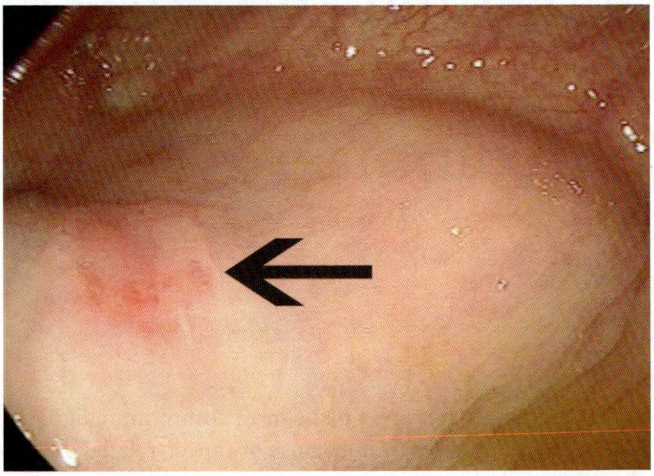

FIGURE 3.1: Flat polyps have a height one-half that of their diameter. They may appear as an erythematous area (*arrow*) and are difficult to detect during routine colonoscopic examination.

Colorectal polyps are classified as sessile, pedunculated, or flat based on their endoscopic appearances. Sessile adenomas are broad-based lesions, whereas pedunculated lesions have a slender fibromuscular stalk connecting the polyp to the colonic wall. There is no clear biologic difference between sessile and pedunculated polyps. However, sessile polyps may require piecemeal removal due to difficulties achieving endoscopic excision, in which case they require follow-up evaluation at very short intervals (2 to 6 months) to confirm complete removal.[15] Flat adenomas have a height that is less than one-half the overall diameter (Figure 3.1). Though less common than raised lesions, flat adenomas are difficult to detect and may behave more aggressively. Flat polyps account for approximately 10% of all adenomas detected by routine colonoscopy compared to 36% of polyps found during colonoscopies enhanced by chromoendoscopy, suggesting that many flat lesions are missed during routine colonoscopy.[16] Flat lesions with central depressions are highly likely to contain invasive adenocarcinoma.[17]

Adenomatous polyps are subdivided into three major types based on the predominant glandular architecture. More than 80% of adenomatous polyps display a tubular growth pattern, whereas tubulovillous and villous adenomas account for the remainder and occur in near equal numbers.[18–20] Tubular, tubulovillous, and villous adenomas vary with respect to their risk for high-grade dysplasia and cancer, and thus, pathologic classification of adenomas affects postpolypectomy surveillance intervals. Adenomas with villous features are more likely to contain high-grade dysplasia and have increased risk of carcinoma. For this reason, they require surveillance at shorter intervals than tubular adenomas (Table 3.1).[21,22]

## SERRATED POLYPS

Serrated polyps comprise a heterogeneous group of nondysplastic and dysplastic polyps with serrated glandular architecture and include hyperplastic polyps, sessile serrated polyps (sessile serrated adenoma), and (traditional) serrated adenomas, as described in Chapter 4. Of these, hyperplastic polyps are most common. They are detected in approximately 10% of routine screening colonoscopies performed among asymptomatic patients over the age of 50 and autopsy data report an overall prevalence of 20% to 35%.[1,23] Sporadic hyperplastic polyps have little, or no, intrinsic malignant potential, and thus, patients with hyperplastic polyps of the distal colon are considered to have normal colonoscopies.[22,24] However, detection of distal hyperplastic polyps during screening sigmoidoscopy may warrant follow-up full colonoscopy since up to 25% of patients with hyperplastic polyps have adenomas in the abdominal colon and 5% have advanced adenomas of the proximal colon.[25] Serrated adenomas comprise approximately 2% of all serrated polyps, are frequently pedunculated, and show a predilection for the left colon.[26,27] Sessile serrated

**Table 3.1** Surveillance Guidelines for Colon Cancer according to the United States Preventive Services Task Force and Multisociety Task Force for Colorectal Cancer

| Patient Characteristics and Surveillance Criteria |
|---|
| Age |
| Regular screening begins at 50 years of age and continues until age of 75 |
| Screening Methods |
| Annual high-sensitivity fecal occult blood testing |
| Flexible sigmoidoscopy repeated every 5 years |
| Colonoscopy as screening tests or follow-up when other screening test are positive |
| Surveillance Protocols[a] |
| Surveillance at 10 years |
| No polyps on initial exam |
| Small (<10 mm) hyperplastic polyps of rectosigmoid colon |
| Surveillance at 5 years |
| One or two small (<10 mm) tubular adenomas |
| Nondysplastic sessile serrated polyp(s) <10 mm |
| Surveillance at 3 years |
| Three to ten tubular adenomas |
| Tubular adenoma ≥10 mm *or* any adenoma with a villous component *or* an adenoma with high-grade dysplasia |
| Nondysplastic sessile serrated polyp(s) ≥10 mm *or* sessile serrated polyp with dysplasia *or* a traditional serrated adenoma |
| Surveillance at <3 years |
| More than 10 tubular adenomas |
| Surveillance at 1 year |
| Serrated polyposis |

[a]Surveillance for patients with inadequate bowel preparation, incomplete or piecemeal removal of polyps is shorter, at discretion of the endoscopist.

Data from Lieberman DA, Rex DK, Winawer SJ, et al. Guidelines for colonoscopy surveillance after screening and polypectomy: a consensus update by the US Multi-Society Task Force on Colorectal Cancer. *Gastroenterology* 2012;143(3):844–857.

polyps occur more commonly in the proximal colon and are often missed during colonoscopy, with a wide variability in their detection rate among endoscopists.[28] This high miss rate is at least partially due to their morphology; sessile serrated polyps are often flat, making them difficult to identify in patients with a poor bowel cleansing preparation (Figure 3.2).[29] Sessile serrated polyps may harbor advanced neoplasia, and large polyps (≥1 cm) have been implicated as potential risk factors for development of colorectal cancer.[30–32] Management of serrated polyps is controversial, although some guidelines recommend that these lesions be managed comparably to adenomatous polyps of similar size.[22,33,34]

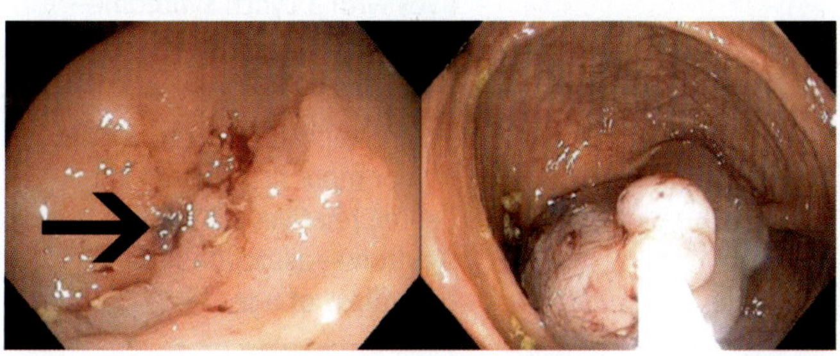

FIGURE 3.2: This sessile serrated polyp of the cecum (*arrow*) is large and flat. Saline injection at the base raises the polyp and aids piecemeal polypectomy.

# HEREDITARY POLYPOSIS SYNDROMES

## Lynch Syndrome

Lynch syndrome (hereditary nonpolyposis colorectal cancer) is the most common colon cancer susceptibility syndrome. As discussed in Chapter 11, it is an autosomal dominant disorder caused by a germline mutation in one of several DNA mismatch repair genes, including MSH2, MLH1, MSH6, PMS1, and PMS2. Patients may have heritable cancers limited to the colorectum or, more classically, an increased risk for a variety of malignancies, including endometrial, ovarian, urologic, gastric, small bowel, pancreatic, and central nervous system tumors. The hallmark of Lynch syndrome is early-onset colorectal cancer with malignancies diagnosed an average of 20 years earlier than in patients with sporadic colorectal cancer. Presumably, patients with Lynch syndrome develop adenomas at rates comparable to healthy controls, but their adenomas progress to cancers more rapidly. Compared to sporadic adenomas, those seen in Lynch syndrome are more often large, flat, proximally located, and display high-grade dysplasia and/or villous histology.[35] Extracolonic cancers also occur earlier than sporadic malignancies.

Multiple strategies have been proposed to identify patients with Lynch syndrome. The International Collaborative Group on Hereditary Non-Polyposis Colorectal Cancer developed the Amsterdam criteria in 1991 to identify patients likely to have Lynch syndrome (Table 3.2).[36] The Amsterdam criteria were later refined and ultimately replaced by guidelines developed in a 1996 workshop sponsored by the National Cancer Institute. The revised Bethesda guidelines recommend microsatellite instability (MSI) testing followed by germline testing of mismatch repair genes when MSI is identified.[37] However, both the Amsterdam criteria and Bethesda guidelines fail to identify some patients with Lynch syndromes, and, thus, many physicians advocate

**Table 3.2 Enumeration of the Amsterdam Criteria and Revised Bethesda Guidelines for Detection of Lynch Syndrome**

| Amsterdam Criteria | Amsterdam II Criteria | Revised Bethesda Guidelines |
|---|---|---|
| Three or more relatives with colorectal cancer, one of whom is a first-degree relative of the other two | Three or more relatives with Lynch syndrome–associated tumors, one of whom is a first-degree relative of the other two | Colorectal cancer diagnosed under age of 50 years |
| At least two successive generations involved | At least two successive generations affected | Synchronous or metachronous Lynch syndrome–associated tumors, regardless of age |
| At least one of the cancers diagnosed before 50 years of age | At least one of the cancers diagnosed before 50 years of age | Colorectal cancer with histologic features of MSI diagnosed in patient <60 years of age |
| | Exclusion of familial adenomatous polyposis | Colorectal cancer diagnosed in one or more first-degree relatives with a Lynch syndrome–associated tumor, one of whom is diagnosed at <50 years of age |
| | Tumors verified by pathologic examination | Colorectal cancer diagnosed in two or more first- or second-degree relatives with Lynch syndrome–associated tumor, regardless of age |

universal testing for MSI on all colorectal cancers. This approach is common at large cancer centers and has been shown to identify a large number of patients who would have been missed by clinical criteria.[38,39]

Once Lynch syndrome is diagnosed, patients require vigilant surveillance for development of both colorectal and extracolonic tumors. Multiple surveillance regimens have been proposed, but these are mostly based on observational data. Current guidelines recommend annual colonoscopy beginning at age 20 to 25 or 10 years prior to the earliest age of colon cancer diagnosis in the family. Detection of an advanced adenoma or invasive adenocarcinoma is generally considered an indication for total or partial colectomy with continued surveillance of any remaining portion of the colorectum. Subtotal colectomy is associated with a higher risk of development of a second colorectal cancer, although patients may prefer this therapeutic option to total proctocolectomy.[40] Surveillance for carcinomas of endometrial, ovarian, and urologic origin as well as the upper gastrointestinal tract is also recommended.[41–44]

## Familial Adenomatous Polyposis

Familial adenomatous polyposis is the second most common inherited colon cancer susceptibility syndrome. Variants include Crail syndrome, Gardner syndrome, and attenuated familial adenomatous polyposis, as discussed in Chapter 11. This autosomal dominant disorder is caused by germline mutations in the adenomatous polyposis coli (*APC*) gene and displays nearly 100% penetrance. Patients with familial adenomatous polyposis develop hundreds to thousands of tubular, villous, or tubulovillous adenomas that become apparent at approximately 10 years of age (Figure 3.3). Although an individual polyp is associated with the same risk of progression to malignancy as sporadic polyps found in the general population, the markedly increased risk of colorectal cancer among familial adenomatous polyposis patients is a function of the number of polyps and the early age at which they develop. Colorectal cancer is considered inevitable approximately 10 to 20 years after the development of polyposis.

Genetic testing for *APC* mutations should be performed when patients are found to have more than 100 adenomas during their lifetimes. Affected family members require very early screening, including sigmoidoscopy beginning at 10 years of age, followed by colectomy in all patients once polyposis is identified.[45] Patients with familial adenomatous polyposis also require surveillance for upper gastrointestinal tumors as well as extraintestinal disease manifestations (Figure 3.4).

Attenuated familial adenomatous polyposis is associated with fewer colonic polyps (usually 10 to 100 lifetime polyps). Patients with attenuated disease have a delayed onset of polyposis and

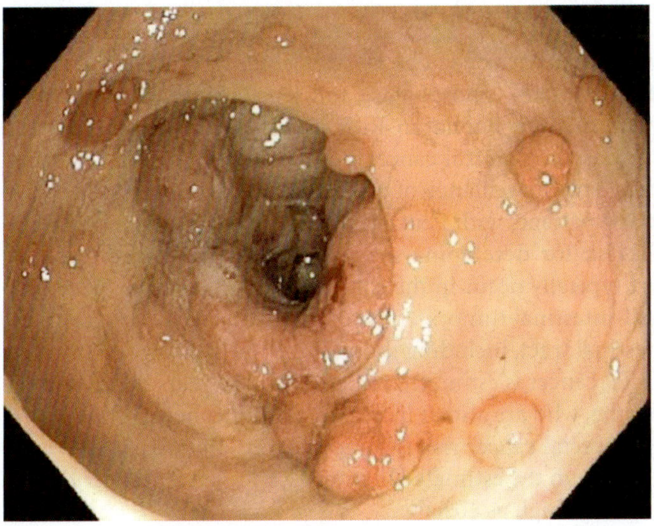

FIGURE 3.3: Numerous adenomatous polyps and a nearly obstructing circumferential carcinoma are present in the colon of a young patient with familial adenomatous polyposis.

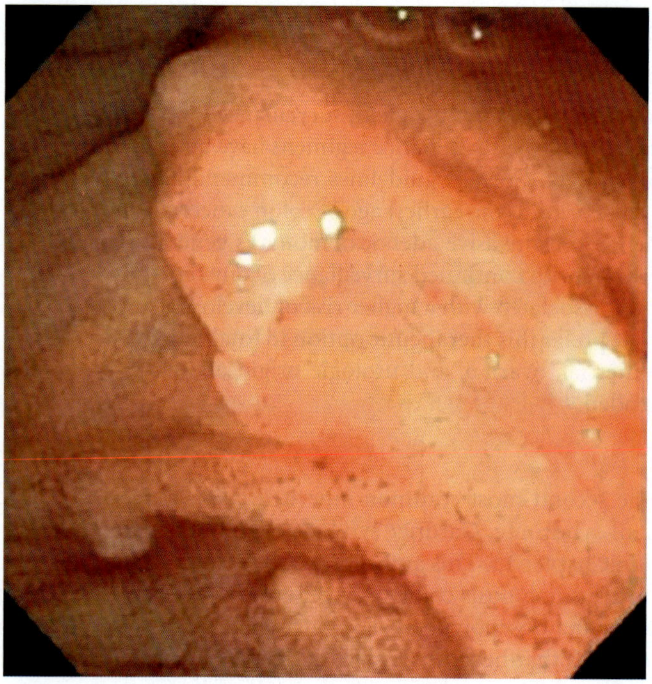

**FIGURE 3.4:** Patients with familial adenomatous polyposis are at risk for duodenal adenomas and adenocarcinomas. This patient had periampullary adenoma identified during screening endoscopy.

colorectal cancer, and, although cancer risk is extremely high, colorectal cancer development is not inevitable.[46–48] Patients with 10 to 100 adenomas should be referred for genetic testing, and, if the diagnosis is confirmed, at risk family members should be tested as well. Early colorectal cancer screening is recommended for patients with attenuated familial adenomatous polyposis, albeit less intensively than that of patients with classic disease. Colonoscopic surveillance every 2 years beginning at the age 20 years is recommended.[45] Some patients may be followed with ongoing surveillance and endoscopic removal of adenomas, whereas those with numerous polyps should be considered for colectomy if endoscopic treatment is not feasible. Upper gastrointestinal malignancies, such as duodenal adenomas and periampullary carcinomas, also develop in patients with attenuated familial adenomatous polyposis, and, thus, upper gastrointestinal screening is recommended.

## Hamartomatous Polyposes

Several hamartomatous polyposis syndromes have been described, including Peutz-Jeghers syndrome, juvenile polyposis syndrome, and PTEN (phosphatase and tensin homologue) hamartoma tumor syndrome (Cowden syndrome and Bannayan-Riley-Ruvalcaba syndrome). All of these disorders are associated with increased colorectal cancer risk as well as a risk for extracolonic malignancies, and, thus, screening and surveillance of affected patients are recommended (Table 3.3). Cancer risk is highest among patients with Peutz-Jeghers syndrome who have a 93% overall lifetime cancer risk and 66% risk for developing malignancies of the gastrointestinal tract.[49,50] Their gastrointestinal tumors typically occur in the colorectum and pancreas, although patients also develop gastric and small-intestinal tumors. Affected individuals develop a variety of malignancies outside the gastrointestinal tract, including those of the testis, ovary, and uterine cervix. The cumulative risk for colorectal cancer is estimated to be 68% by 60 years of age among patients with juvenile polyposis syndrome, who are also at increased risk for cancers of the stomach, small intestine, and pancreas.[51] Colorectal cancer risk is somewhat less among patients with PTEN hamartoma tumor syndrome, although the estimated lifetime risk for breast cancer is 25% to 50% and that of thyroid cancer may be as high as 10%.[52–55]

**Table 3.3 Proposed Guidelines for Surveillance of Patients with Hamartomatous Polyposis Syndromes**

| Organ Evaluated | Peutz-Jeghers Syndrome | Juvenile Polyposis Syndrome | PTEN Hamartoma Tumor Syndrome |
|---|---|---|---|
| Gastrointestinal Tract | | | |
| Esophagus | Upper endoscopy every 2 years | None | None |
| Stomach | Upper endoscopy every 2 years | Endoscopy with onset of symptoms or in late teens; repeat every 3 years | Not defined |
| Small Intestine | Imaging every 2 years beginning at age 10 | Endoscopy with onset of symptoms or in late teens; repeat every 3 years | Not defined |
| Colon | Colonoscopy with onset of symptoms or in late teens; repeat every 3 years | Colonoscopy with onset of symptoms or in late teens; repeat every 3 years | Not defined |
| Pancreas | Ultrasound every 2 years beginning at age 30 | | |
| Other Organ Systems | | | |
| Breast | Mammogram and examination every 2–3 years beginning at age 25 | | Annual examination beginning at age 25; annual mammography beginning at age 30 |
| Ovary, Cervix, Uterus | Annual Pap smear, ultrasound, and uterine washings beginning at age 20 | | Evaluation with biopsies for endometrial cancer every 5–10 years beginning at age 35 |
| Testis | Annual examination and ultrasound beginning at age 10 | | |
| Lung | Uncertain | | |
| Thyroid | | | Annual examination beginning in teens |

Data from Eng C. PTEN Hamartoma Tumor Syndrome (PHTS). In: Pagon RA, Bird TD, Dolan CR, et al., eds. *GeneReviews*. Seattle, WA: University of Washington; 1993. http://www.ncbi.nlm.nih.gov/books/NBK1116/. Updated 2012.

## SUMMARY AND CONCLUSIONS

Colorectal carcinoma is a global health problem and a leading cause of cancer-related morbidity and mortality in the United States. Virtually all of these tumors develop from noninvasive dysplastic precursor lesions amenable to endoscopic removal. Indeed, the goal of screening and surveillance programs is detection and removal of these cancer precursors. Screening methods and surveillance intervals vary depending on perceived cancer risk in individual patients, which is determined by a number of factors. Important issues to consider when assessing patient risk include the number and type of colorectal polyps encountered during colonoscopy, polyp size, the presence or absence of high-risk features (e.g., villous architecture and high-grade dysplasia), family history of colorectal polyps or cancer, and features suggestive of an underlying heritable syndrome.

## ACKNOWLEDGMENT

The authors would like to acknowledge Jasmine Paulino, of the Ethical Culture Fieldston School in the Bronx, New York, for her contributions to this chapter.

# References

1. Williams AR, Balasooriya BA, Day DW. Polyps and cancer of the large bowel: a necropsy study in Liverpool. *Gut* [Research Support, Non-U.S. Gov't] 1982;23(10):835–842.
2. Pendergrass CJ, Edelstein DL, Hylind LM, et al. Occurrence of colorectal adenomas in younger adults: an epidemiologic necropsy study. *Clin Gastroenterol Hepatol* [Comparative Study Research Support, N.I.H., Extramural Research Support, Non-U.S. Gov't] 2008;6(9):1011–1015.
3. Betes M, Munoz-Navas MA, Duque JM, et al. Use of colonoscopy as a primary screening test for colorectal cancer in average risk people. *Am J Gastroenterol* 2003;98(12):2648–2654.
4. Nguyen SP, Bent S, Chen YH, et al. Gender as a risk factor for advanced neoplasia and colorectal cancer: a systematic review and meta-analysis. *Clin Gastroenterol Hepatol* [Meta-Analysis Review] 2009;7(6): 676–681; e1–e3.
5. Ben Q, An W, Jiang Y, et al. Body mass index increases risk for colorectal adenomas based on meta-analysis. *Gastroenterology* [Meta-Analysis Research Support, Non-U.S. Gov't] 2012;142(4):762–772.
6. Rex DK, Khan AM, Shah P, et al. Screening colonoscopy in asymptomatic average-risk African Americans. *Gastrointest Endosc* 2000;51(5):524–527.
7. Penn E, Garrow D, Romagnuolo J. Influence of race and sex on prevalence and recurrence of colon polyps. *Arch Intern Med* [Comparative Study Research Support, Non-U.S. Gov't] 2010;170(13):1127–1132.
8. Weston AP, Campbell DR. Diminutive colonic polyps: histopathology, spatial distribution, concomitant significant lesions, and treatment complications. *Am J Gastroenterol* 1995;90(1):24–28.
9. Church JM. Clinical significance of small colorectal polyps. *Dis Colon Rectum* 2004;47(4):481–485.
10. Spencer RJ, Melton LJ III, Ready RL, et al. Treatment of small colorectal polyps: a population-based study of the risk of subsequent carcinoma. *Mayo Clin Proc* [Research Support, U.S. Gov't, P.H.S.] 1984;59(5):305–310.
11. Hoff G, Foerster A, Vatn MH, et al. Epidemiology of polyps in the rectum and colon. Recovery and evaluation of unresected polyps 2 years after detection. *Scand J Gastroenterol* [Research Support, Non-U.S. Gov't] 1986;21(7):853–862.
12. Hofstad B, Vatn M. Growth rate of colon polyps and cancer. *Gastrointest Endosc Clin N Am* [Review] 1997;7(3):345–363.
13. Kessler WR, Imperiale TF, Klein RW, et al. A quantitative assessment of the risks and cost savings of forgoing histologic examination of diminutive polyps. *Endoscopy* [Research Support, N.I.H., Extramural] 2011;43(8):683–691.
14. Shinya H, Wolff WI. Morphology, anatomic distribution and cancer potential of colonic polyps. *Ann Surg* 1979;190(6):679–683.
15. Walsh RM, Ackroyd FW, Shellito PC. Endoscopic resection of large sessile colorectal polyps. *Gastrointest Endosc* 1992;38(3):303–309.
16. Kubota O, Kino I, Kimura T, et al. Nonpolypoid adenomas and adenocarcinomas found in background mucosa of surgically resected colons. *Cancer* 1996;77(4):621–626.
17. Sakashita M, Aoyama N, Maekawa S, et al. Flat-elevated and depressed, subtypes of flat early colorectal cancers, should be distinguished by their pathological features. *Int J Colorectal Dis* 2000;15(5–6):275–281.
18. Imperiale TF, Wagner DR, Lin CY, et al. Results of screening colonoscopy among persons 40 to 49 years of age. *N Engl J Med* [Research Support, U.S. Gov't, P.H.S.] 2002;346(23):1781–1785.

19. Konishi F, Morson BC. Pathology of colorectal adenomas: a colonoscopic survey. *J Clin Pathol* [Research Support, Non-U.S. Gov't] 1982;35(8):830–841.
20. O'Brien MJ, Winawer SJ, Zauber AG, et al. The National Polyp Study. Patient and polyp characteristics associated with high-grade dysplasia in colorectal adenomas. *Gastroenterology* [Clinical Trial Multicenter Study Randomized Controlled Trial Research Support, U.S. Gov't, P.H.S.]. 1990;98(2):371–379.
21. Screening for colorectal cancer: U.S. Preventive Services Task Force recommendation statement. *Ann Intern Med* [Practice Guideline Research Support, U.S. Gov't, P.H.S.] 2008;149(9):627–637.
22. Lieberman DA, Rex DK, Winawer SJ, et al. Guidelines for colonoscopy surveillance after screening and polypectomy: a consensus update by the US Multi-Society Task Force on Colorectal Cancer. *Gastroenterology* [Practice Guideline Review Webcasts] 2012;143(3):844–857.
23. Eide TJ, Stalsberg H. Polyps of the large intestine in Northern Norway. *Cancer* 1978;42(6):2839–2848.
24. Imperiale TF, Glowinski EA, Lin-Cooper C, et al. Five-year risk of colorectal neoplasia after negative screening colonoscopy. *N Engl J Med* [Research Support, N.I.H., Extramural] 2008;359(12): 1218–1224.
25. Dave S, Hui S, Kroenke K, et al. Is the distal hyperplastic polyp a marker for proximal neoplasia? *J Gen Intern Med* [Research Support, U.S. Gov't, P.H.S. Review] 2003;18(2):128–137.
26. Groff RJ, Nash R, Ahnen DJ. Significance of serrated polyps of the colon. *Curr Gastroenterol Rep* [Review] 2008;10(5):490–498.
27. Noffsinger AE, Hart J. Serrated adenoma: a distinct form of non-polypoid colorectal neoplasia?. *Gastrointest Endosc Clin N Am* [Review] 2010;20(3):543–563.
28. Kahi CJ, Hewett DG, Norton DL, et al. Prevalence and variable detection of proximal colon serrated polyps during screening colonoscopy. *Clin Gastroenterol Hepatol* [Evaluation Studies] 2011;9(1):42–46.
29. Parra-Blanco A, Nicolas-Perez D, Gimeno-Garcia A, et al. The timing of bowel preparation before colonoscopy determines the quality of cleansing, and is a significant factor contributing to the detection of flat lesions: a randomized study. *World J Gastroenterol* [Randomized Controlled Trial Research Support, Non-U.S. Gov't] 200614;12(38):6161–6166.
30. Hiraoka S, Kato J, Fujiki S, et al. The presence of large serrated polyps increases risk for colorectal cancer. *Gastroenterology* [Comparative Study Multicenter Study] 2010;139(5):1503–1510, 1510 e1–3.
31. Li D, Jin C, McCulloch C, et al. Association of large serrated polyps with synchronous advanced colorectal neoplasia. *Am J Gastroenterol* 2009;104(3):695–702.
32. Schreiner MA, Weiss DG, Lieberman DA. Proximal and large hyperplastic and nondysplastic serrated polyps detected by colonoscopy are associated with neoplasia. *Gastroenterology* [Comparative Study Multicenter Study Research Support, U.S. Gov't, Non-P.H.S.] 2010;139(5):1497–1502.
33. East JE, Saunders BP, Jass JR. Sporadic and syndromic hyperplastic polyps and serrated adenomas of the colon: classification, molecular genetics, natural history, and clinical management. *Gastroenterol Clin North Am* [Review] 2008;37(1):25–46, v.
34. Terdiman JP, McQuaid KR. Surveillance guidelines should be updated to recognize the importance of serrated polyps. *Gastroenterology* [Comment Editorial] 2010;139(5):1444–1447.
35. Barrow E, Alduaij W, Robinson L, et al. Colorectal cancer in HNPCC: cumulative lifetime incidence, survival and tumour distribution. A report of 121 families with proven mutations. *Clin Genet* 2008;74(3):233–242.
36. American Gastroenterological Association. American Gastroenterological Association medical position statement: hereditary colorectal cancer and genetic testing. *Gastroenterology* [Research Support, Non-U.S. Gov't] 2001;121(1):195–197.
37. Umar A, Boland CR, Terdiman JP, et al. Revised Bethesda Guidelines for hereditary nonpolyposis colorectal cancer (Lynch syndrome) and microsatellite instability. *J Natl Cancer Inst* [Congresses] 2004;96(4):261–268.
38. Beamer LC, Grant ML, Espenschied CR, et al. Reflex immunohistochemistry and microsatellite instability testing of colorectal tumors for Lynch syndrome among US cancer programs and follow-up of abnormal results. *J Clin Oncol* [Research Support, N.I.H., Extramural] 2012;30(10):1058–1063.
39. Hampel H, Frankel WL, Martin E, et al. Screening for the Lynch syndrome (hereditary nonpolyposis colorectal cancer). *N Engl J Med* [Multicenter Study Research Support, Non-U.S. Gov't Research Support, U.S. Gov't, P.H.S.] 2005;352(18):1851–1860.
40. Kalady MF, McGannon E, Vogel JD, et al. Risk of colorectal adenoma and carcinoma after colectomy for colorectal cancer in patients meeting Amsterdam criteria. *Ann Surg* 2010;252(3):507–511; discussion 11–13.
41. Burke W, Petersen G, Lynch P, et al. Recommendations for follow-up care of individuals with an inherited predisposition to cancer. I. Hereditary nonpolyposis colon cancer. Cancer Genetics Studies Consortium.

*JAMA* [Consensus Development Conference Guideline Practice Guideline Review] 1997;277(11): 915–919.
42. Hirota WK, Zuckerman MJ, Adler DG, et al. ASGE guideline: the role of endoscopy in the surveillance of premalignant conditions of the upper GI tract. *Gastrointest Endosc* [Practice Guideline] 2006;63(4): 570–580.
43. Lindor NM, Petersen GM, Hadley DW, et al. Recommendations for the care of individuals with an inherited predisposition to Lynch syndrome: a systematic review. *JAMA* [Research Support, N.I.H., Extramural Research Support, N.I.H., Intramural Review] 2006;296(12):1507–1517.
44. Schulmann K, Brasch FE, Kunstmann E, et al. HNPCC-associated small bowel cancer: clinical and molecular characteristics. *Gastroenterology* [Research Support, Non-U.S. Gov't] 2005;128(3):590–599.
45. Vasen HF, Moslein G, Alonso A, et al. Guidelines for the clinical management of familial adenomatous polyposis (FAP). *Gut* [Practice Guideline] 2008;57(5):704–713.
46. Galiatsatos P, Foulkes WD. Familial adenomatous polyposis. *Am J Gastroenterol* [Review] 2006;101(2):385–398.
47. Knudsen AL, Bisgaard ML, Bulow S. Attenuated familial adenomatous polyposis (AFAP). A review of the literature. *Fam Cancer* [Review] 2003;2(1):43–55.
48. Lynch HT, Smyrk T, McGinn T, et al. Attenuated familial adenomatous polyposis (AFAP). A phenotypically and genotypically distinctive variant of FAP. *Cancer* [Research Support, Non-U.S. Gov't] 1995;76(12):2427–2433.
49. Giardiello FM, Brensinger JD, Tersmette AC, et al. Very high risk of cancer in familial Peutz-Jeghers syndrome. *Gastroenterology* [Meta-Analysis Research Support, Non-U.S. Gov't Research Support, U.S. Gov't, P.H.S.] 2000;119(6):1447–1453.
50. Lim W, Olschwang S, Keller JJ, et al. Relative frequency and morphology of cancers in STK11 mutation carriers. *Gastroenterology* [Research Support, Non-U.S. Gov't] 2004;126(7):1788–1794.
51. Murday V, Slack J. Inherited disorders associated with colorectal cancer. *Cancer Surv* 1989;8(1):139–157.
52. Starink TM, van der Veen JP, Arwert F, et al. The Cowden syndrome: a clinical and genetic study in 21 patients. *Clin Genet* 1986;29(3):222–233.
53. Pilarski R, Eng C. Will the real Cowden syndrome please stand up (again)? Expanding mutational and clinical spectra of the PTEN hamartoma tumour syndrome. *J Med Genet* [Review] 2004;41(5):323–326.
54. Wirtzfeld DA, Petrelli NJ, Rodriguez-Bigas MA. Hamartomatous polyposis syndromes: molecular genetics, neoplastic risk, and surveillance recommendations. *Ann Surg Oncol* [Review] 2001;8(4):319–327.
55. Eng C. PTEN Hamartoma Tumor Syndrome (PHTS). In: Pagon RA, Bird TD, Dolan CR, et al., eds. *GeneReviews*. Seattle, WA: University of Washington; 1993. http://www.ncbi.nlm.nih.gov/books/NBK1116/. Updated 2012.

SECTION

# II

# Cancer Precursors: Colorectal Polyps and Chronic Colitis

# Epithelial Polyps and Inflammatory Bowel Disease–Related Dysplasia

# 4

Nicole C. Panarelli

Colorectal epithelial polyps comprise a heterogeneous group of dysplastic and nondysplastic neoplasms, many of which confer risk of metachronous or subsequent colorectal adenocarcinoma. Dysplastic polyps (i.e., adenomas) are widely recognized precursors to adenocarcinoma, but until recently, nondysplastic serrated polyps were believed to lack malignant potential. Better characterization of serrated polyps and emerging molecular evidence have improved our understanding of the biologic potential of serrated polyps and led to changes in their clinical management. This chapter discusses the clinical, pathologic, immunohistochemical, and molecular features of epithelial colorectal polyps and reviews current evidence regarding their biologic importance.

## HYPERPLASTIC POLYPS

### Clinical and Endoscopic Features of Hyperplastic Polyps

Nondysplastic serrated polyps are classified in two broad groups: hyperplastic polyps without proliferative abnormalities and sessile serrated polyps (sessile serrated adenomas) with proliferative abnormalities. Hyperplastic polyps are the most common type of polyps in the colorectum, are small (usually <0.5 cm), and show a predilection for the distal colorectum. They develop earlier than adenomas and are found in 23% of patients 20 to 54 years old, but their prevalence also increases with age.[1] Alcohol consumption, smoking, obesity, and low dietary folate are all associated with an increased risk of hyperplastic polyps.[2] Hyperplastic polyps have been historically considered to be nonneoplastic, and prospective data indicate that their presence does not confer an increased risk for colorectal cancer, despite the frequent detection of specific molecular changes in these lesions.[3] Hyperplastic polyps are pale, sessile polyps with a smooth contour that may flatten upon air insufflation or show a layer of mucus on the surface.[4] They display a crypt pattern of orderly circular dots by chromoendoscopy, which distinguishes them from adenomatous polyps.[5]

### Pathologic Features of Hyperplastic Polyps

Hyperplastic polyps are composed of crypts that show prominent infolding of the epithelium, producing a "sawtooth" or serrated appearance in histologic sections (Figure 4.1A). Crypts tend to be narrower at their bases compared to the surface and contain a mixed population of goblet cells, nongoblet mucinous columnar cells, and endocrine cells in varying proportions. Mild cytologic atypia may be seen, but is limited to the basal proliferative crypt region, and dysplasia is absent. Multinucleated cells are also occasionally observed and likely represent a degenerative phenomenon (Figure 4.1B). They do not reflect viral infection or abnormal proliferation.[6] Some left-sided hyperplastic polyps also contain a thickened basement membrane.

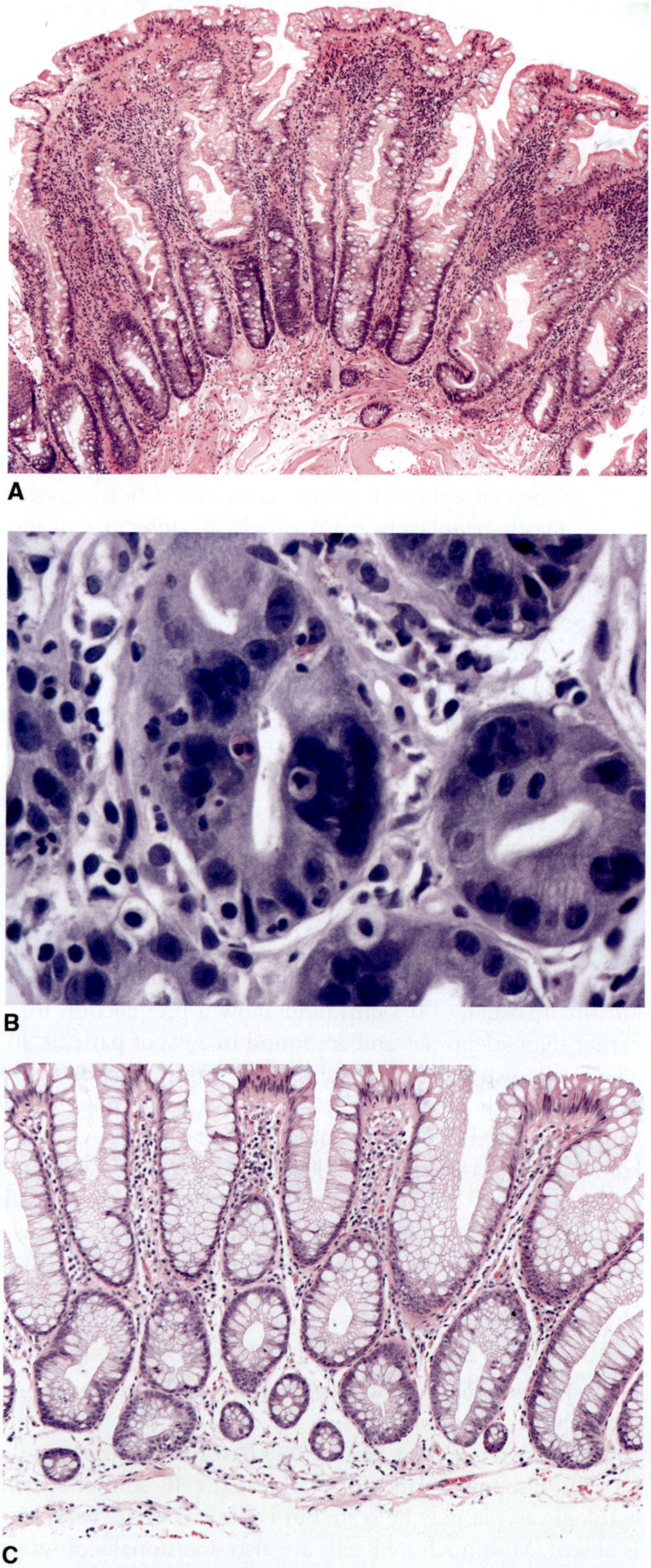


**FIGURE 4.1:** Microvesicular hyperplastic polyps are composed of serrated crypts that are narrow at their bases with wide openings at the surface. The crypts contain goblet and nongoblet mucinous cells with abundant cytoplasm and small basally oriented nuclei (**A**). Cytologic atypia, including multinucleated cells, is occasionally encountered (**B**). Goblet cell–rich hyperplastic polyps display serration mostly on the surface and are largely composed of goblet cells (**C**).

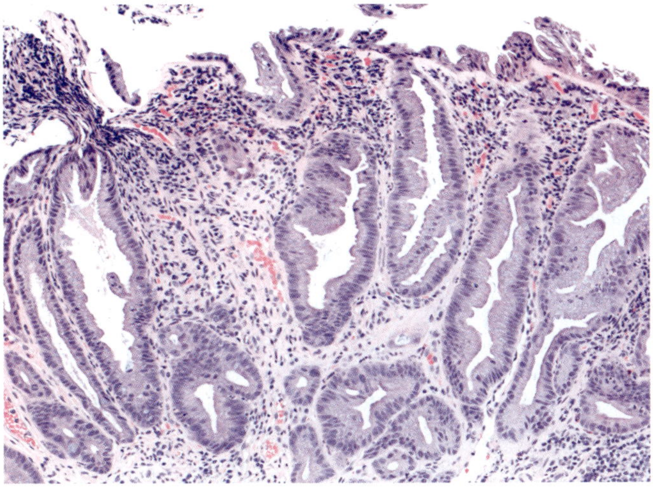

D

**FIGURE 4.1:** (*Continued*) Mucin-poor hyperplastic polyps display a serrated architecture similar to microvesicular hyperplastic polyps, but contain somewhat mucin-depleted epithelial cells and decreased goblet cells (**D**).

Three morphologic subtypes of hyperplastic polyp are described: microvesicular, goblet cell rich, and mucin poor. Microvesicular hyperplastic polyps are most common and display prominent crypt and surface serration. They contain a dual population of goblet cells and more numerous nongoblet mucinous epithelial cells with "microvesicular" cytoplasm (Figure 4.1A). Goblet cell–rich hyperplastic polyps expand the mucosa and display minimal crypt serration with numerous goblet cells (Figure 4.1C). Mucin-poor hyperplastic polyps are architecturally similar to microvesicular hyperplastic polyps and contain numerous nongoblet mucin-depleted epithelial cells with hyperchromatic nuclei and rare goblet cells (Figure 4.1D).[7] These lesions share immunohistochemical and molecular features with microvesicular hyperplastic polyps and likely represent the latter with superimposed regenerative features. Notably, subclassification of hyperplastic polyps has not been shown to be clinically important and is not recommended at this time.

## Immunohistochemical and Molecular Features of Hyperplastic Polyps

Immunohistochemical Ki-67 staining of hyperplastic polyps reveals a symmetrically expanded proliferative zone that extends approximately 1/3 to 1/2 up the crypt length.[8–10] Cytokeratin 20 staining is present in deep and surface epithelium compared to superficial staining of the normal colon, and uniform nuclear immunostaining for the intestine-specific caudal homeobox protein, CDX2, is limited to the basal 1/3 to 2/3 of crypt epithelial cells.[10,11] Hyperplastic polyps stain for colon-specific apomucin (MUC2) and gastric mucin (MUC5AC) and are reportedly negative for pyloric mucin (MUC6). However, a substantial number of hyperplastic polyps of the abdominal colon show MUC6 positivity, thereby limiting the utility of this marker in the distinction between hyperplastic polyps and sessile serrated polyps.[7,11]

Many hyperplastic polyps have mutually exclusive *KRAS* and *BRAF* mutations, challenging the notion that they are nonneoplastic and lack malignant potential. *KRAS* mutations occur in up to 47% of hyperplastic polyps and are more frequent among distally located and goblet cell–rich examples.[12–14] *BRAF* mutations are detected in 40% to 76% of hyperplastic polyps, particularly those of the proximal colon with microvesicular morphology.[12,14] Approximately 40% to 60% of hyperplastic polyps reportedly show the CpG island methylator phenotype (CIMP), which is more common among microvesicular (70%) than goblet cell–rich (40%) hyperplastic polyps.[14] The CIMP is inversely correlated with *KRAS* mutations, as discussed in Chapter 11.[15] Loss of immunohistochemical staining for $O^6$-methylguanine-methyltransferase (MGMT) and MLH1 is sometimes present in the nonproliferative superficial epithelium of hyperplastic polyps, but does not reflect underlying mutations, promoter methylation, or silencing of these genes from transcription.[14]

# SESSILE SERRATED POLYPS

## Clinical and Endoscopic Features of Sessile Serrated Polyps

Sessile serrated polyps are nondysplastic polyps that show a predilection for the abdominal colon and, unlike most hyperplastic polyps, are more common among women. These polyps have been termed "serrated polyps with abnormal proliferation," "giant hyperplastic polyps," and "sessile serrated adenomas," but are now classified as "sessile serrated adenomas/polyps" by the World Health Organization in order to avoid confusion with hyperplastic polyps and serrated adenomas.[16] Sessile serrated polyps represent 2% to 9% of all endoscopically resected polyps and 7% to 21% of all nondysplastic serrated polyps.[7,17] Sessile serrated polyps are plaques that merge imperceptibly with the adjacent nonlesional mucosa, and, thus, their size may be difficult to appreciate endoscopically. They are often covered with a thick layer of mucus and contain round dilated crypts that are visible by chromoendoscopy. A growing body of evidence indicates that these polyps represent precursors to some sporadic colonic adenocarcinomas characterized by a high degree of microsatellite instability (MSI-H). They are believed to confer a biologic risk approaching that of conventional adenomas of comparable size. Thus, screening guidelines parallel those for conventional adenomas with overt dysplasia.

## Pathologic Features of Sessile Serrated Polyps

Sessile serrated polyps are broad-based polyps that contain numerous elongated crypts with prominent infolding of the crypt epithelium (Figure 4.2A). The crypts of a sessile serrated polyp show persistent dilatation at their bases, often with branching or budding above the muscularis mucosae (Figure 4.2B). The crypts contain variable numbers of goblet cells and nongoblet mucinous columnar cells, similar to hyperplastic polyps, but they tend to show a greater degree of cytologic atypia that extends in an asymmetric fashion from the crypt bases (Figure 4.2C).[7,18] Distinction of sessile serrated polyp from hyperplastic polyp is subject to a high degree of interobserver variability, particularly when polyps are smaller than 1 cm in diameter and occur in the left colon. Diagnostic challenges stem from the fact that there are no "hard" criteria for a diagnosis of sessile serrated polyp. Rather, the diagnosis is based on a constellation of seven findings, four or more of which should be present in order to classify a polyp as a sessile serrated polyp (Table 4.1).[7,18] Unfortunately, quantifying these features is somewhat subjective, and many are frequently present to a variable extent among small, serrated polyps of the descending colon and rectum, resulting in substantial overlap between the diagnostic criteria for hyperplastic polyp and sessile serrated polyp.[8] Indeed, hyperplastic polyps of the abdominal colon also show immunohistochemical and molecular features that substantially overlap with those of sessile serrated polyps, as discussed subsequently.[19]

## Immunohistochemical and Molecular Features of Sessile Serrated Polyps

Sessile serrated polyps show Ki-67 nuclear staining of approximately 33% of the nuclei, which is slightly more than hyperplastic polyps, but less than that of conventional adenomas. Ki-67–labeled nuclei are not confined to the basal epithelial cells, but are randomly distributed within the crypts, reflecting abnormal proliferation.[10] Cytokeratin 20 and CDX2 immunostains demonstrate randomly distributed positive cells within the crypts.[10] Sessile serrated polyps show immunostaining for MUC2, MUC5AC, and MUC6.[11,17,20] Early studies suggested that MUC6 positivity may be a helpful marker to distinguish between sessile serrated polyps and hyperplastic polyps, but better designed studies have since refuted this notion.[20] MUC6 immunostains are often positive in hyperplastic polyps of the abdominal colon, suggesting that it is a marker of location (i.e., proximal colon) rather than phenotype among serrated polyps.[21]

Seventy-eight to 100% of sessile serrated polyps harbor *BRAF* mutations, whereas *KRAS* mutations are uncommon, being observed in less than 10% of cases.[8,13,14,22] These polyps frequently

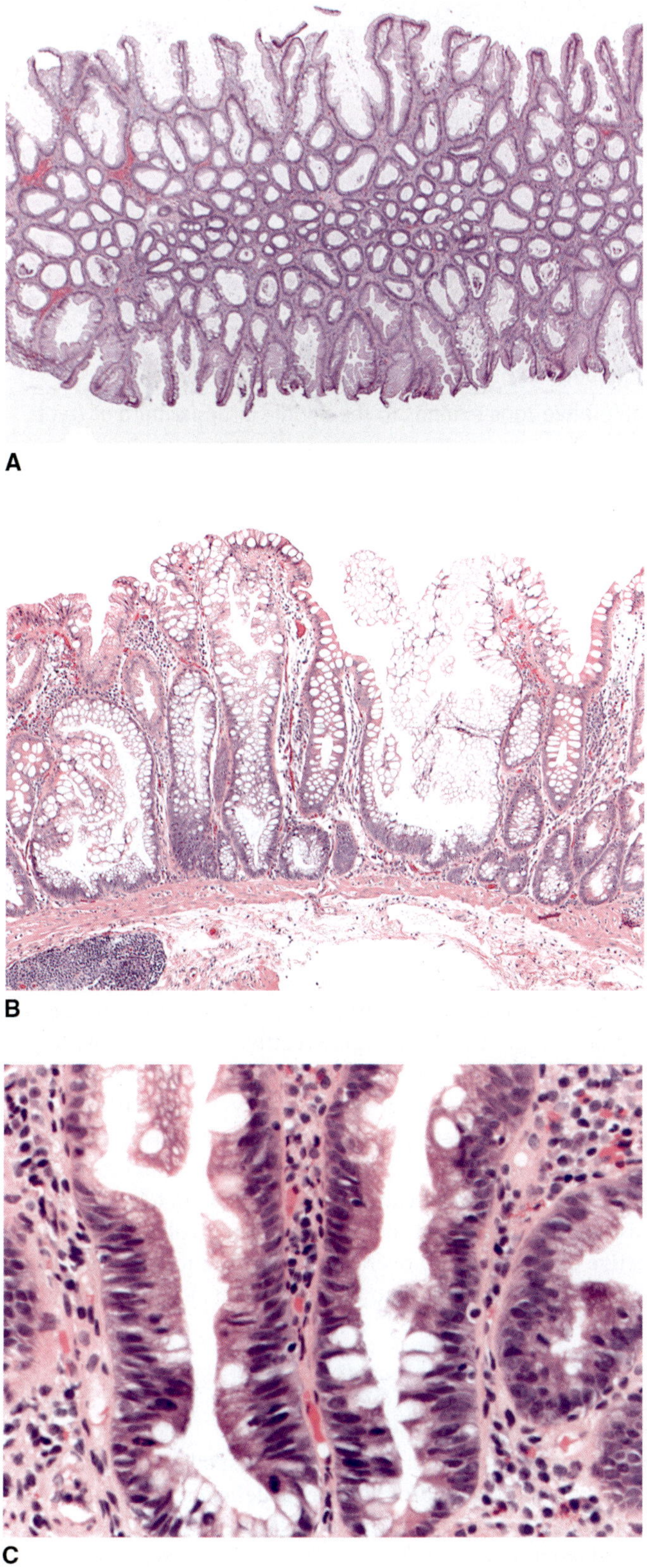

FIGURE 4.2: Sessile serrated polyps are broad-based plaques composed of elongated crypts that show persistent dilatation at their bases (**A**). They also display architectural abnormalities, including laterally branched, or budding, crypts oriented parallel to the muscularis mucosae (**B**). Atypical, hyperchromatic nuclei with pseudostratification may extend beyond the crypt bases into the midcrypt region (**C**).

**Table 4.1 Diagnostic Criteria of Sessile Serrated Polyp**

| Feature | Description |
|---|---|
| Crypt dilatation | Elongated crypts with exaggerated luminal serration<br>Persistent dilatation of crypts into the deep mucosa<br>Inverted L- or T-shaped crypts |
| Crypt orientation | Horizontally oriented crypts above the muscularis mucosae |
| Mucin production | Extracellular mucin in crypt lumina and on polyp surface |
| Cytoplasmic eosinophilia | Clusters of cells with eosinophilic cytoplasm within irregularly shaped, mucin-poor crypts |
| Decreased endocrine cells | Contiguous crypts with absent or rare endocrine cells |
| Abnormal proliferation | Proliferative zone extends to the middle or upper third of crypts |
| Nuclear atypia | Enlarged, oval or round, basally located nuclei<br>Hyperchromasia<br>Prominent nucleoli |

Data from Torlakovic E, Snover DC. Serrated adenomatous polyposis in humans. *Gastroenterology* 1996;110(3):748–755.

(60% to 70%) show the CIMP.[14,22] Loss of MGMT and MLH1 immunoexpression is limited to the superficial epithelial cells, but reflects the nonproliferative nature of the polyp surface, rather than underlying microsatellite instability (MSI). Early investigations reported *MGMT* and *MLH1* promoter methylation in 40% and 72% of sessile serrated polyps, respectively.[7,14,17,23] Unfortunately, these studies utilized qualitative, rather than quantitative, assays, and more recent data indicate that sessile serrated polyps are microsatellite stable with preserved MLH1 function.[24]

# SERRATED (HYPERPLASTIC) POLYPOSIS

Serrated (hyperplastic) polyposis is defined by the presence of (1) at least five hyperplastic polyps located proximal to the sigmoid colon, two of which span at least 1 cm, (2) twenty or more hyperplastic polyps of any size distributed throughout the colorectum, or (3) any number of hyperplastic polyps proximal to the sigmoid colon in a first-degree relative of a patient with serrated (hyperplastic) polyposis.[25] The molecular features of these phenotypes are variable. Patients with large polyps of the abdominal colon tend to have fewer serrated polyps that harbor *BRAF* mutations and show the CIMP. They also have a variety of other types of dysplastic colorectal polyps with, or without, serrated morphology. In contrast, other patients have numerous small polyps with *KRAS* mutations and, possibly lower overall cancer risk. Approximately 5% of serrated polyposis cases have a familial association, although the precise genes involved and modes of inheritance are not clear. Retrospective data suggest an overall colorectal cancer prevalence of 35% to 50%, although prospective data estimate cancer risk to be 5% to 10% at 7 years.[26]

# CONVENTIONAL ADENOMAS

## Clinical and Endoscopic Features of Conventional Adenomas

Conventional adenomas occur throughout the colorectum and are usually asymptomatic, although large polyps may ulcerate causing rectal bleeding and iron deficiency anemia. They account for 40% to 60% of all endoscopically removed colorectal polyps, and their incidence increases with age, such that they are detected in approximately 12% of adults over 50 years of age.[27] The number and size of adenomatous polyps is associated with a risk of future cancer

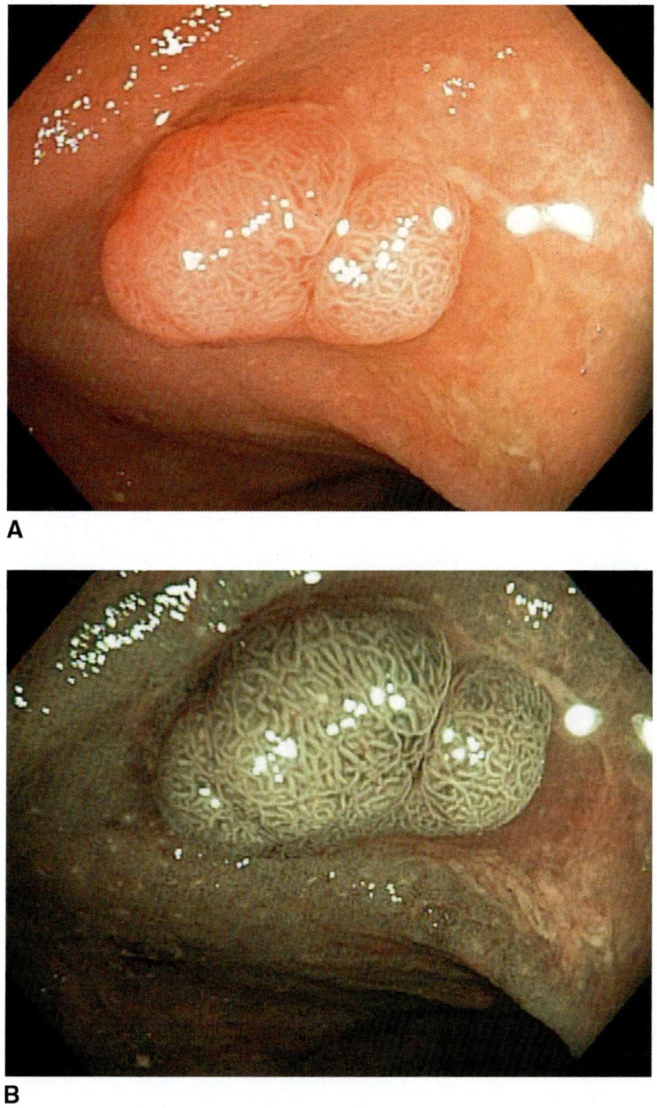

FIGURE 4.3: A sessile tubular adenoma of the right colon is slightly more erythematous than the background mucosa (**A**). Narrow band imaging accentuates the irregular pit pattern characteristic of dysplastic (adenomatous) polyps (**B**).

development, as discussed in Chapter 3. Patients with a few, small adenomas are at low cancer risk, whereas those with more numerous adenomas, large polyps (>1 cm), or high-grade dysplasia are at a higher risk for cancer development and undergo more rigorous surveillance.

Adenomas are red, multilobulated masses that are either plaque-like (sessile) or pedunculated (Figure 4.3A). Magnifying colonoscopy and chromoendoscopy reveal variably sized tubular glands with irregular, cerebriform configurations (Figure 4.3B). Some adenomas appear as small erythematous plaques with central depressions and have been reported to rapidly progress to invasive carcinoma. However, recent data indicate that they are not associated with increased risk during surveillance.[28]

## Pathologic Features of Conventional Adenomas

Conventional adenomas are classified as tubular, villous, and tubulovillous adenomas based on their morphologic appearances. Straight tubular or branched crypts comprise at least 75% of the volume of tubular adenomas, whereas villous adenomas contain slender fronds of neoplastic epithelium that account for at least 75% of the polyp volume (Figure 4.4A and B). Polyps with a

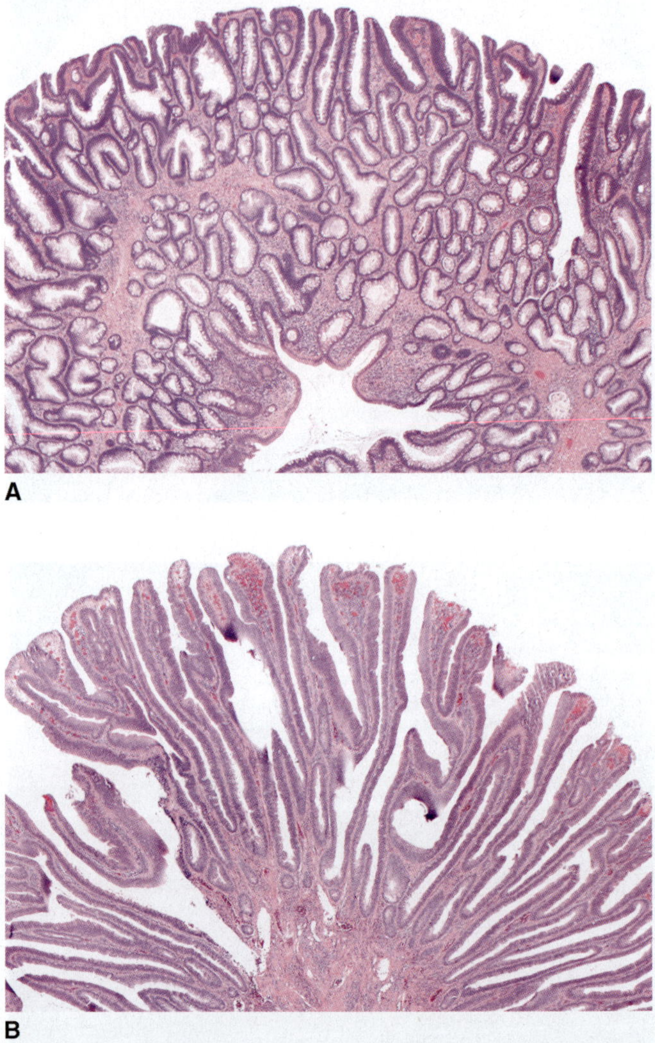

**FIGURE 4.4:** Tubular adenomas have smooth, rounded surfaces and contain tubular crypts lined by dysplastic epithelial cells. The crypts are irregularly spaced and crowded (**A**). A villous adenoma contains frond-like projections of mucosa lined by neoplastic epithelial cells. Small crypts are present at the bases of the villi (**B**).

limited villous component (25% to 75%) are classified as tubulovillous adenomas. All adenomas are, by definition, dysplastic. The degree of dysplasia is classified as low grade or high grade based on a combination of cytologic and architectural features. Low-grade dysplasia is characterized by a proliferation of crowded, variably sized crypts that lack orientation to the muscularis mucosae. The cells contain elongated, large nuclei with small nucleoli. Nuclei maintain their relationships to the basement membrane and are located in the bases of the cells. Apoptotic epithelial cells are easily detected in the deep and superficial crypt regions, and a neutrophil-rich inflammatory infiltrate is sometimes present (Figure 4.5A). High-grade dysplasia shows complex architectural features, including cribriform growth, irregular crypt budding, and loss of the relationship between epithelial cells and the basement membrane, the latter of which is manifest by cellular stratification. High-grade cytologic features include a markedly increased nuclear-to-cytoplasmic ratio, loss of cell polarity, prominent nucleoli, frequent mitotic figures, and luminal necrosis (Figure 4.5B).

Some adenomas contain adenocarcinomas that breach the basement membrane, but are confined to the lamina propria or muscularis mucosae. These tumors have no potential for metastases and are termed intramucosal adenocarcinoma, as discussed in Chapter 9. The biologic behavior of intramucosal carcinoma has been attributed to a paucity of lymphatic channels in the lamina propria, although this explanation is likely overly simplistic since inflammation

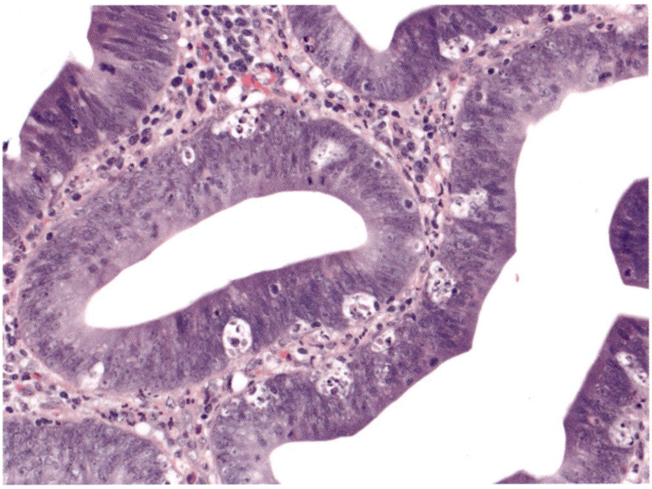

A

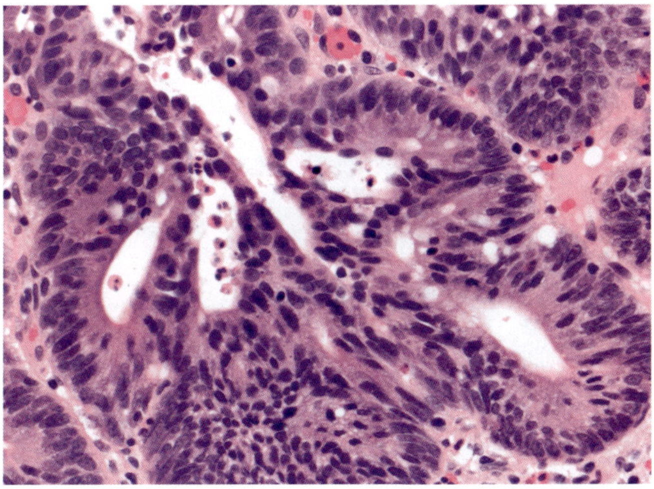

B

FIGURE 4.5: Adenomas with low-grade dysplasia contain crypts with single lumina lined by mucin-poor columnar cells with dense cytoplasm and elongated, hyperchromatic nuclei. Each nucleus is confined to the lower half of the cell and maintains its relationship to the basement membrane. Apoptotic cellular debris is universally present in the crypt epithelium (**A**). High-grade dysplasia is characterized by fused crypts that contain large nuclei, some of which are located in the superficial cytoplasm (**B**).

and neoplasia can certainly induce neovascularization of the lamina propria.[29] Regardless, intramucosal adenocarcinoma is managed similarly to high-grade dysplasia.[30] Intramucosal adenocarcinoma consists of an expansile proliferation of neoplastic glands with irregular or back-to-back, interanastomosing configurations (Figure 4.6A). Small clusters of cells infiltrate around larger glands (Figure 4.6B). Notably, intramucosal adenocarcinoma does not generally elicit desmoplasia in the lamina propria.

Some adenomas are classified as "advanced adenomas" by clinicians because they are associated with an increased risk of subsequent colon cancer. Advanced adenomas are defined as adenomas that are large (>1 cm), contain a villous component comprising at least 25% of the polyp, or display high-grade dysplasia. Unfortunately, the morphologic criteria inherent in this definition are highly subjective, resulting in considerable interobserver variability regarding assessment of villous architecture and dysplasia. Polyp size remains the only reliable criterion for this designation.[31]

Large pedunculated adenomas of the distal colorectum are subject to luminal trauma that may cause displacement or herniation of dysplastic epithelium into the submucosa. Displaced benign epithelium has been termed "epithelial misplacement" and "pseudoinvasion." Displaced epithelium appears as lobules of adenomatous glands surrounded by a rim of lamina propria

**FIGURE 4.6:** Intramucosal adenocarcinoma expands the lamina propria (*arrow*) of a villous adenoma (**A**). Small nests of tumor cells infiltrate between larger adenomatous crypts, but do not elicit a desmoplastic response (**B**).

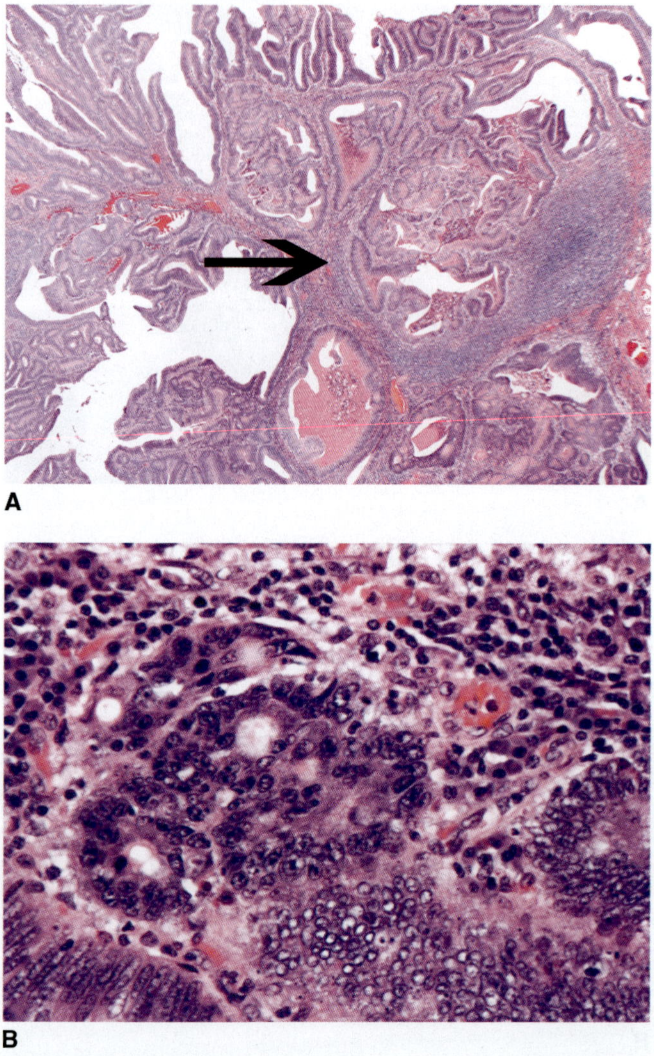

(Figure 4.7A). Some of the glands may become cystically dilated or rupture, and extrude mucin into the submucosa, where it elicits an inflammatory response. Fresh hemorrhage and hemosiderin are often found in the vicinity of misplaced epithelium, providing evidence of its trauma-induced, rather than invasive, nature (Figure 4.7B).[32] The differential diagnosis of displaced epithelium in adenomas is discussed in Chapter 10.

Approximately 2% to 5% of endoscopically removed colorectal adenomas contain submucosally invasive adenocarcinoma.[33] Most of these "malignant polyps" are pedunculated lesions that are adequately managed by complete endoscopic resection, provided they do not contain high-grade invasive carcinoma, lack lymphovascular invasion, and are resected with a margin of at least 0.1 cm.[34,35] However, endoscopists commonly inject the base of a sessile polyp with saline to lift it off the muscularis propria, thereby creating a wheal that simulates a stalk in histologic sections. Thus, the distinction between pedunculated and sessile polyps is best left to endoscopists. The histologic features of superficially invasive adenocarcinoma and its differential diagnoses are fully discussed in Chapters 9 and 10. Invasive adenocarcinomas are the most common malignancies to complicate adenomas; however, other types of tumors develop in these lesions on rare occasions. Small series describe low-grade and high-grade (neuro)endocrine tumors,

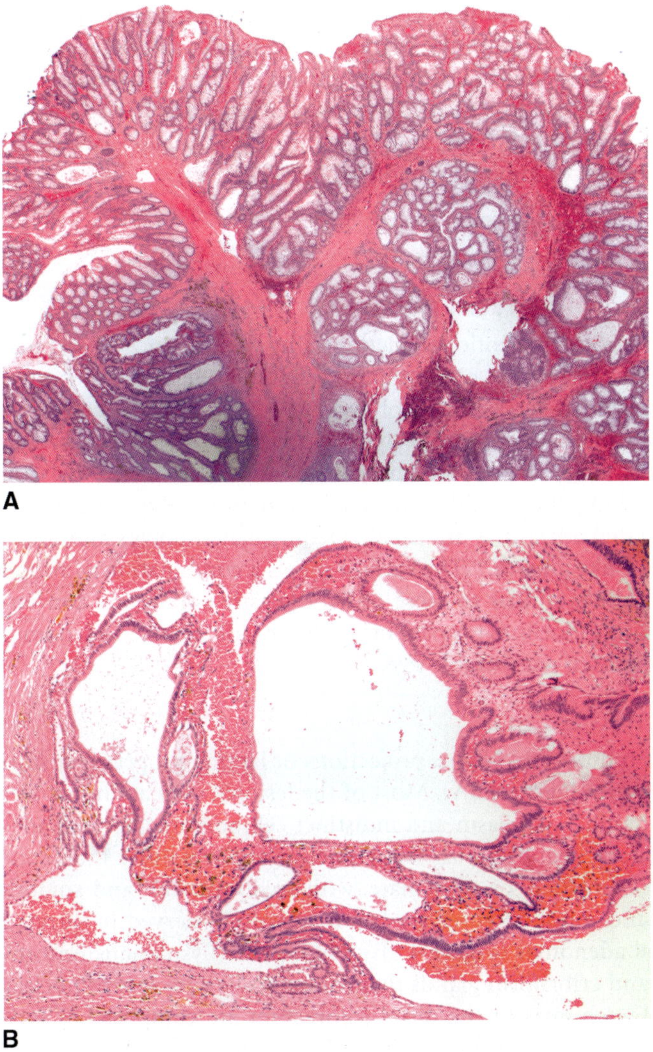

**FIGURE 4.7:** Displaced lobules of mucosa are present in the submucosa of a traumatized adenoma (**A**). Some of the displaced adenomatous glands are cystically dilated and associated with hemorrhage and hemosiderin (**B**).

although the latter are quite rare.[36,37] Adenomas rarely harbor metastases from extracolonic sites, including carcinomas, sarcomas, and malignant melanoma.[38–40]

## Immunohistochemical and Molecular Features of Conventional Adenomas

Conventional adenomas are proliferative lesions and show an increased number of Ki-67–labeled cells in the neoplastic crypts and surface epithelium.[10] Staining for cytokeratin 20 is randomly distributed in adenomatous epithelium, and CDX2 shows strong and diffuse nuclear staining.[11] Immunostains for MUC2 and MUC5AC are usually positive, whereas MUC6 is negative.[11]

Most colorectal adenocarcinomas develop from preexisting adenomas *via* the adenoma–carcinoma sequence, as discussed in Chapter 11. This mechanism of carcinogenesis is initiated by biallelic inactivating mutations in *adenomatous polyposis coli (APC)*. Dysfunctional APC fails to participate in the multiprotein complex that normally sequesters β-catenin and facilitates its cytoplasmic degradation. The net effect of *APC* inactivation is constitutive APC/β-catenin/Wnt signaling that allows cytoplasmic accumulation of β-catenin. β-catenin is translocated to the nucleus, where it facilitates transcription of protooncogenes, driving cell proliferation. Although only 80% of conventional adenomas have detectable inactivating *APC* mutations, nearly all show aberrant nuclear β-catenin immunoexpression, indicating that Wnt signaling pathway abnormalities are essentially universal in these lesions.[41] Lower rates of *APC* mutation detection likely reflect a tendency for most laboratories to limit evaluation to the mutation cluster region, rather than evaluating the entire gene. Other molecular changes are less frequent. Approximately 20% of adenomas have *KRAS* mutations, and loss of heterozygosity affecting *MTS1* (*p16*) and chromosome 3p occurs in up to 20% of cases.[41] Mutations affecting *TP53* develop late in the adenoma–carcinoma sequence and are uncommon in adenomas.[41]

## SERRATED ADENOMAS

### Clinical and Endoscopic Features of Serrated Adenomas

Serrated adenomas are distinguished from conventional adenomas by the presence of serrated architecture. They show overt dysplasia, similar to conventional adenomas. Serrated adenomas are uncommon and account for approximately 1% to 2% of endoscopically removed colorectal adenomas.[42] They also show a predilection for the sigmoid colon and rectum of older adults and, thus, display clinical features distinct from sessile serrated polyps.[42] Most serrated adenomas are sporadic, but they have been described in patients with familial adenomatous polyposis and serrated (hyperplastic) polyposis.[43] Serrated adenomas are usually pedunculated polyps and infrequently display broad-based or carpet-like growth.[44] The surface shows a combination of round crypt openings and cerebriform infoldings similar to those of hyperplastic polyps and conventional adenomas, respectively. Screening guidelines for patients with sporadic serrated adenomas parallel those for conventional adenomas of comparable size.

### Pathologic Features of Serrated Adenomas

Serrated adenomas are composed of tubules and villous projections of lamina propria that support crypts with convoluted architecture (Figure 4.8A). Most of the lesional cells are nongoblet epithelial cells with abundant eosinophilic cytoplasm and indistinct cell borders. Serrated adenomas usually show low-grade cytologic features with fewer nuclear abnormalities than conventional adenomas. The nuclei are elongated, or penicillate, with small nucleoli and smooth contours. Apoptotic epithelial cells and mitotic figures are less frequently observed in serrated adenomas compared to conventional adenomas (Figure 4.8B). High-grade dysplasia is uncommon, but manifest by back-to-back and cribriform glands that contain cells with loss of nuclear polarity. Some traumatized serrated adenomas of the distal colorectum are composed of bulbous finger-like projections lined by serrated epithelium (Figure 4.9A). These "filiform" serrated adenomas often show prominent lamina propria edema or ulceration (Figure 4.9B).[45]

**FIGURE 4.8:** Serrated adenomas are composed of serrated crypts with diffuse cytologic dysplasia (**A**).

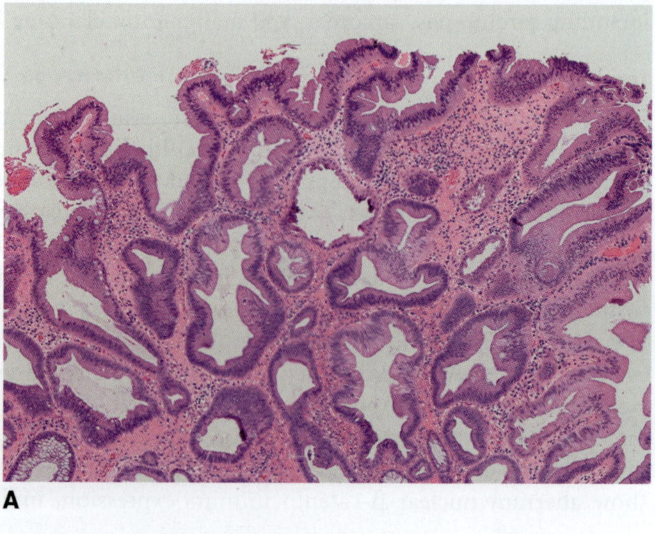

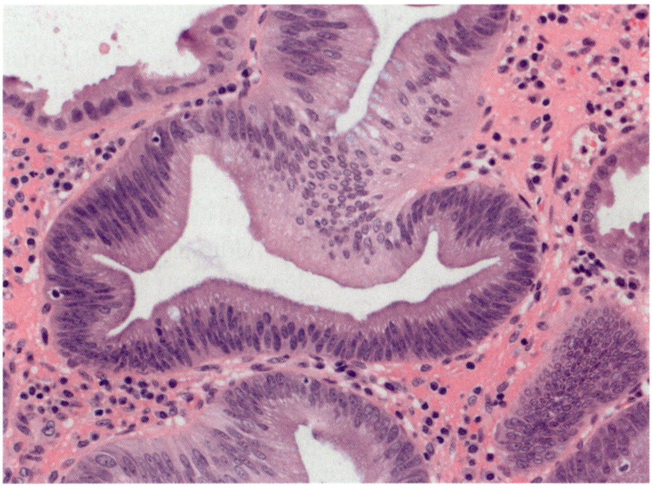

B

FIGURE 4.8: (*Continued*) Most cells contain dense, eosinophilic cytoplasm with elongated, slightly hyperchromatic nuclei (**B**).

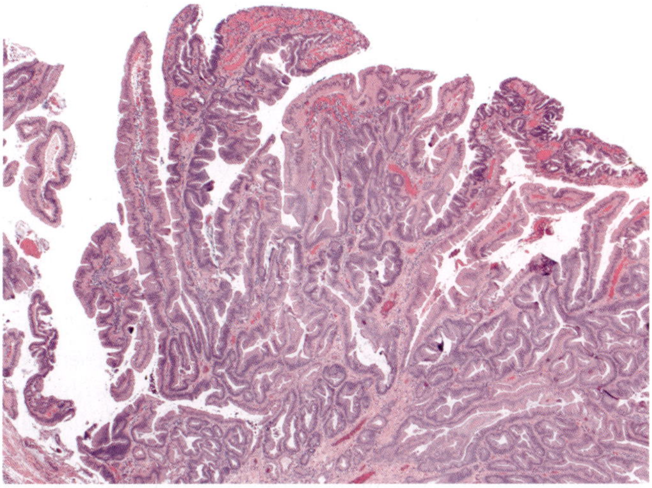

A

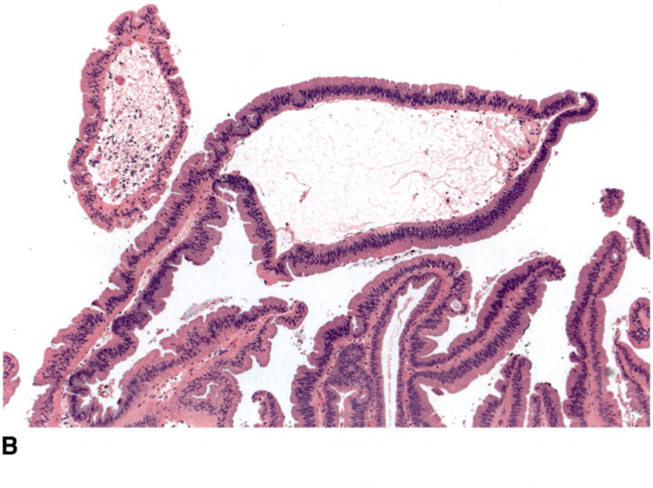

B

FIGURE 4.9: Filiform serrated adenomas contain finger-like projections that are longer than the villi of a villous adenoma (**A**). These projections are lined by serrated epithelium and often show striking mucosal edema (**B**).

### Immunohistochemical and Molecular Features

Serrated adenomas share immunohistochemical staining characteristics with conventional adenomas. Immunostains for Ki-67 show increased numbers of positive nuclei in the basal and surface epithelial cells compared to normal colonic epithelium. Serrated adenomas are positive for CDX2.[45] Most examples show staining for MUC2 and MUC5AC, but serrated adenomas are negative for MUC6.[11]

Reports describing the molecular features of serrated adenomas are conflicting because many evaluate them together with other types of dysplastic and serrated polyps, although it is likely that true molecular heterogeneity exists within this group. Some serrated adenomas show abnormalities in APC/β-catenin/Wnt signaling similar to conventional adenomas. *APC* mutations are found in 13% to 20% of serrated adenomas, and nuclear immunostaining for β-catenin is frequent. Up to 70% of serrated adenomas harbor *KRAS* mutations.[13,14,41,46] Loss of heterozygosity at *TP53, MTS1 (p16)*, and 3p occur at rates comparable to those of conventional adenomas.[41] The CIMP has been reported in 43% to 90% of serrated adenomas, although higher frequencies are reported in studies that combine these polyps with sessile serrated polyps with dysplasia for purposes of analysis. *MGMT* promoter methylation and *BRAF* mutations occur in a minority of cases, suggesting that serrated adenomas are not involved in the serrated neoplastic pathway, as discussed subsequently.[14,41]

## SESSILE SERRATED POLYPS WITH DYSPLASIA

### Clinical and Endoscopic Features of Sessile Serrated Polyps with Dysplasia

Sessile serrated polyps with dysplasia were, until recently, classified as mixed hyperplastic/adenomatous polyps in the literature. They are uncommon and account for approximately 1% of all endoscopically removed polyps. Most occur in the right colons of older adults (>50 years) and are more frequent in women than men. Their endoscopic appearance is similar to sessile serrated polyps.

### Pathologic Features of Sessile Serrated Polyps with Dysplasia

Sessile serrated polyps with dysplasia likely represent an intermediate stage in the progression of sessile serrated polyps to invasive carcinoma rather than a collision of separate neoplasms. They contain areas of serrated polyp that may resemble either a hyperplastic polyp or sessile serrated polyp admixed with areas of overt dysplasia that show a tubular, villous, or serrated morphology and display low- or high-grade cytologic dysplasia. Dysplastic areas usually contain epithelial cells with penicillate, hyperchromatic, pseudostratified nuclei, although high-grade dysplasia typically shows a serrated architecture and contains cells with eosinophilic cytoplasm and round nuclei with open chromatin and prominent nucleoli.

### Immunohistochemical and Molecular Features of Sessile Serrated Polyps with Dysplasia

The reported immunohistochemical and molecular features of sessile serrated polyps with dysplasia are conflicting, reflecting different criteria for diagnoses, interpretation of immunohistochemistry, and variable molecular techniques.[47,48] Approximately 60% of these polyps display loss of MLH1 immunostaining and MSI in their dysplastic areas, but not in the nondysplastic components.[49] *BRAF* mutations are identified in 40% to 89% of mixed polyps, whereas alterations in *KRAS* are present in less than 10%.[46] Unlike serrated adenomas, sessile serrated polyps with dysplasia represent a putative intermediate step in the serrated neoplastic pathway, as described below.

## THE SERRATED NEOPLASTIC PATHWAY

Serrated polyps do not display abnormalities in APC/Wnt/β-catenin signaling, but harbor mutations in *BRAF* and show variable DNA methylation. Presumably, a subset of serrated polyps with *BRAF* mutations and the CIMP develop progressive methylation and silencing of mismatch

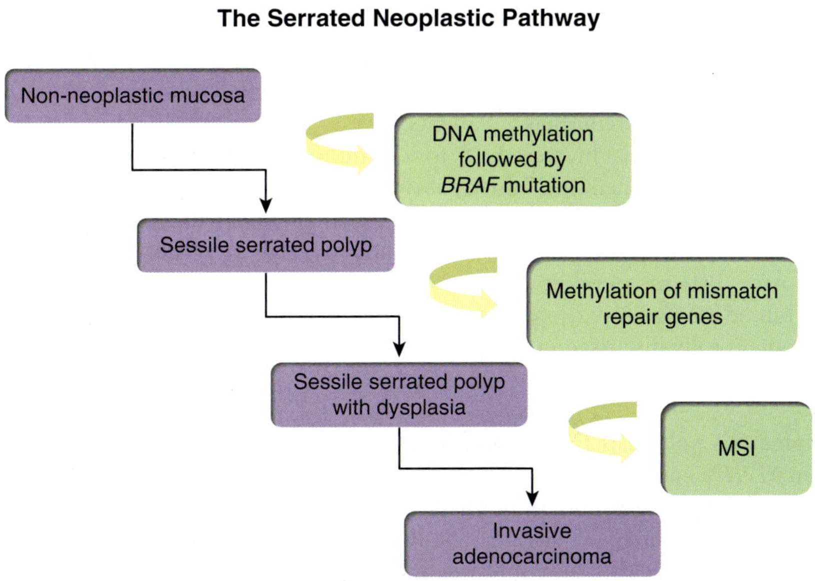


FIGURE 4.10: Hypermethylation of CpG-rich islands in gene promoters facilitates mutations in *BRAF* and inhibition of apoptosis, resulting in development of nondysplastic sessile serrated polyps. These polyps are subject to further promoter methylation and silencing of DNA mismatch repair genes, which coincide with the onset of cytologic dysplasia. Silencing of MLH1 *via* methylation results in MSI that promotes development of adenocarcinoma.

repair genes, including *MGMT* and *MLH1*. Loss of DNA mismatch repair function coincides with onset of dysplasia in serrated polyps (sessile serrated polyps with dysplasia) and causes accumulation of mutations in genomic microsatellite regions, leading to development of invasive adenocarcinomas. Progression of serrated polyps to invasive adenocarcinoma *via* DNA methylation and MSI has been termed the "serrated neoplastic pathway" and is further discussed in Chapter 11 (Figure 4.10).

## POLYPOSIS SYNDROMES ASSOCIATED WITH CONVENTIONAL ADENOMAS

### Familial Adenomatous Polyposis

Familial adenomatous polyposis is an autosomal dominant condition caused by hereditary or sporadic germline mutations affecting *APC* on chromosome 5q. The syndrome is characterized by numerous adenomatous polyps in the colorectum and confers a colorectal cancer risk of nearly 100% by 30 years of age. Although most patients undergo proctocolectomy upon reaching skeletal maturity, surgery does not entirely eliminate cancer risk in these individuals, since they are at risk for a number of extracolonic cancers of the gastrointestinal tract as well as extraintestinal malignancies.[43] Several variant syndromes are described. Gardner syndrome is characterized by intestinal fibromatoses, osteomas, epidermoid cysts, dental abnormalities, and congenital hyperpigmentation of the retinal pigmented epithelium, in addition to adenomatous polyps. Crail syndrome is the eponym applied to the combination of adenomatous polyposis and specific central nervous system tumors, namely, medulloblastomas, ependymomas, and astrocytomas.[43] Attenuated forms of familial adenomatous polyposis are associated with fewer than 100 polyps and lifetime colorectal cancer risk of 80%. Attenuated phenotypes are attributed to mutational differences that result in variably functional APC protein, as discussed in Chapter 11.

### Lynch Syndrome (Hereditary Nonpolyposis Colon Cancer)

Lynch syndrome is caused by germline mutations affecting one of four DNA mismatch repair genes (*MLH1, MSH2, MSH6*, and *PMS2*) and is associated with development of gastrointestinal and extragastrointestinal carcinomas.[43] Patients have a 50% to 80% lifetime risk of colorectal cancer development and are at increased risk for carcinomas of the endometrium, pancreas, small intestine, stomach, and urothelium. Named subtypes of Lynch syndrome include Muir-Torre syndrome and Turcot syndrome.[43] The former is applied to patients with sebaceous neoplasms and colorectal neoplasia, whereas the latter describes individuals with Lynch syndrome and glioblastoma multiforme. Patients develop conventional adenomas at rates comparable to the general population, but adenomas rapidly progress to carcinoma, presumably due to the onset of MSI. Lynch syndrome is fully discussed in Chapters 11 and 12.

### MYH Adenomatous Polyposis

*MYH* adenomatous polyposis (MAP syndrome) is an autosomal recessive disorder caused by mutations in *MYH*, a base excision repair gene located on chromosome 1. Defects in MYH function promote *APC* mutations, and, thus, the phenotype mimics familial adenomatous polyposis, particularly attenuated forms of disease. The lifetime risk of colorectal cancer development is estimated to be 80%. Some evidence indicates that monoallelic *MYH* mutation carriers are also at increased risk for colorectal cancer development.[43]

## INFLAMMATORY BOWEL DISEASE–ASSOCIATED DYSPLASIA

### Clinical and Endoscopic Features

Patients with idiopathic inflammatory bowel disease are at increased risk for development of colorectal adenocarcinoma. Risk factors include prolonged disease duration (>8 to 10 years), extensive mucosal involvement (pancolitis), concomitant primary sclerosing cholangitis, and a family history of colorectal dysplasia. Dysplasia risk is estimated to be 5% to 20% after 10 years of disease.[50]

Dysplasia is classified as either flat or elevated. Flat dysplasia is endoscopically undetectable and comprises less than 5% of dysplasias discovered by endoscopic surveillance. Elevated lesions appear as nodules, ulcers, or strictures and are termed "dysplasia-associated lesion or masses (DALMs)," which are further subcategorized into nonadenoma-like and adenoma-like types. Nonadenoma-like DALMs are broad-based, sessile, irregular, ulcerated, or constricting masses that are highly associated with metachronous or synchronous adenocarcinoma. Nonadenoma-like DALMs and flat dysplasia, whether low or high grade, are considered strong indications for colectomy as discussed in Chapter 15.[51] Adenoma-like dysplasia appears as a well-circumscribed, sessile, or pedunculated polyp that is essentially indistinguishable from a sporadic adenoma. Features that favor a sporadic adenoma include polyp occurrence in nondiseased mucosa and older patient age. Patients with adenoma-like DALMs may develop additional polyps during surveillance, but are not at increased risk for flat dysplasia or carcinoma (Figure 4.11).[52]

### Pathologic Features

Pathologic evaluation for inflammatory bowel disease–associated dysplasia requires classification of samples as negative for dysplasia, positive for dysplasia, or indefinite for dysplasia. Cases that are deemed positive for dysplasia are further classified as low-grade or high-grade. The criteria for low- and high-grade dysplasia are the same for flat and raised lesions and closely parallel those applied to sporadic adenomas. Low-grade dysplasia is characterized crowded crypts, some of which may be dilated (Figure 4.12A). Cytologic abnormalities include nuclear elongation, hyperchromasia, and pseudostratification and are present on the surface as well as the crypt region (Figure 4.12B). High-grade dysplasia is marked by increased architectural complexity, including fused or cribriform glands with irregular budding (Figure 4.13A). Lesional cells display loss of polarity and contain large round to ovoid nuclei with mitotic figures (Figure 4.13B). Some cases of dysplasia appear as irregular, branching crypts with distended goblet cells and large, atypical nuclei (Figure 4.14). The presence of intimately admixed dysplastic and nondysplastic crypts generally favors a diagnosis of inflammatory bowel disease–related dysplasia over a sporadic adenoma, but classification of dysplasia should be performed based on all available information, rather than histologic assessment alone (Figure 4.15).

Reparative and inflammatory changes in active inflammatory bowel disease produce reactive epithelial cell changes that simulate dysplasia. These findings are often classified as indefinite for dysplasia when the cytologic and architectural abnormalities are concerning, but insufficient for a diagnosis of low-grade dysplasia. Regenerating colonic epithelial cells at sites of recent injury often have cytologic features that simulate low-grade dysplasia. The cells contain small

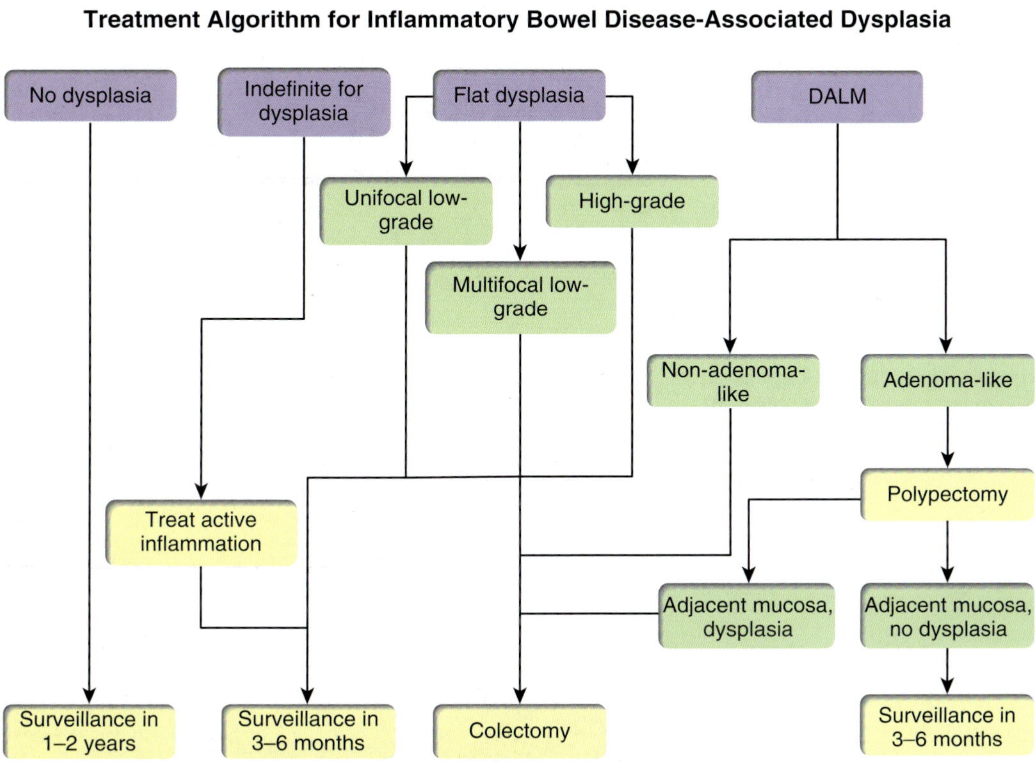


**FIGURE 4.11:** Algorithm for management of dysplasia in patients with inflammatory bowel disease. (DALM, dysplasia-associated lesion or mass.)

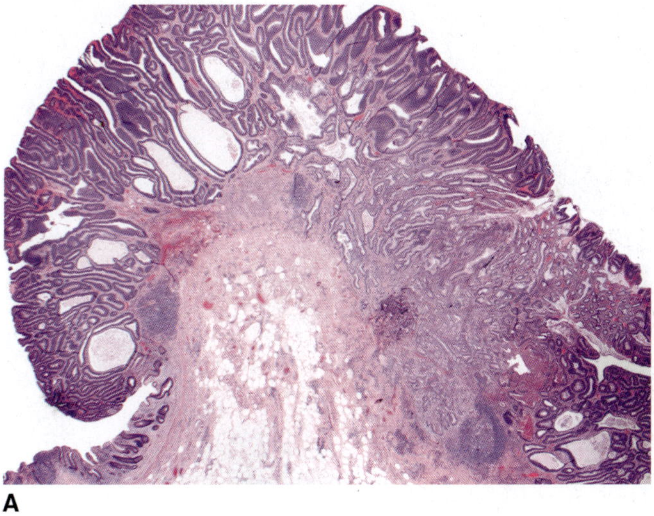


**FIGURE 4.12:** An adenoma-like DALM protrudes into the colonic lumen and comprises branched and dilated crypts (**A**).

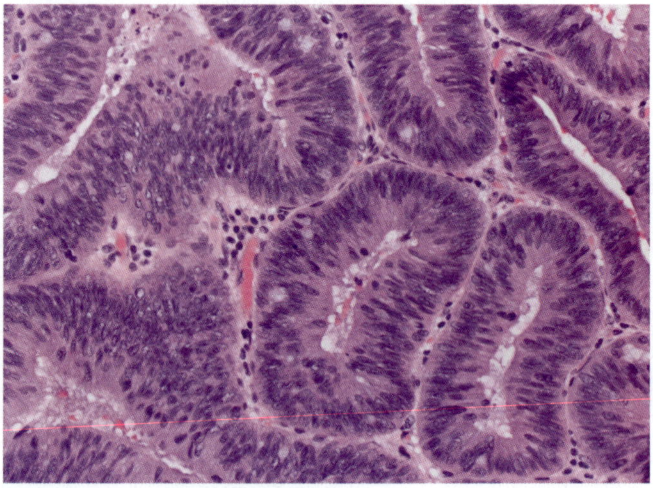

B

**FIGURE 4.12:** (*Continued*) Low-grade cytologic features, including basally located polarized nuclei with hyperchromasia and apoptotic cellular debris, are indistinguishable from those of a sporadic adenoma (**B**).

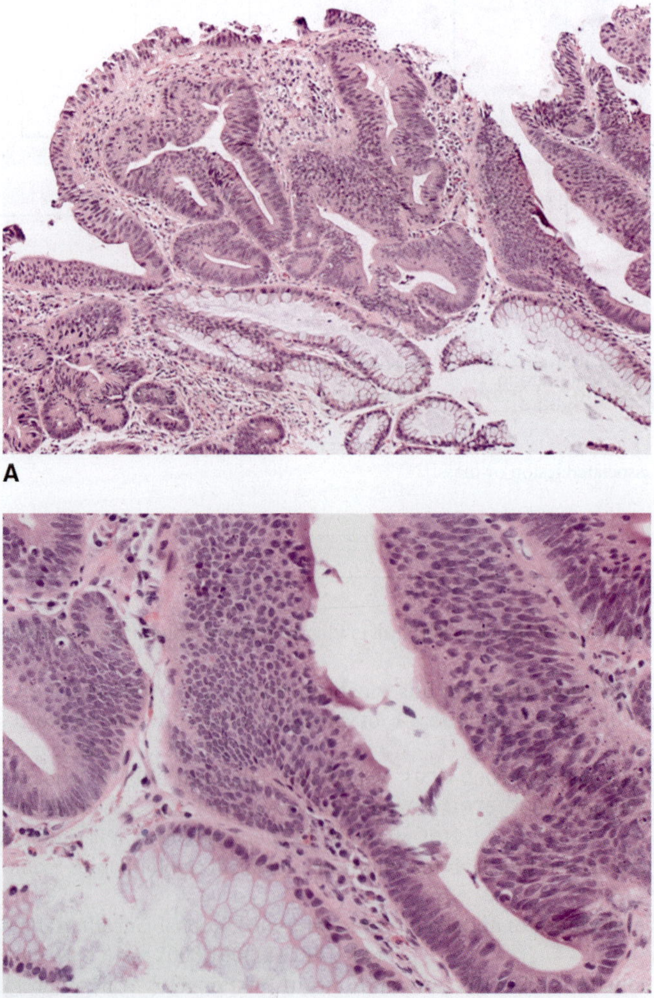

A

B

**FIGURE 4.13:** Flat high-grade dysplasia is composed of fused, mucin-depleted crypts (**A**). The cells show loss of polarity with round, hyperchromatic nuclei (**B**).

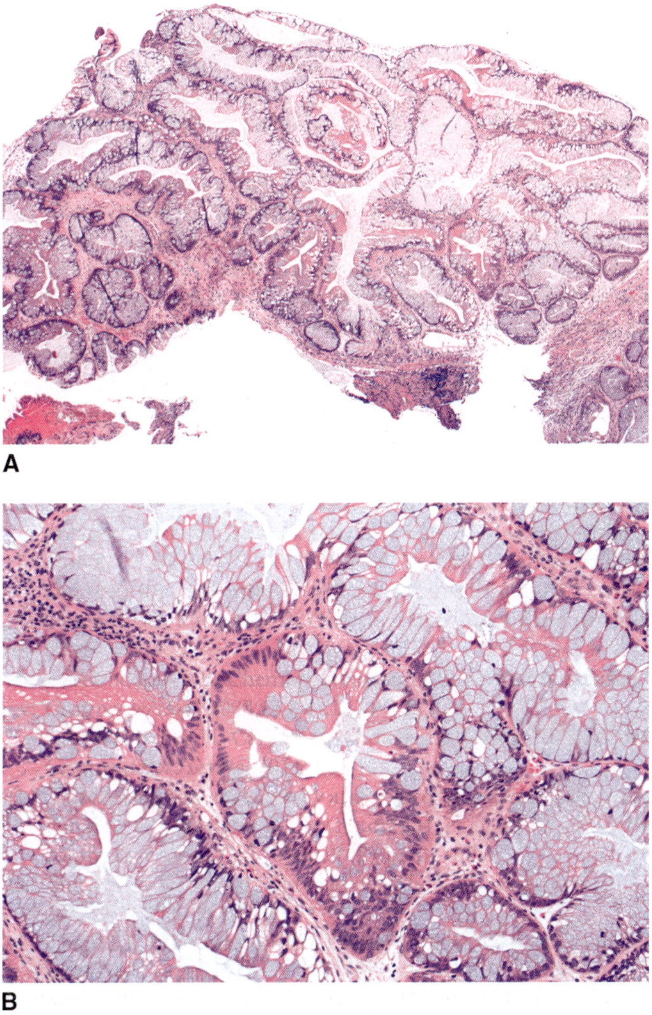

FIGURE 4.14: This patient with ulcerative colitis has low-grade dysplasia characterized by a proliferation of crowded crypts (**A**). The crypts contain distended goblet cells and nongoblet columnar cells with hyperchromatic, pseudostratified nuclei (**B**).

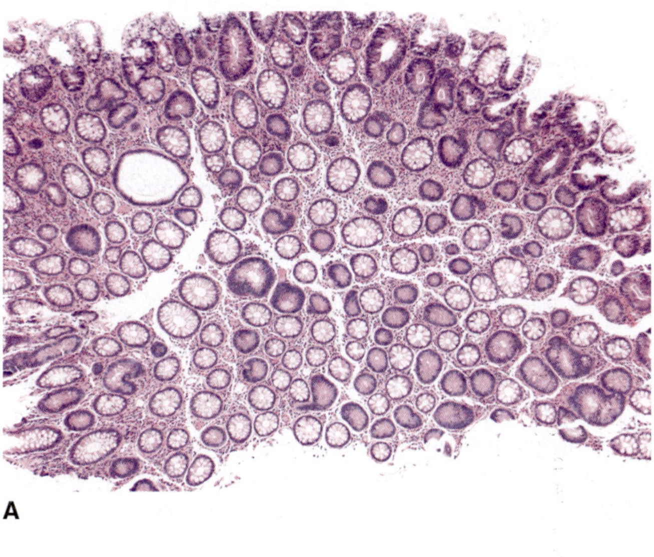

A

FIGURE 4.15: A polypoid dysplastic lesion contains two populations of crypts (**A**).

**FIGURE 4.15:** (*Continued*) Dysplastic crypts interspersed between nondysplastic crypts (**B**).

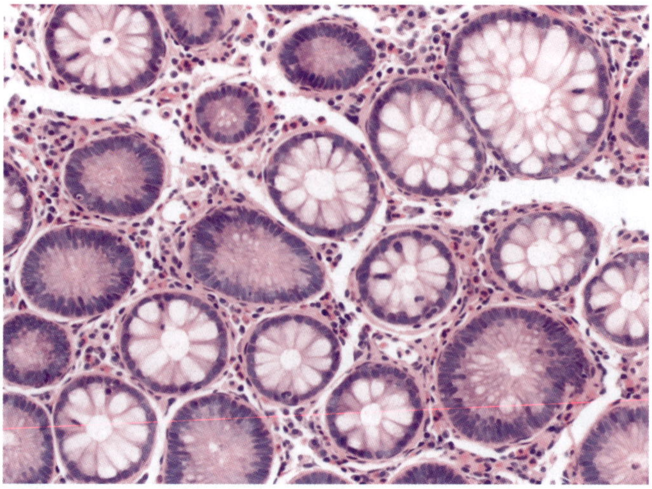


amounts of cytoplasm and slightly large nuclei that may be elongated and contain prominent nucleoli. A provisional diagnosis of indefinite for dysplasia is appropriate when epithelial cells appear dysplastic, but cytologic abnormalities are associated with neutrophil-rich infiltrates and when cytologic abnormalities are observed in the colonic crypts, but not the surface (Figure 4.16). Reevaluation following treatment of inflammatory activity is suggested in these cases.

## Immunohistochemical and Molecular Features

Immunohistochemical stains that distinguish inflammatory bowel disease–associated dysplasia from reactive epithelial cell atypia are not useful in most cases. Although Ki-67, $\alpha$-methylacyl-CoA racemase (AMACR), and TP53 stains have been identified as potential dysplasia markers, they usually confirm cases that are clearly dysplastic or reactive by morphologic assessment alone and are not definitive in challenging cases. For example, restricted basal Ki-67 staining supports a reactive, rather than dysplastic, process, but some cases with reactive atypia show surface Ki-67 staining, especially in areas of healed erosion.[53] Cytoplasmic staining for AMACR is common in high-grade dysplastic foci, but is of no utility in distinguishing between low-grade dysplasia and reactive atypia, which is more often the diagnostically challenging situation.[54] Low- and high-grade dysplastic foci may show strong nuclear TP53 staining, but staining is less intense in low-grade dysplasia and overlaps substantially with the staining quality of reactive epithelium.[53]

A similar spectrum of molecular aberrations occurs in inflammatory bowel disease–associated dysplasia and conventional adenomas, including mutations in *APC, TP53, KRAS, DPC4,* and *MTS1 (p16),* although the sequence of events may be different between the two groups.[55] For example, *TP53* mutations are likely late events in the adenoma–carcinoma sequence, but may be found in inflammatory bowel disease–associated low-grade dysplasia. Immunostains for TP53 are more commonly positive in adenoma-like DALMs, whereas β-catenin immunoexpression is more frequent in sporadic adenomas.[56] Unfortunately, these features are not universal and, thus, cannot be entirely relied upon to distinguish between dysplasia due to chronic colitis and sporadic adenomas.

## Serrated Neoplasia in Inflammatory Bowel Disease

Some patients with inflammatory bowel disease develop serrated neoplasia in the form of hyperplastic polyps, sessile serrated polyps, and serrated adenomas. In fact, inflammatory bowel disease–associated adenocarcinomas are often associated with adjacent mucosal hyperplasia or serrated polyps, raising the possibility that serrated neoplasms sometimes represent carcinoma precursors in this patient population.[57] Rare patients with inflammatory bowel disease have innumerable serrated polyps that simulate serrated polyposis and may be associated with increased cancer risk.[58]

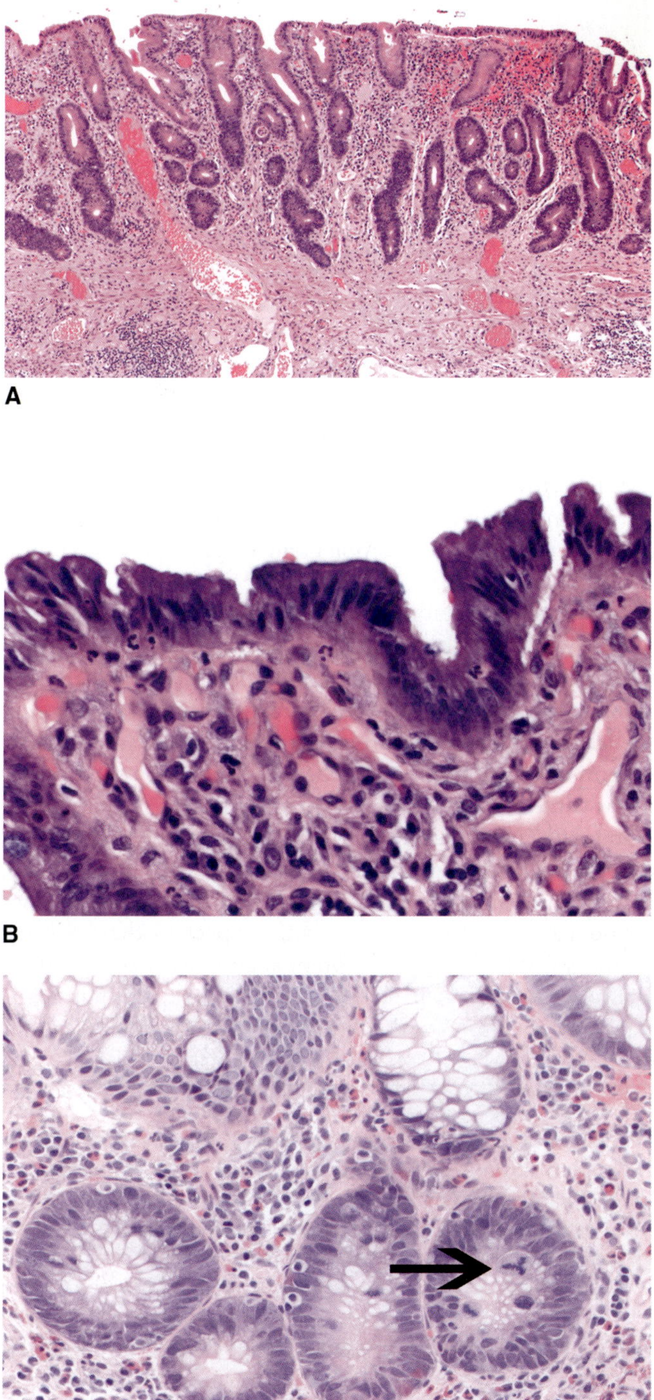


**FIGURE 4.16:** Regenerating crypts in an area of erosion have irregular contours and an uneven distribution in the lamina propria (**A**). Surface epithelial cells are mucin depleted with hyperchromatic nuclei, but intraepithelial neutrophils are present (**B**). Crowded clusters of crypts contain hyperchromatic, enlarged nuclei with an atypical mitotic figure (*arrow*), raising concern for dysplasia (**C**).

FIGURE 4.16: (*Continued*) However, surface maturation, neutrophil-rich infiltrates, and crypt destruction deep in the mucosa all raise the possibility of a reparative process, so a diagnosis of indefinite for dysplasia was rendered (**D**). Subsequent biopsies of the area were negative for dysplasia.

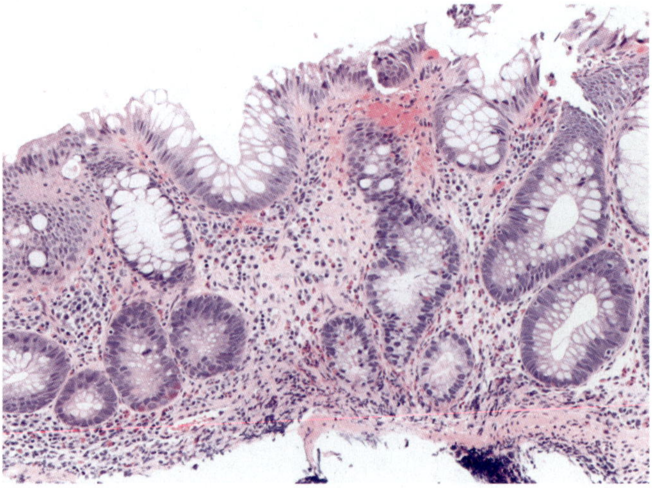

D

Most serrated lesions in inflammatory bowel disease are similar to nonserrated DALMs in that they display abnormalities in *KRAS, APC, MTS1 (p16)*, and chromosome 3p, although others harbor *BRAF* mutations.[58] Only a minority of inflammatory bowel disease–associated neoplasms shows MSI, which usually reflects hypermethylation of the *MLH1* promoter and loss of MLH1 function.[59]

## SUMMARY AND CONCLUSIONS

Pathologists play a major role in guiding patient management and endoscopic surveillance by histologically classifying epithelial colorectal polyps. Morphologic characterization and emerging molecular analyses of colorectal epithelial polyps improve cancer prevention by elucidating their clinical importance and neoplastic potential. Recent correlations between morphologic features and molecular characteristics reveal that some polyps that were initially thought to be innocuous may, in fact, harbor malignant potential. These observations have led to recognition of the serrated neoplastic pathway, important groups of sporadic colorectal cancers, and their precursors. The spectrum of invasive colorectal neoplasms that result from epithelial polyps is further discussed in Sections III and IV of this book.

# References


1. Clark JC, Collan Y, Eide TJ, et al. Prevalence of polyps in an autopsy series from areas with varying incidence of large-bowel cancer. *Int J Cancer* 1985;36(2):179–186.
2. Kearney J, Giovannucci E, Rimm EB, et al. Diet, alcohol, and smoking and the occurrence of hyperplastic polyps of the colon and rectum (United States). *Cancer Causes Control* 1995;6(1):45–56.
3. Winawer SJ, Zauber AG, Fletcher RH, et al. Guidelines for colonoscopy surveillance after polypectomy: a consensus update by the US Multi-Society Task Force on Colorectal Cancer and the American Cancer Society. *CA Cancer J Clin* 2006;56(3):143–59; quiz 84–85.
4. Waye JD, Bilotta JJ. Rectal hyperplastic polyps: now you see them, now you don't—a differential point. *Am J Gastroenterol* 1990;85(12):1557–1559.
5. Huang Q, Fukami N, Kashida H, et al. Interobserver and intra-observer consistency in the endoscopic assessment of colonic pit patterns. *Gastrointest Endosc* 2004;60(4):520–526.
6. Kambham N, Troxell M, Longacre TA. Multinucleated epithelial giant cells in colorectal polyps: a potential mimic of viropathic and/or dysplastic changes. *Am J Surg Pathol* 2005;29(7):912–919.
7. Torlakovic E, Skovlund E, Snover DC, et al. Morphologic reappraisal of serrated colorectal polyps. *Am J Surg Pathol* 2003;27(1):65–81.

8. Chung SM, Chen YT, Panczykowski A, et al. Serrated polyps with "intermediate features" of sessile serrated polyp and microvesicular hyperplastic polyp: a practical approach to the classification of non-dysplastic serrated polyps. *Am J Surg Pathol* 2008;32(3):407–412.
9. Higuchi T, Jass JR. My approach to serrated polyps of the colorectum. *J Clin Pathol* 2004;57(7):682–686.
10. Torlakovic EE, Gomez JD, Driman DK, et al. Sessile serrated adenoma (SSA) vs. traditional serrated adenoma (TSA). *Am J Surg Pathol* 2008;32(1):21–29.
11. Mochizuka A, Uehara T, Nakamura T, et al. Hyperplastic polyps and sessile serrated 'adenomas' of the colon and rectum display gastric pyloric differentiation. *Histochem Cell Biol* 2007;128(5):445–455.
12. Spring KJ, Zhao ZZ, Karamatic R, et al. High prevalence of sessile serrated adenomas with BRAF mutations: a prospective study of patients undergoing colonoscopy. *Gastroenterology* 2006;131(5):1400–1407.
13. Jass JR, Baker K, Zlobec I, et al. Advanced colorectal polyps with the molecular and morphological features of serrated polyps and adenomas: concept of a 'fusion' pathway to colorectal cancer. *Histopathology* 2006;49(2):121–131.
14. O'Brien MJ, Yang S, Mack C, et al. Comparison of microsatellite instability, CpG island methylation phenotype, BRAF and KRAS status in serrated polyps and traditional adenomas indicates separate pathways to distinct colorectal carcinoma end points. *Am J Surg Pathol* 2006;30(12):1491–1501.
15. Otori K, Oda Y, Sugiyama K, et al. High frequency of K-ras mutations in human colorectal hyperplastic polyps. *Gut* 1997;40(5):660–663.
16. Snover DC, Ahnen DJ, Burt RW, et al. Serrated polyps of the colon and rectum and serrated polyposis. In: Bosman FT, Carneiro F, Hruban RH, et al., eds. *WHO Classification of Tumours of the Digestive System*. Lyon, France: IARC Press; 2010.
17. Higuchi T, Sugihara K, Jass JR. Demographic and pathological characteristics of serrated polyps of colorectum. *Histopathology* 2005;47(1):32–40.
18. Torlakovic E, Snover DC. Serrated adenomatous polyposis in humans. *Gastroenterology* 1996;110(3): 748–755.
19. Park SJ, Rashid A, Lee JH, et al. Frequent CpG island methylation in serrated adenomas of the colorectum. *Am J Pathol* 2003;162(3):815–822.
20. Owens SR, Chiosea SI, Kuan SF. Selective expression of gastric mucin MUC6 in colonic sessile serrated adenoma but not in hyperplastic polyp aids in morphological diagnosis of serrated polyps. *Mod Pathol* 2008;21(6):660–669.
21. Bartley AN, Thompson PA, Buckmeier JA, et al. Expression of gastric pyloric mucin, MUC6, in colorectal serrated polyps. *Mod Pathol* 2010;23(2):169–176.
22. Wynter CV, Walsh MD, Higuchi T, et al. Methylation patterns define two types of hyperplastic polyp associated with colorectal cancer. *Gut* 2004;53(4):573–580.
23. Oh K, Redston M, Odze RD. Support for hMLH1 and MGMT silencing as a mechanism of tumorigenesis in the hyperplastic-adenoma-carcinoma (serrated) carcinogenic pathway in the colon. *Hum Pathol* 2005;36(1):101–111.
24. Yantiss RK, Panczykowski A, Misdraji J, et al. A comprehensive study of non-dysplastic and dysplastic serrated polyps of the vermiform appendix. *Am J Surg Pathol* 2007;31(11):1742–1753.
25. Jass JR, Burt RW. Hyperplastic polyposis. In: Hamilton SR, Altonnen L, eds. *WHO International Classification of Tumors: Pathology and Genetics of Tumors of the Digestive System*. Berlin, Germany: Springer-Verlag; 2000:135–136.
26. Leggett BA, Devereaux B, Biden K, et al. Hyperplastic polyposis: association with colorectal cancer. *Am J Surg Pathol* 2001;25(2):177–184.
27. Winawer SJ, Zauber AG, Ho MN, et al. The National Polyp Study. *Eur J Cancer Prev* 1993;2(suppl 2):83–87.
28. O'Brien MJ, Winawer SJ, Zauber AG, et al. Flat adenomas in the National Polyp Study: is there increased risk for high-grade dysplasia initially or during surveillance? *Clin Gastroenterol Hepatol* 2004;2(10):905–911.
29. Fenoglio CM, Kaye GI, Lane N. Distribution of human colonic lymphatics in normal, hyperplastic, and adenomatous tissue. Its relationship to metastasis from small carcinomas in pedunculated adenomas, with two case reports. *Gastroenterology* 1973;64(1):51–66.
30. Kim MN, Kang JM, Yang JI, et al. Clinical features and prognosis of early colorectal cancer treated by endoscopic mucosal resection. *J Gastroenterol Hepatol* 2011;26(11):1619–1625.
31. van Putten PG, Hol L, van Dekken H, et al. Inter-observer variation in the histological diagnosis of polyps in colorectal cancer screening. *Histopathology* 2011;58(6):974–981.
32. Tanizawa T, Seki T, Nakano M, et al. Pseudoinvasion of the colorectal polypoid tumors: serial section study of problematic cases. *Pathol Int* 2003;53(9):584–590.
33. Markowitz AJ, Winawer SJ. Management of colorectal polyps. *CA Cancer J Clin* 1997;47(2):93–112.

34. Cooper GS, Xu F, Barnholtz Sloan JS, et al. Management of malignant colonic polyps: a population-based analysis of colonoscopic polypectomy versus surgery. *Cancer* 2012;118(3):651–659.
35. Waye JD, Haggitt RC. Controversies, dilemmas, and dialogues. When is colonoscopic resection of an adenomatous polyp containing a "malignancy" sufficient? *Am J Gastroenterol* 1990;85(12):1564–1568.
36. Ispas C, Yu J, Tarantino DR, et al. Pathologic quiz case: a 44-year-old woman with a tubulovillous adenoma of the colon and liver and bone lesions. Small cell (neuroendocrine) carcinoma of the colon with metastasis and an associated, overlying villous adenoma. *Arch Pathol Lab Med* 2005;129(3):412–414.
37. Pulitzer M, Xu R, Suriawinata AA, et al. Microcarcinoids in large intestinal adenomas. *Am J Surg Pathol* 2006;30(12):1531–1536.
38. Ozuner G. Colonoscopic detection of a malignant melanoma metastatic to a tubular adenoma of the colon: report of a case. *Dis Colon Rectum* 2002;45(12):1681–1684.
39. Ricchetti T, Paci M, Cavazza A, et al. A case of metastatic epithelioid angiosarcoma in the lamina propria of a sigmoid tubulovillous adenoma. *Tumori* 2005;91(2):210–212.
40. Bismar TA, Maluf H, Wang HL. Metastatic foci of signet ring cell carcinoma in a tubular adenoma of the colon. *Arch Pathol Lab Med* 2003;127(11):1509–1512.
41. Sawyer EJ, Cerar A, Hanby AM, et al. Molecular characteristics of serrated adenomas of the colorectum. *Gut* 2002;51(2):200–206.
42. Longacre TA, Fenoglio-Preiser CM. Mixed hyperplastic adenomatous polyps/serrated adenomas. A distinct form of colorectal neoplasia. *Am J Surg Pathol* 1990;14(6):524–537.
43. Gala M, Chung DC. Hereditary colon cancer syndromes. *Semin Oncol* 2011;38(4):490–499.
44. Matsumoto T, Mizuno M, Shimizu M, et al. Serrated adenoma of the colorectum: colonoscopic and histologic features. *Gastrointest Endosc* 1999;49(6):736–742.
45. Yantiss RK, Oh KY, Chen YT, et al. Filiform serrated adenomas: a clinicopathologic and immunophenotypic study of 18 cases. *Am J Surg Pathol* 2007;31(8):1238–1245.
46. Chan TL, Zhao W, Leung SY, et al. BRAF and KRAS mutations in colorectal hyperplastic polyps and serrated adenomas. *Cancer Res* 2003;63(16):4878–4881.
47. Konishi K, Yamochi T, Makino R, et al. Molecular differences between sporadic serrated and conventional colorectal adenomas. *Clin Cancer Res* 2004;10(9):3082–3090.
48. Iino H, Jass JR, Simms LA, et al. DNA microsatellite instability in hyperplastic polyps, serrated adenomas, and mixed polyps: a mild mutator pathway for colorectal cancer? *J Clin Pathol* 1999;52(1):5–9.
49. Sheridan TB, Fenton H, Lewin MR, et al. Sessile serrated adenomas with low- and high-grade dysplasia and early carcinomas: an immunohistochemical study of serrated lesions "caught in the act." *Am J Clin Pathol* 2006;126(4):564–571.
50. Friedman S, Rubin PH, Bodian C, et al. Screening and surveillance colonoscopy in chronic Crohn's colitis. *Gastroenterology* 2001;120(4):820–826.
51. Ullman T, Croog V, Harpaz N, et al. Progression of flat low-grade dysplasia to advanced neoplasia in patients with ulcerative colitis. *Gastroenterology* 2003;125(5):1311–1319.
52. Kisiel JB, Loftus EV Jr, Harmsen WS, et al. Outcome of sporadic adenomas and adenoma-like dysplasia in patients with ulcerative colitis undergoing polypectomy. *Inflamm Bowel Dis* 2012;18(2):226–235.
53. Wong NA, Mayer NJ, MacKell S, et al. Immunohistochemical assessment of Ki-67 and p53 expression assists the diagnosis and grading of ulcerative colitis-related dysplasia. *Histopathology* [Research Support, Non-U.S. Gov't] 2000;37(2):108–114.
54. Dorer R, Odze RD. AMACR immunostaining is useful in detecting dysplastic epithelium in Barrett's esophagus, ulcerative colitis, and Crohn's disease. *Am J Surg Pathol* 2006;30(7):871–877.
55. Odze RD, Brown CA, Hartmann CJ, et al. Genetic alterations in chronic ulcerative colitis-associated adenoma-like DALMs are similar to non-colitic sporadic adenomas. *Am J Surg Pathol* [Comparative Study] 2000;24(9):1209–1216.
56. Walsh SV, Loda M, Torres CM, et al. P53 and beta catenin expression in chronic ulcerative colitis—associated polypoid dysplasia and sporadic adenomas: an immunohistochemical study. *Am J Surg Pathol* 1999;23(8):963–969.
57. Rubio CA. Serrated neoplasias and de novo carcinomas in ulcerative colitis: a histological study in colectomy specimens. *J Gastroenterol Hepatol* 2007;22(7):1024–1031.
58. Srivastava A, Redston M, Farraye FA, et al. Hyperplastic/serrated polyposis in inflammatory bowel disease: a case series of a previously undescribed entity. *Am J Surg Pathol* 2008;32(2):296–303.
59. Fleisher AS, Esteller M, Harpaz N, et al. Microsatellite instability in inflammatory bowel disease-associated neoplastic lesions is associated with hypermethylation and diminished expression of the DNA mismatch repair gene, hMLH1. *Cancer Res* 2000;60(17):4864–4868.

# Hamartomatous Polyps and Polyposis Syndromes

# 5

Rhonda K. Yantiss

Hamartomatous polyps of the colorectum develop sporadically or in patients with hamartomatous polyposis syndromes, such as Peutz-Jeghers syndrome, juvenile polyposis, and phosphatase and tensin homologue (PTEN) hamartoma tumor syndrome. Although hamartomatous polyps are benign lesions comprising a variable admixture of nonneoplastic epithelial and stromal elements, syndromic polyps are associated with cancer risk, and, thus, clinicians and pathologists endeavor to identify at-risk patients and their family members. Recent advances in molecular pathology have provided important insight into the pathogenesis of hamartomatous polyposes and their relationships to cancer. However, application of pathologic, clinical, and molecular criteria still fails to identify all patients with hamartomatous syndromes. Despite recent advances in molecular techniques, a substantial number of patients with multiple gastrointestinal hamartomas lack detectable mutations, and up to 50% of patients do not have afflicted family members. With the exception of Peutz-Jeghers polyps, most gastrointestinal hamartomas are sporadic and do not reflect the presence of an underlying syndrome. Furthermore, most nonneoplastic polyps of the gastrointestinal tract are hyperplastic or inflammatory lesions that may be indistinguishable from hamartomas, particularly juvenile polyps. Pathologists play an important role in the detection and classification of hamartomatous polyposis syndromes, as well as distinguishing them from inflammatory conditions that require specific therapies. The purpose of this chapter is to discuss the clinicopathologic features and differential diagnoses of the most common hamartomatous polyps of the colorectum.

## SPORADIC HAMARTOMAS

Sporadic hamartomas show a spectrum of morphologic features and contain nondysplastic epithelium, lamina propria, lymphoid tissue, and submucosal elements in various combinations. They may comprise some, or mostly, mesenchymal elements, in which case they show overlapping features with ganglioneuromas, Schwann cell hamartomas, lipomas, and perineuriomas. Polyps that consist of abundant inflamed stroma and cystically dilated glands are generally considered to represent inflammatory-type polyps in adults, whereas similar-appearing polyps among children are usually classified as juvenile polyps, as discussed subsequently. Most other sporadic hamartomas are asymptomatic, subcentimeter polyps that are incidentally discovered during screening or surveillance colonoscopy. They contain well-organized elements and show subtle abnormalities, such as distorted, thick-walled blood vessels, abnormal fat deposits, and irregularly distributed ganglion cells (Figure 5.1). Indeed, they may be overlooked and interpreted to represent normal mucosa in polypectomy specimens.

### Peutz-Jeghers Syndrome

#### *Clinical and Endoscopic Features*

Virtually all Peutz-Jeghers hamartomatous polyps occur in the setting of the Peutz-Jeghers syndrome. Morphologically similarly polyps are rarely encountered as sporadic lesions, especially in the small intestine. Indeed, limited data suggest a relationship between sporadic Peutz-Jeghers

**FIGURE 5.1:** This hamartomatous polyp was found in the ascending colon of a middle-aged female during screening colonoscopy. It contains many elements native to the colon, but they are disorganized. Dense lymphoid inflammation is subjacent to colonic crypts and superficial to large, irregular smooth muscle bundles contiguous with the muscularis mucosae (**A**). Numerous ganglion cells are present singly and in clusters (*arrows*) within an abnormally thick muscularis mucosae (**B**).

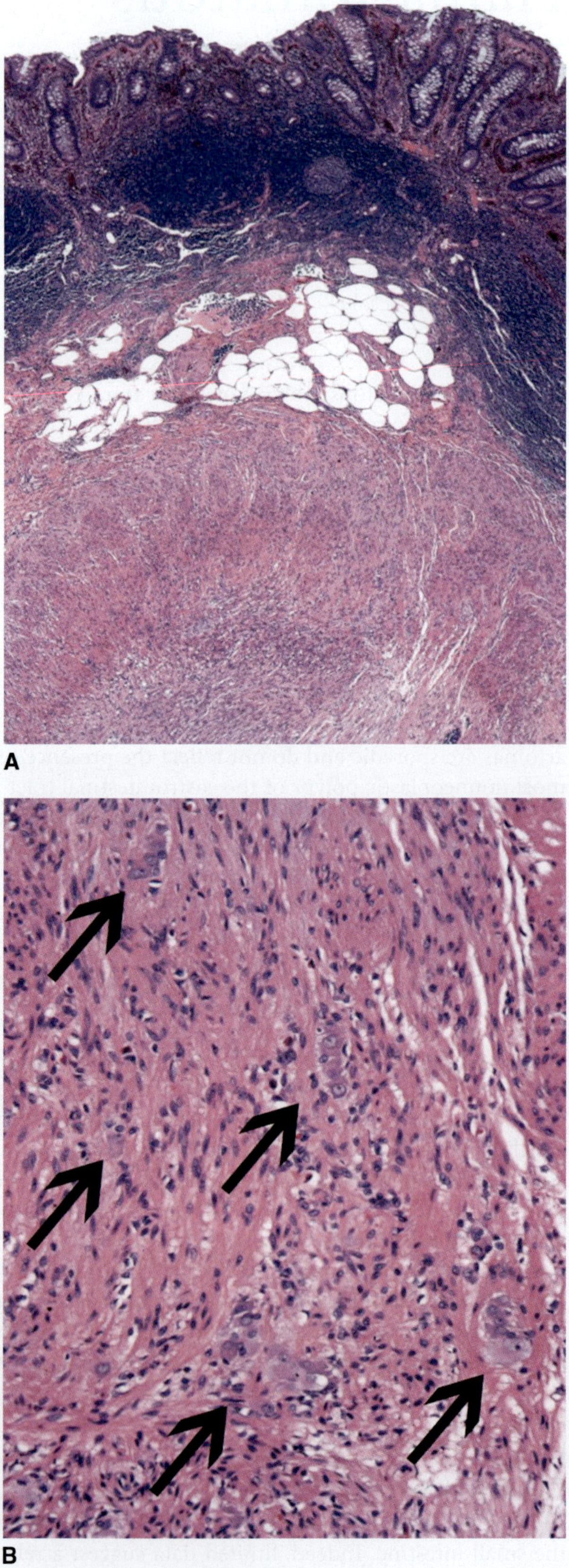

polyps and a variety of malignancies typically associated with the syndrome, suggesting that "isolated" Peutz-Jeghers polyps simply represent a *forme fruste* of the syndrome.[1] Thus, detection of polyps that show morphologic features of Peutz-Jeghers hamartomatous lesions should prompt evaluation for a heritable syndrome and assessment for possible malignancy, particularly when they are multiple or encountered in the small intestine.

Peutz-Jeghers syndrome is an autosomal dominant hereditary polyposis syndrome affecting 1 in 200,000 persons in the United States. It is characterized by the presence of numerous gastrointestinal hamartomatous polyps, mucocutaneous pigmentation, and an increased risk for developing a variety of malignancies in multiple organ systems (Table 5.1).[2] Diagnostic criteria for the syndrome include (1) three or more Peutz-Jeghers polyps, (2) any number of Peutz-Jeghers polyps in a patient with a family history of the syndrome, (3) characteristic mucocutaneous pigmentation in a patient with a family history of the syndrome, or (4) any number of Peutz-Jeghers polyps in association with mucocutaneous pigmentation.[3]

The overall risk of gastrointestinal and extraintestinal malignancy among patients with Peutz-Jeghers syndrome is estimated to be 93% by 65 years of age. Up to 12% of patients with the disorder have dysplasia and/or invasive carcinoma in their polyps, but the adjacent, nonpolypoid mucosa is also at risk for malignancy. The lifetime risk of colorectal cancer among patients with Peutz-Jeghers syndrome is 35% to 40%, followed in frequency by pancreatic cancer (35%) and gastric cancer (28%). Despite the frequent occurrence of small-intestinal polyps in Peutz-Jeghers syndrome, the lifetime risk of small bowel cancer is only 10% to 15%.[4–7]

Peutz-Jeghers polyps show a predilection for the small intestine, but may occur anywhere in stomach, colon, or small intestine, as well as the gallbladder, bladder, and nasopharynx.[3] These polyps have a characteristic endoscopic appearance. They are multilobulated or rounded with a smooth surface that is similar in color to the background mucosa. Colorectal polyps may be pedunculated or sessile, and, when present, the stalk is usually thicker and longer than that of an adenoma (Figure 5.2). Patients with colorectal polyps almost always have small bowel polyps as well, the latter of which tend to produce clinical symptoms of recurrent abdominal pain secondary to intussusception. Individuals less than 30 years of age typically present with symptoms reflecting benign complications of disease, such as abdominal pain or bleeding, whereas malignant complications are more common presenting manifestations among older adults.

### *Pathologic Features*

Peutz-Jeghers polyps are composed of nondysplastic mucosal aggregates and smooth muscle bundles that emanate in an arborizing fashion from the muscularis mucosae (Figure 5.3). Polyps contain lobules of mature-appearing colonic epithelium supported by lamina propria (Figure 5.4). Crypts are normal or display mildly serrated epithelium and occasional cystic dilatation. Up to 10% of small-intestinal Peutz-Jeghers polyps are associated with displaced mucosa in the submucosa, muscularis propria, or subserosa of the subjacent bowel wall. This finding likely reflects a developmental phenomenon related to their hamartomatous nature, rather than trauma-related epithelial misplacement, and is usually lacking in colorectal hamartomatous polyps.

The differential diagnosis of Peutz-Jeghers polyps includes other types of hamartomatous polyps, mucosal prolapse polyps, adenoma with misplaced (displaced) epithelium, and invasive adenocarcinoma. The morphologic features of some Peutz-Jeghers polyps overlap with those of juvenile polyps, the latter of which may be seen in association with juvenile polyposis and PTEN hamartoma tumor syndrome. Overlapping features are particularly problematic among gastric and colonic Peutz-Jeghers polyps that do not show well-developed arborizing bundles of smooth muscle cells characteristic of small bowel polyps. Indeed, colonic and gastric Peutz-Jeghers hamartomas often display superimposed inflammatory changes more typically seen in juvenile polyps (Figure 5.5).[8] Sporadic mucosal prolapse-type polyps contain abundant smooth muscle bundles extending into the lamina propria that simulate arborizing muscle

**Table 5.1** Clinicopathologic and Molecular Features of Hamartomatous Polyposis Syndromes

| | Peutz-Jeghers Syndrome | Juvenile Polyposis Syndrome | PTEN Hamartoma Tumor Syndrome |
|---|---|---|---|
| **Affected Gene** | *LKB1 (STK11)* | *SMAD4 and BMBR1A* | *PTEN* |
| **Gene Location** | 19p13.3 | 18q21.1 (*SMAD4*)<br>10q22.3 (*BMBR1A*) | 10q22.3 (*PTEN*)<br>1p35-36 (*SDHB*)<br>11q23 (*SDHD*) |
| **Gene Function** | Serine threonine kinase | TGF-β–mediated signal transduction | Tumor suppressor gene |
| **Prevalence in Affected Patients** | 70% | 35%–60% | 85% |
| **Dermatologic Manifestations** | Perioral, buccal, and conjunctival pigmentation | | Oral papillomas, tricholemmomas, acral keratoses |
| **Other Abnormalities** | | Cranial and cardiac abnormalities<br>Cleft palate<br>Polydactyly<br>Intestinal malrotation<br>Hereditary hemorrhagic telangiectasia | Autoimmune thyroiditis<br>Macrocephaly<br>Mental impairment<br>Fibrocystic breast disease<br>Glycogenic acanthosis |
| **Distribution of Polyps** | 1. Small intestine<br>2. Colon<br>3. Stomach | 1. Colon<br>2. Stomach<br>3. Small intestine | 1. Colon<br>2. Stomach<br>3. Small intestine |
| **Gastrointestinal Carcinomas** | Carcinomas of colon, stomach, pancreas, small intestine | Carcinomas of colorectum, pancreas, stomach, duodenum | Carcinomas of colorectum and stomach |
| **Other Malignancies** | Ovarian sex cord–stromal tumor with annular tubules<br>Adenoma malignum of cervix<br>Testicular large cell calcifying<br>Sertoli cell tumor<br>Carcinoma of breast | | Breast cancer<br>Thyroid cancer, follicular |

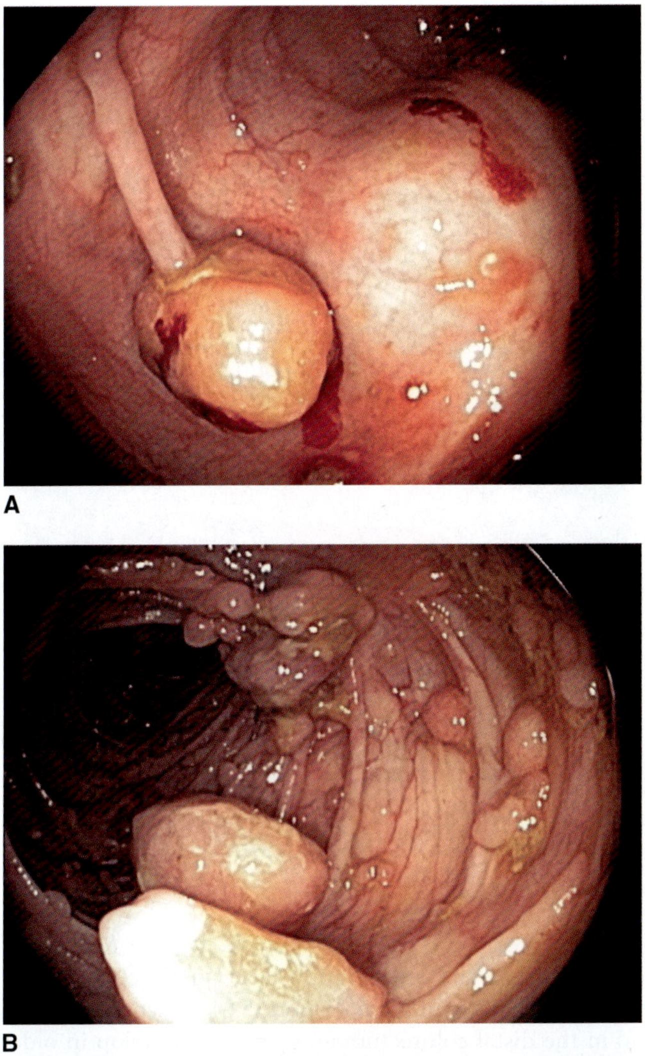


FIGURE 5.2: Colonoscopic examination of a patient with Peutz-Jeghers syndrome demonstrates innumerable colonic polyps. One colonic polyp contains a long slender stalk composed of normal mucosal and submucosal elements (**A**), whereas others are sessile with a multinodular appearance (**B**). (Photographs courtesy of Dr. Randall Burt, University of Utah School of Medicine, Salt Lake City, UT.)

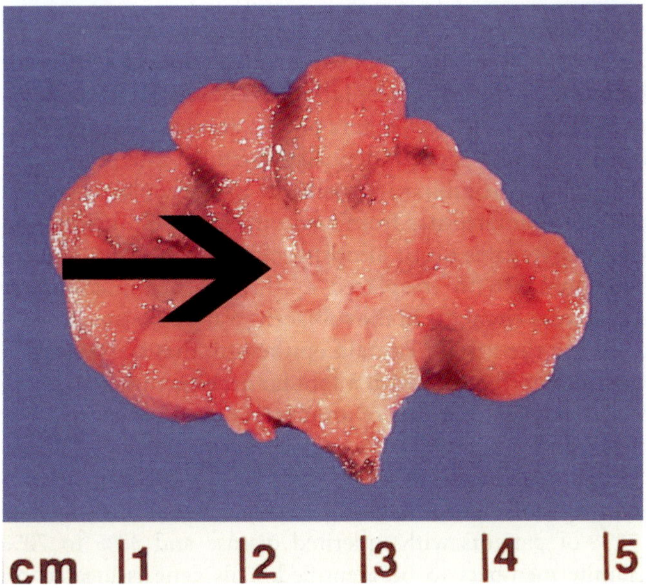


FIGURE 5.3: A cross-section through a Peutz-Jeghers polyp demonstrates a multinodular polyp head and dense stalk, reflecting smooth muscle cells emanating from the muscularis mucosae. The stalk shows some arborizing muscle bundles that extend into the head of the polyp (*arrow*).

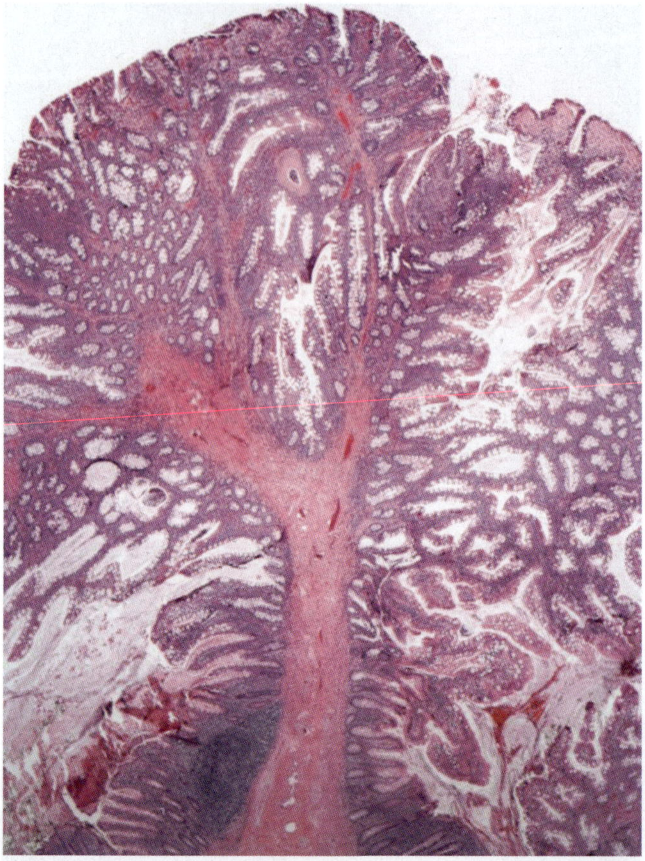

**FIGURE 5.4:** Peutz-Jeghers polyps of the colorectum contain round aggregates of mucosal elements that are more numerous at the surface. Splayed bundles of smooth muscle cells fill the polyp stalk.

bundles in Peutz-Jeghers polyps. However, prolapse-type polyps also show other features of luminal trauma, including erosions, hyperplasia and regeneration of crypts associated with ischemic-type surface epithelial changes, and inflammation (Figure 5.6). Mucosal prolapse polyps are most commonly observed in the distal colorectum and generally develop in older adults.

Peutz-Jeghers polyps that show epithelium in the subjacent bowel wall may simulate epithelial misplacement in adenomas as well as well-differentiated adenocarcinoma. Although both Peutz-Jeghers polyps and adenomas with epithelial misplacement contain lobules of epithelium surrounded by lamina propria, those of Peutz-Jeghers polyps are unassociated with features suggestive of polyp trauma, such as hemosiderin deposits, extruded mucin, hemorrhage, or scarring. A lack of these findings, in combination with the non-neoplastic nature of the epithelium, facilitates distinction of hamartomas from adenomas with epithelial misplacement. Importantly, mural mucosal aggregates occur almost exclusively in Peutz-Jeghers polyps of the small bowel where adenomas with misplaced epithelium are uncommon. Peutz-Jeghers polyps associated with mucosal elements in the subjacent wall may also simulate invasive adenocarcinoma, particularly with the former contain epithelium that is dysplastic.[9] However, the Peutz-Jeghers polyps contain epithelium with a lobular architecture associated with lamina propria, rather than the desmoplastic stroma of an invasive carcinoma.

### *Molecular Alterations*

More than half of patients with Peutz-Jeghers syndrome have detectable mutations in *LKB1* (*STK11*), including approximately 70% of patients with inherited disease and 30% to 70% of those who are the first affected family members to be identified. This gene is located on

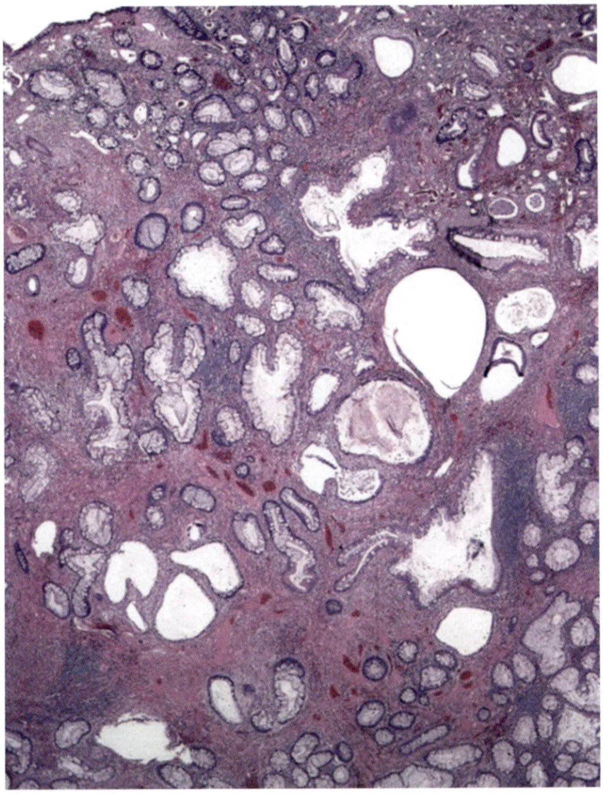

A

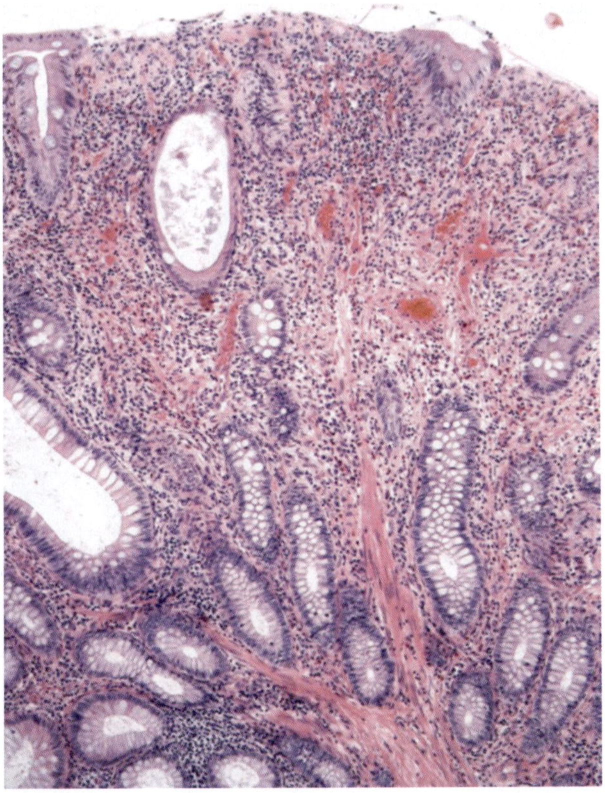

B

FIGURE 5.5: A Peutz-Jeghers polyp of the colon is composed of numerous cystically dilated glands, some of which contain inspissated secretions. The lobular architecture of mucosal elements is lacking and smooth muscle bundles are not prominent (**A**). The lamina propria contains granulation tissue, eosinophils, and dilated crypts reminiscent of a juvenile polyp (**B**).

**FIGURE 5.6:** A mucosal prolapse polyp is eroded and contains cystically dilated crypts, some of which are serrated (**A**). Bundles of smooth muscle cells emanate from the muscularis mucosae into the polyp head, simulating the appearance of a Peutz-Jeghers polyp (**B**).

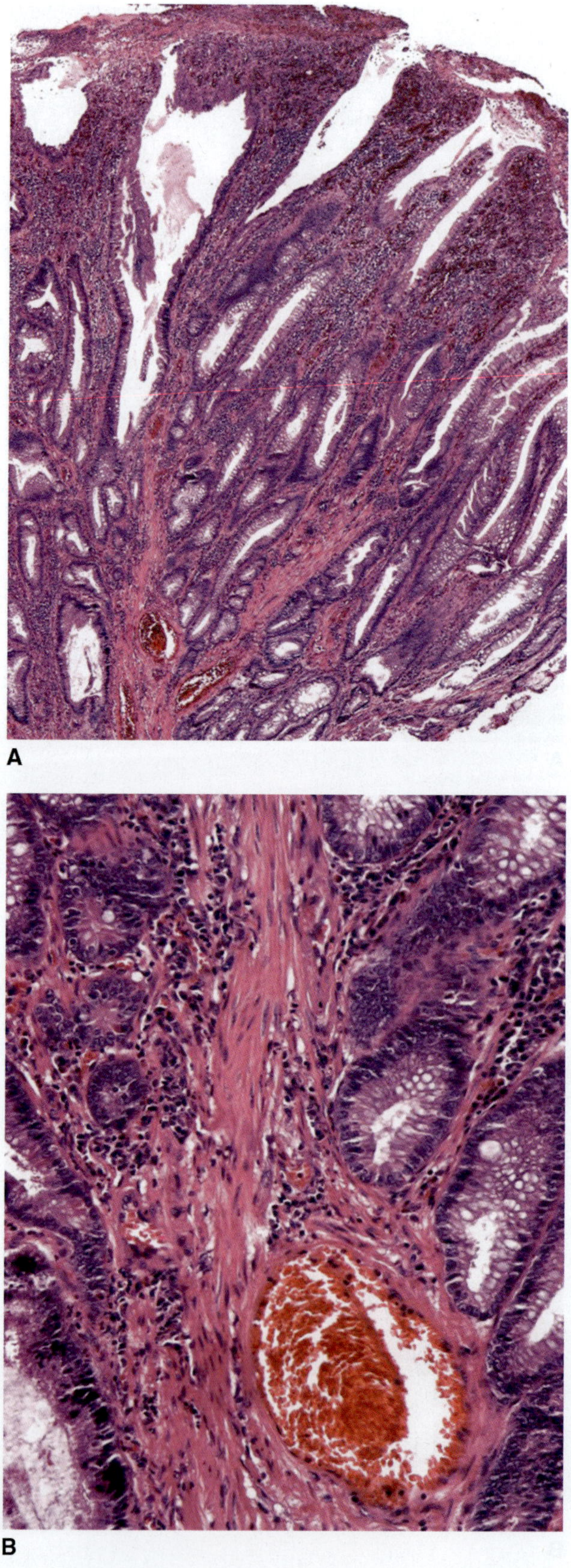

A

B

chromosome 19p13.3 and encodes a nuclear serine threonine kinase that normally inhibits cell growth by stimulating the promoter activity of *p27*.[10–13] The disease phenotype tends to be more severe in patients with truncating mutations compared to missense mutations.[11]

## Juvenile Polyposis Syndrome

### *Clinical and Endoscopic Features*

Unlike Peutz-Jeghers polyps, juvenile polyps may develop sporadically or in association with one of several polyposis syndromes, including juvenile polyposis syndrome, Cowden syndrome, and Bannayan-Riley-Ruvalcaba syndrome, as discussed in the next section. Isolated juvenile polyps of childhood show a predilection for the rectum and affect approximately 1% to 2% of children and adolescents.[14] They are smooth, pedunculated, or sessile mucosal lesions that are somewhat friable and readily autoamputate in the fecal stream. Thus, juvenile polyps produce signs and symptoms related to gastrointestinal bleeding, including occult blood loss, hematochezia, anemia, passage of tissue per rectum, and mucosal prolapse.

Juvenile polyposis syndrome is an autosomal dominant hereditary polyposis syndrome affecting 1 in 100,000 persons in the United States. Phenotypic variants include infantile juvenile polyposis, juvenile polyposis coli, and generalized juvenile polyposis. Infantile juvenile polyposis is least common and unassociated with a family history of juvenile polyposis syndrome. It typically presents within the first 2 years of life with gastrointestinal polyposis, gastrointestinal bleeding, diarrhea, malnutrition, and protein-losing enteropathy and may result in early death.[15] Patients with juvenile polyposis coli develop colorectal hamartomas, whereas those with generalized juvenile polyposis have numerous gastrointestinal polyps affecting the colon, stomach, and small intestine. Diagnostic criteria for juvenile polyposis include (1) three or more colorectal juvenile polyps, (2) any number of extracolonic juvenile polyps, or (3) any number of juvenile polyps in patients with a family history of the syndrome.[16] However, only 20% to 50% of patients with syndromic disease have a family history of juvenile polyposis.

Approximately 15% of patients with juvenile polyposis syndrome also have congenital anomalies that include cranial and cardiac abnormalities, cleft palate, polydactyly, and intestinal malrotation (Table 5.1).[17] The syndrome has also been reported in association with hereditary hemorrhagic telangiectasia characterized by vascular malformations affecting multiple organs, including those of the gastrointestinal tract.[18] Reports have described patients with juvenile polyposis syndrome and pulmonary arteriovenous malformations as well as hypertrophic osteoarthropathy.[19] Patients with juvenile polyposis are at increased risk for the development of colorectal carcinoma, the cumulative risk of which is estimated to be 68% by 60 years of age.[20] These individuals also suffer a higher incidence of carcinomas of the stomach, pancreas, and proximal small intestine.

More than 50% of isolated juvenile polyps develop in the rectum, although they may also occur proximal to the splenic flexure.[21] Most patients with juvenile polyposis syndrome have numerous (3 to 200) colorectal polyps, and those with generalized juvenile polyposis develop lesions in the stomach and small intestine as well. Small juvenile polyps are sessile, erythematous lesions that simulate the endoscopic appearance of hyperplastic polyps. Larger polyps may be pedunculated and frequently display erythema and adherent fibrin on the polyp head reflecting erosions or ulcers (Figure 5.7). Syndromic polyps often have a mulberry-like multilobular appearance and have been termed "atypical juvenile polyps" (Figure 5.8).

### *Pathologic Features*

Sporadic juvenile polyps are spherical, smooth lesions with an erythematous surface and numerous cysts (Figure 5.9). The gross findings reflect the presence of dilated crypts enmeshed in markedly inflamed, edematous stroma that contains a mixed inflammatory cell infiltrate rich in eosinophils (Figure 5.10). These lesions may also harbor aberrant components in the lamina propria, including ganglion cells and neuromatous elements. Small syndromic juvenile polyps

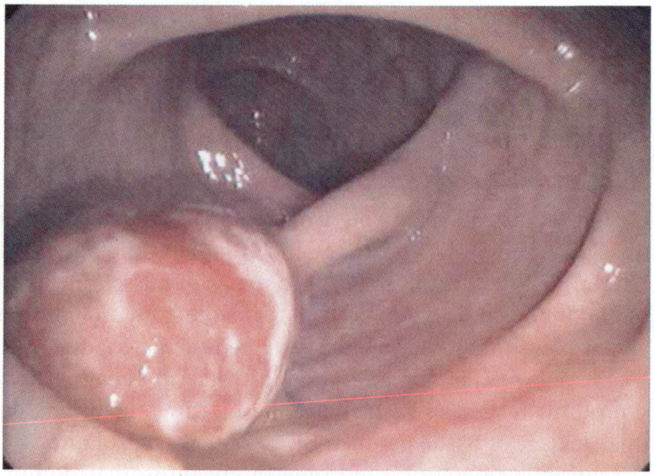

FIGURE 5.7: Polyps that occur in patients with juvenile polyposis syndrome are more common in the colon and are multiple. They may resemble sporadic juvenile polyps and display a smooth, pedunculated surface with ulcer debris on the surface. (Reprinted from Burt RW, Jacoby RF. Polyposis syndromes. In: Yamada T, ed. *Atlas of Gastroenterology*. 4th ed. Oxford, UK: Wiley-Blackwell; 2009:449–464, with permission.)

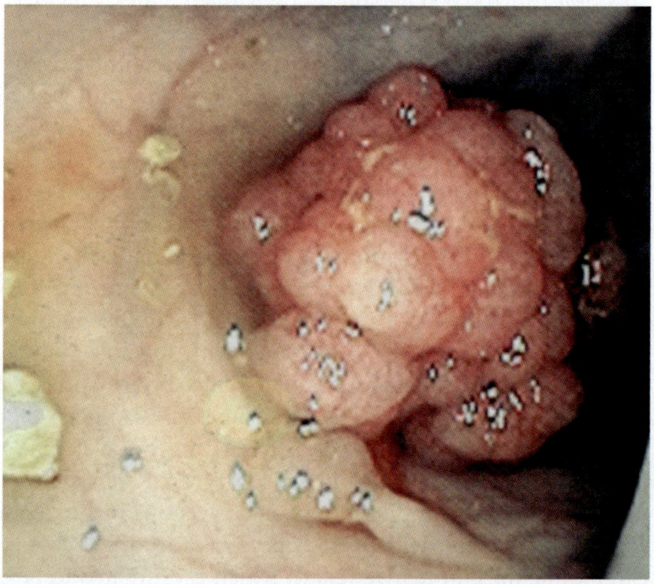

FIGURE 5.8: Large syndromic polyps have a multilobulated "mulberry-like" appearance, particularly when they are large or contain areas of dysplasia. (Photograph courtesy of Dr. Randall Burt, University of Utah School of Medicine, Salt Lake City, UT.)

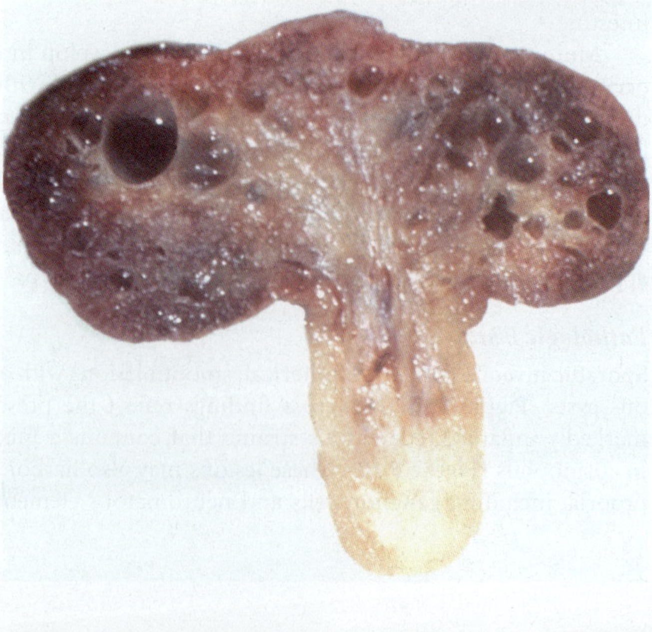

FIGURE 5.9: A sporadic juvenile polyp has a smooth surface and erythematous head, reflecting an abundance of inflamed granulation tissue. Numerous cysts correspond to dilated crypts. (Photograph courtesy of Dr. Harvey Goldman, Beth Israel Deaconess Medical Center, Harvard Medical School, Boston, MA.)

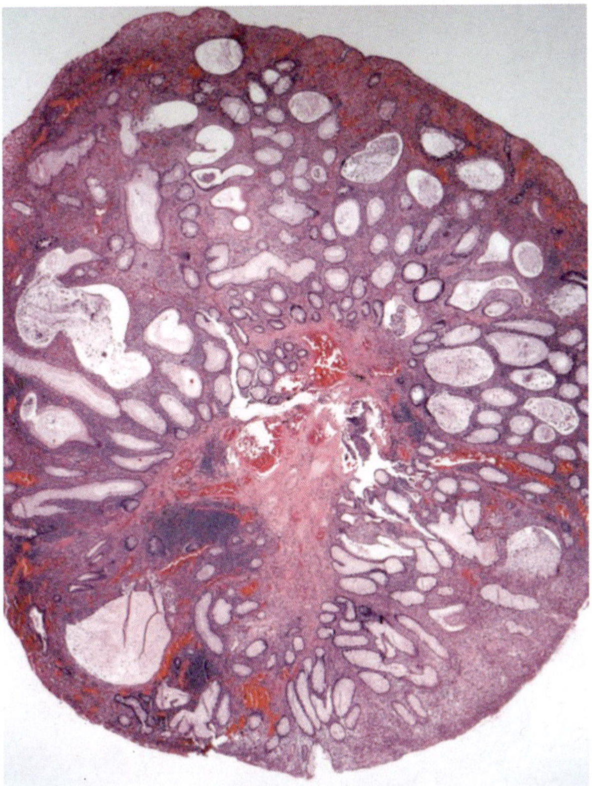

A

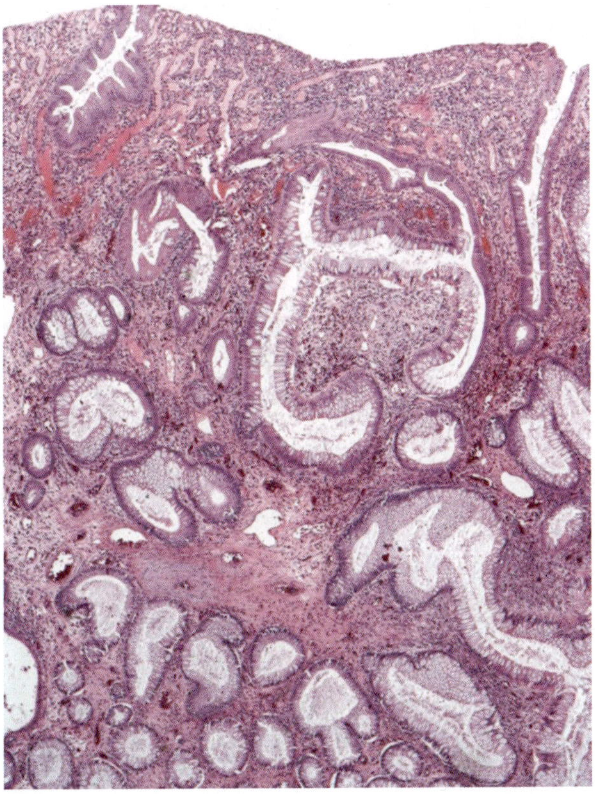

B

FIGURE 5.10: A sporadic juvenile polyp is composed of cystically dilated crypts embedded in inflamed granulation tissue (**A**). The lamina propria contains dilated, thin-walled vessels perpendicularly oriented to the surface, which is eroded (**B**).

**FIGURE 5.10:** *(Continued)* Some of the crypts are entirely denuded and extrude pools of mucin in the lamina propria, but intact crypts are not dysplastic (**C**). Numerous eosinophils and dilated capillaries are present in granulation tissue between crypts (**D**).

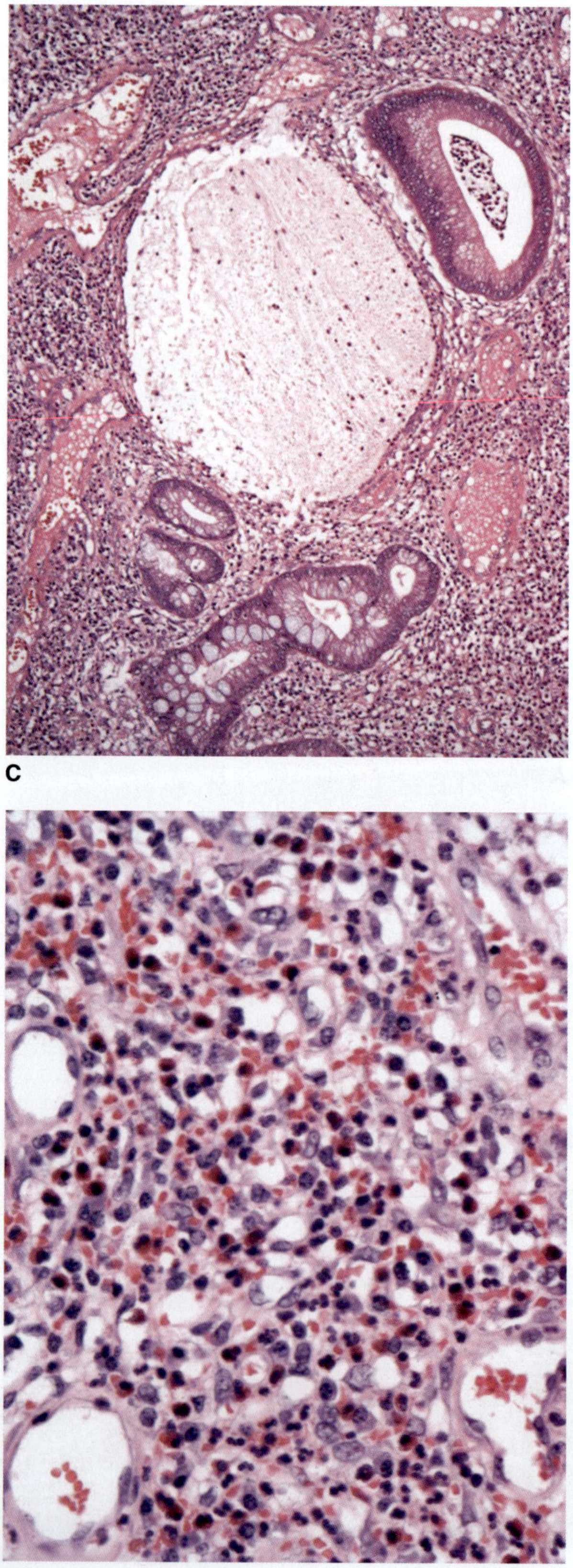

C

D

are morphologically similar to sporadic lesions, although they often display a lesser degree of crypt dilatation and edema of the lamina propria (Figure 5.11). Atypical juvenile polyps contain crowded, irregularly shaped crypts with little intervening stroma (Figure 5.12). Dysplasia may develop in syndromic juvenile polyps or appear as concomitant colorectal adenomas.[22,23]

The differential diagnosis of juvenile polyposis syndrome includes other hamartomatous syndromes and inflammatory conditions. Traumatized juvenile polyps may contain prominent fascicles of smooth muscle cells that simulate the appearance of Peutz-Jeghers polyps, and, conversely, Peutz-Jeghers polyps with prominent inflammatory changes mimic juvenile polyps (Figure 5.13). Inflammatory bowel disease, inflammatory "cap" polyposis, and Cronkhite-Canada syndrome all produce inflammatory-type polyps that are indistinguishable from juvenile polyps in some cases. Juvenile polyposis of the stomach produces thickened mucosal folds in combination with numerous polyps that can be mistaken for multiple hyperplastic polyps or Ménétrier disease, as discussed subsequently. Sampling of the intervening, nonpolypoid mucosa is necessary to distinguish these inflammatory conditions from juvenile polyposis syndrome: inflammatory-type polyps due to these disorders are associated with similar changes in the nonpolypoid mucosa, whereas the intervening mucosa is normal in patients with juvenile polyposis syndrome.

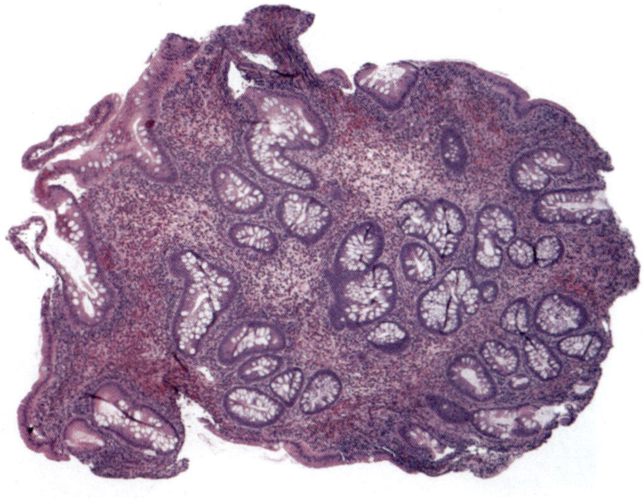

**FIGURE 5.11:** A 28-year-old patient presented with rectal bleeding secondary to juvenile polyposis syndrome. He was found to have approximately 50 colorectal polyps, some of which spanned up to 2 cm in diameter. Most of the polyps resembled inflammatory-type polyps and contained crypts with mild architectural distortion supported by inflamed lamina propria. Cystically dilated crypts were not prominent.

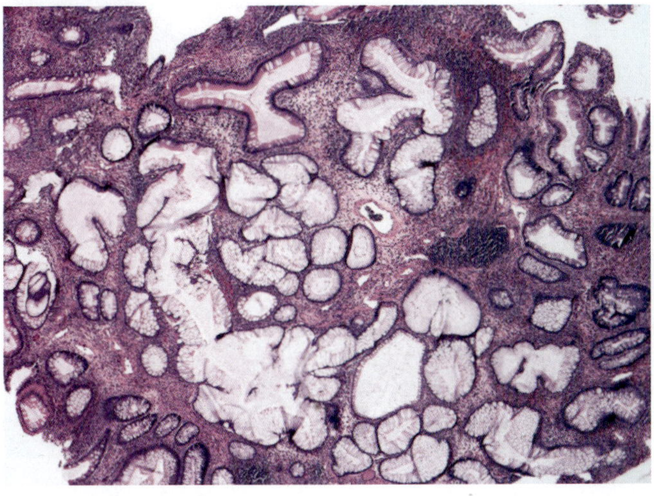

**FIGURE 5.12:** "Atypical juvenile polyps" contain increased numbers of architecturally distorted crypts that show branching and mild dilatation. The lamina propria is mildly inflamed, but does not display the same degree of eosinophilia and edema as is typical of sporadic juvenile polyps.

FIGURE 5.13: A traumatized juvenile polyp of the distal colorectum contains bundles of smooth muscle cells surrounding aggregates of mucosal elements, thereby simulating the appearance of a Peutz-Jeghers polyp (**A**). An ulcerated Peutz-Jeghers polyp contains cystically dilated glands and inflamed stroma that mimic features of a juvenile polyp (**B**).

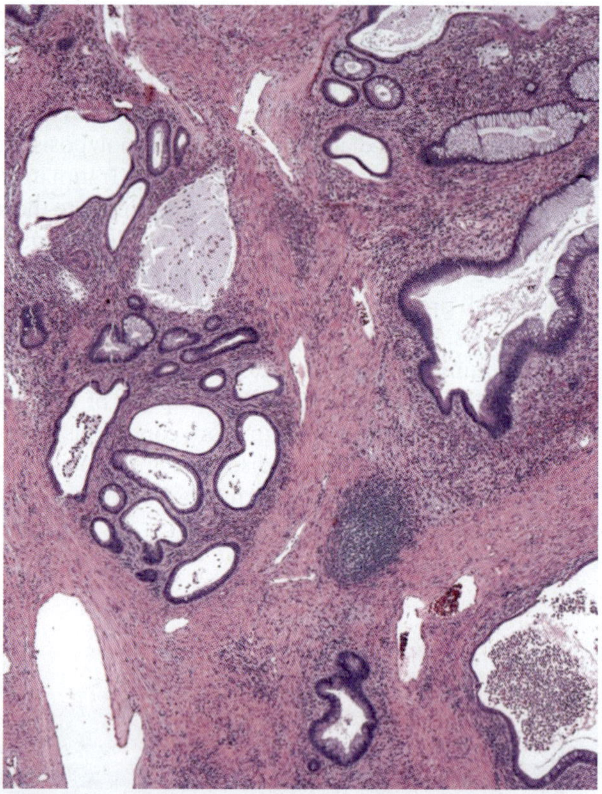

A

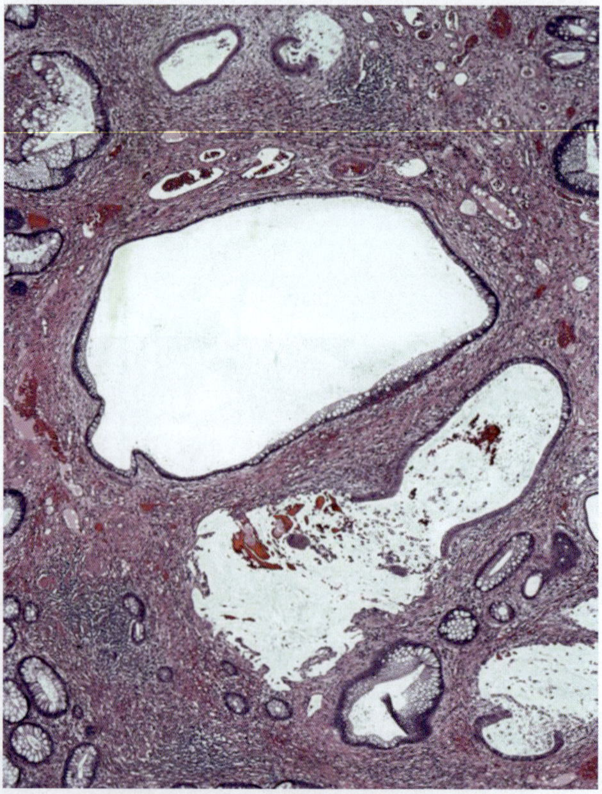

B

### *Molecular Alterations*

The development of juvenile polyposis has been linked to abnormalities in the signal transduction pathway initiated by transforming growth factor-β. Large deletions involving contiguous tumor suppressor genes, namely, *BMBR1A* and *PTEN* (phosphatase and tensin homologue [mutated in multiple advanced cancers 1]), have been described in infantile juvenile polyposis.[24] Alterations in *SMAD4* located on chromosome 18q21.1 occur in 15% to 20% of cases, and another 20% to 25% of cases show abnormalities in *BMBR1A* (bone morphogenetic protein receptor 1A) located on chromosome 10q22.3.[24–26] Specific molecular alterations may also produce phenotypically different patterns of disease: *SMAD4* mutations are associated with polyps and cancers of the upper gastrointestinal tract and hereditary hemorrhagic telangiectasia, whereas *BMPR1A* mutations are more frequent among patients with cardiac defects.

## PTEN Hamartoma Tumor Syndrome

### *Clinical and Endoscopic Features*

PTEN hamartoma tumor syndrome is a recently proposed term that encompasses Cowden syndrome, Bannayan-Ruvalcaba-Riley syndrome, and related disorders that share in common underlying mutations affecting the *PTEN* gene (Table 5.1).[27] Cowden syndrome is an autosomal dominant disorder named after the family in which it was first described and affects approximately 1 in 200,000 persons.[28] It is characterized by the presence of numerous hamartomatous polyps throughout the gastrointestinal tract in combination with oral and cutaneous hamartomatous lesions (e.g., oral papillomas, tricholemmomas, and acral keratoses), carcinomas of the breast and thyroid, autoimmune thyroiditis, macrocephaly, and mental impairment. Lhermitte-Duclos disease is a phenotypic variant characterized by the abovementioned constellation of findings in addition to dysplastic gangliocytoma of the cerebellum. Patients with Bannayan-Ruvalcaba-Riley syndrome have similar manifestations, but also develop a variety of soft tissue tumors, including multiple lipomatosis, hemangiomata, and mixed vascular and fatty tumors involving skin and viscera.[29–31] Patients with Bannayan-Ruvalcaba-Riley syndrome may have down-slanting palpebral fissures, ocular hypertelorism, pseudopapilledema, and prominent corneal nerves. Café au lait spots, acanthosis nigricans, and wart-like lesions of the face have been described, and most affected males have cutaneous pigmented macules on the shaft and glans penis. More than half of patients with Bannayan-Ruvalcaba-Riley syndrome have some degree of hypotonia secondary to a lipid storage myopathic process of the proximal muscles. Skeletal abnormalities, including joint hyperextensibility, scoliosis, and pectus excavatum, are also common. Other disorders that have been linked to *PTEN* abnormalities include autism spectrum disorder with macrocephaly, Proteus syndrome, and VATER with macrocephaly.[32–34]

The International Cowden Consortium enumerated common diagnostic criteria for the PTEN hamartoma tumor syndrome based on review of the literature and anecdotal experience (Table 5.2).[35] Virtually all patients have mucocutaneous lesions by the third decade of life, but only 35% to 40% develop gastrointestinal hamartomatous polyps. Other common manifestations include thyroid abnormalities, fibrocystic breast disease and mammary carcinoma, uterine leiomyomata of early onset, macrocephaly, and mental impairment.[36] Estimated lifetime risk for breast cancer is 25% to 50% among women with Cowden syndrome, compared to approximately 10% among women in the general population, and disease onset is probably a decade earlier among patients with the disorder. The lifetime risk for thyroid cancer may be as high as 10%, and follicular carcinomas are more common than papillary neoplasms.[37–39]

The endoscopic features of PTEN hamartoma tumor syndrome are variable, reflecting the spectrum of polyp types observed in patients with this disorder. Multifocal glycogenic acanthosis of the esophageal mucosa is virtually pathognomonic of PTEN hamartoma tumor syndrome. Hamartomas similar to juvenile polyps develop in the stomach, small intestine, and colon and appear as erythematous nodules or pedunculated polyps. Lesions that contain more abundant mesenchymal elements may be small sessile lesions that vary depending on the types and amounts of connective tissue present in the lesions.

**Table 5.2** Criteria for Diagnosis of Cowden Syndrome and Operational Diagnoses in Affected Patients

| Diagnostic Criteria | Operational Diagnosis in Individual | Operational Diagnosis in Family with an Individual Who Has Cowden Syndrome |
|---|---|---|
| 1. Pathognomonic criteria<br>Mucocutaneous lesions<br>Facial tricholemmomas<br>Acral keratosis<br>Papillomatous papules<br>Mucosal lesions<br>2. Major criteria<br>Breast cancer<br>Thyroid cancer<br>Macrocephaly (>97th percentile)<br>Lhermitte-Duclos disease<br>3. Minor criteria<br>Thyroid adenomas or goiter<br>Mental retardation (IQ <75)<br>Gastrointestinal hamartomas | 1. Mucocutaneous lesions alone, if<br>Six or more facial papules, including three or more tricholemmomas<br>Cutaneous facial papules and oral mucosal papillomatosis<br>Oral mucosal papillomatosis and acral keratosis<br>Six or more palmoplantar keratoses<br>2. Two major criteria, including macrocephaly or Lhermitte-Duclos disease<br>3. One major and three minor criteria<br>4. Four minor criteria | 1. At least one pathognomonic criterion<br>2. Any major criterion<br>3. Two minor criteria |

### *Pathologic Features*

Patients with PTEN hamartoma tumor syndrome develop hamartomatous polyps throughout the gastrointestinal tract, particularly the stomach and colorectum. Gastric lesions often appear as inflammatory-type hyperplastic polyps with cystically dilated glands or regenerative-appearing pits enmeshed in an inflamed lamina propria. Intestinal lesions closely simulate the features of juvenile polyps, in that they contain cystically dilated colonic crypts within an expanded and inflamed lamina propria. However, hamartomatous polyps that develop in combination with PTEN hamartoma tumor syndrome tend to display slightly more numerous myofibroblastic spindle cells within the lamina propria compared to juvenile polyps and commonly contain scattered ganglion cells as well (Figure 5.14). Patients with this disorder may also develop lipomas, ganglioneuromas, lymphoid nodules, and colonic adenomas.

### *Molecular Alterations*

Approximately 85% of patients with Cowden syndrome and 60% of those with Bannayan-Riley-Ruvalcaba syndrome have detectable germline *PTEN* mutations.[34,35,40] This gene encodes a 403 amino acid phosphatase that functions as a tumor suppressor and lipid phosphatase integral to the cell cycle, apoptosis, cell migration, and genomic stability. Phosphatidylinositol-3,4,5-trisphosphate (PIP3) is the primary substrate of PTEN and represents one component of the PI3 kinase pathway, which mediates cell survival *via* AKT/PKB.[41] Patients without germline *PTEN* mutations have been found to harbor mutations affecting dehydrogenase complex subunits B (*SDHB*) or D (*SDHD*) located on 1p35-36 and 11q23, respectively.[42]

## Cronkhite-Canada Syndrome

### *Clinical and Endoscopic Features*

Cronkhite-Canada syndrome is a nonhereditary gastrointestinal polyposis disorder associated with ectodermal changes that was first described in 1955.[43] Unlike previously described

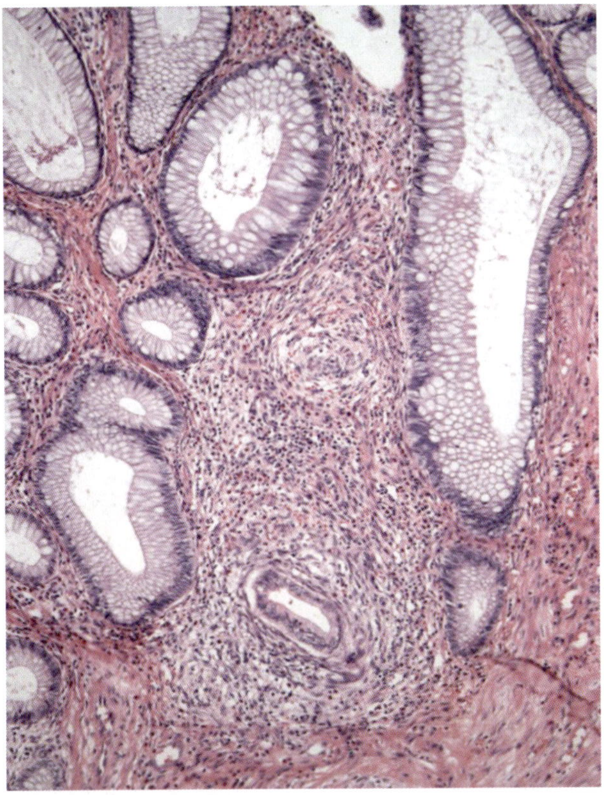

A

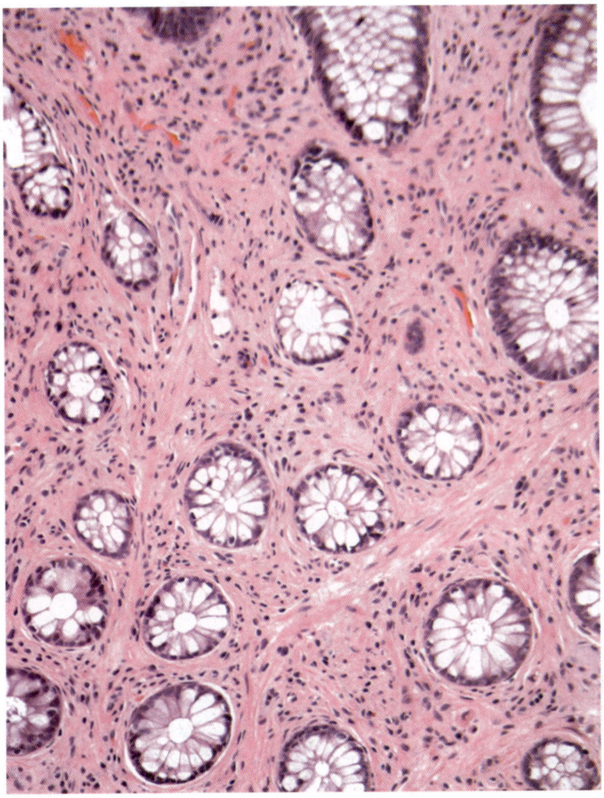

B

FIGURE 5.14: Hamartomatous polyps that develop in association with PTEN hamartoma tumor syndrome contain hyperplastic, or cystically dilated, crypts in cellular stroma (**A**). This hamartomatous polyp contains lamina propria enriched in myofibroblastic spindle cells (**B**).

**FIGURE 5.14:** (*Continued*) Clusters of ganglion cells associated with neuromatous elements are present in a polyp from a patient with PTEN hamartoma tumor syndrome (**C**). Another polyp from the same patient contains mature fat (**D**). (Photograph [*B*] courtesy of Dr. Wade Samowitz, University of Utah School of Medicine, Salt Lake City, UT.)

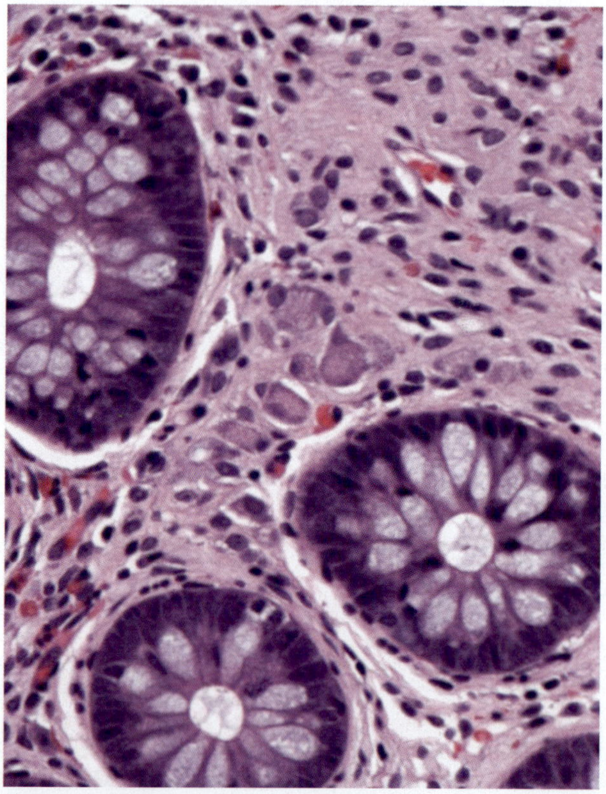

C

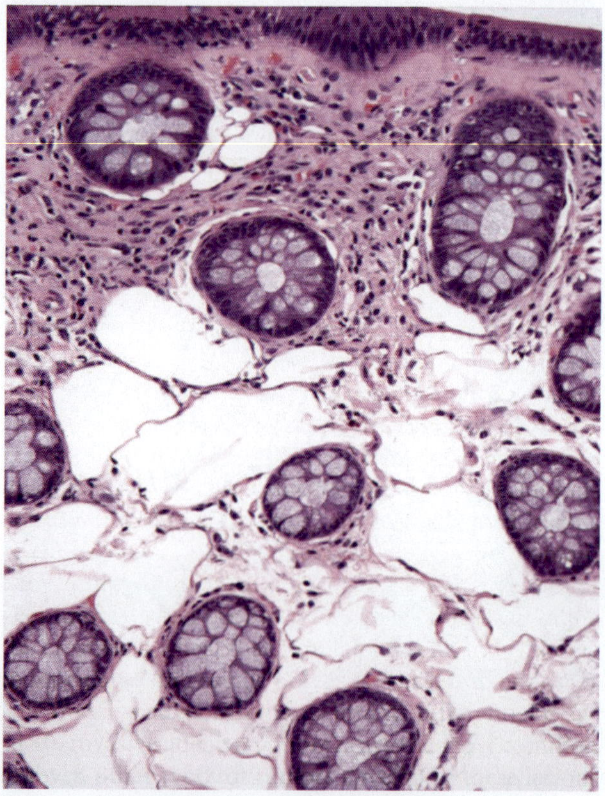

D

hamartomatous polyposes, Cronkhite-Canada syndrome is best considered an inflammatory polyposis disorder in which most of the nongastrointestinal manifestations of disease result from mucosal abnormalities in the gastrointestinal tract. Most patients are older adults who present with symptoms of diarrhea, abdominal discomfort, anorexia, weight loss, protein-losing enteropathy, or edema followed by ectodermal changes such as hyperpigmentation, nail dystrophy, and alopecia.[44] Paresthesias, seizures, and tetany are likely related to fluid and electrolyte imbalances. Other manifestations include vitiligo, glossitis, thrombosis, schizophrenia, eosinophilic gastroenteritis, hypothyroidism, arthritis, and cataracts.[45]

Cronkhite-Canada is historically associated with high mortality rates related to severe malnutrition, bleeding from the gastrointestinal tract, infection, and fluid or electrolyte imbalances. Treatment consists of a combination of supportive care (e.g., rehydration, correction of electrolyte imbalances, and nutritional supplementation) combined with immunosuppressive agents, antibiotics, and antihistamines.[46,47] Although the polyps associated with Cronkhite-Canada syndrome are not dysplastic, patients seem to have an increased risk of adenomas and carcinomas in the stomach and colon. Approximately 15% to 25% of patients have a gastrointestinal malignancy at the time of diagnosis, although these values may, in part, be attributed to an overall increased cancer risk in the older population as well as a reporting bias among patients with a relatively rare disorder.[44,48–53]

The etiology of Cronkhite-Canada syndrome is unknown. It is unassociated with a heritable genetic alteration, but tends to be more common among patients of Asian or European descent. Some investigators suggest that it may represent an immune-mediated disease. A subset of patients have elevated serum IgG4 and/or antinuclear autoantibodies, as well as other immune-mediated disorders, such as systemic lupus erythematosus, thyroiditis, and rheumatoid arthritis.[54,55]

Cronkhite-Canada syndrome affects the stomach, small bowel, and colon in the form of multiple gastrointestinal polyps, but generally spares the esophagus. The polyps are somewhat translucent, reflecting the presence of striking mucosal edema that is invariably present. They vary in size from a few millimeters to a few centimeters in largest diameter and may produce thickened mucosal folds, particularly in the stomach.

### *Pathologic Features*

The polyps of Cronkhite-Canada syndrome display edematous stroma and cystically dilated glands and most show a variable amount of inflammation in the lamina propria (Figure 5.15). Gastric lesions typically display some degree of surface epithelial hyperplasia and are indistinguishable from sporadically occurring hyperplastic/regenerative gastric polyps. Importantly, the intervening, nonpolypoid mucosa also shows edematous, inflamed lamina propria and cystically dilated glands similar to that of the polyps. The tendency for Cronkhite-Canada syndrome to

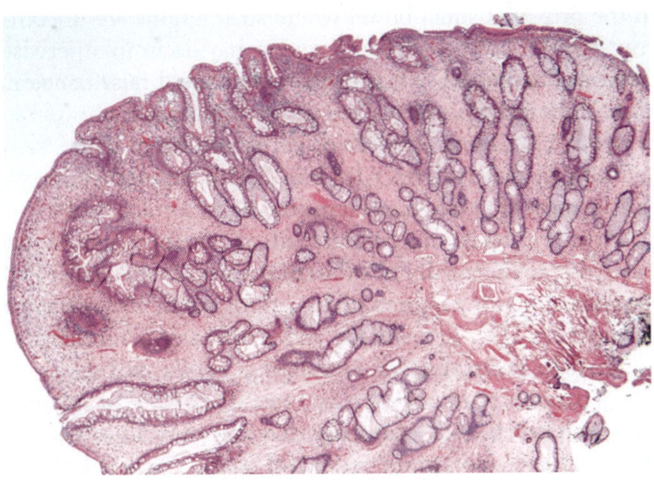

**FIGURE 5.15:** A colonic polyp from a patient with Cronkhite-Canada syndrome consists of tortuous, somewhat dilated crypts enmeshed in inflamed, edematous lamina propria. (Photograph courtesy of Dr. Lisa Yerian, Cleveland Clinic Foundation, Cleveland, OH.)

affect the nonpolypoid mucosa is an important distinguishing feature that aids the pathologic distinction of this entity from other hamartomatous polyposis syndromes.

### Differential Diagnosis of Hamartomatous Polyps

Polyps that show hyperplastic and/or inflammatory changes develop in association with juvenile polyposis, PTEN hamartoma tumor syndrome, and Cronkhite-Canada syndrome.[15,44,56] These polyps show a high degree of morphologic overlap with each other as well as with inflammatory-type polyps that are not associated with polyposis syndromes. For example, isolated gastric hyperplastic polyps can be difficult to distinguish from juvenile polyps, polyps of PTEN hamartoma tumor syndrome, and lesions that develop in association with Cronkhite-Canada syndrome. The diffuse mucosal abnormalities of Ménétrier disease simulate the features of gastric hamartomatous polyposis, particularly juvenile polyposis. Colorectal inflammatory-type polyps that mimic hamartomatous polyps develop in patients with mucosal prolapse, inflammatory cap polyposis, or inflammatory bowel disease and may be detected in asymptomatic patients undergoing routine screening colonoscopy.

Clues to the underlying diagnosis of a polyposis disorder include the absence of intestinal and colonic involvement in patients with sporadic, isolated gastric hyperplastic polyps and Ménétrier disease, as well as the lack of upper gastrointestinal involvement in patients with isolated juvenile polyps. The presence of similar histologic changes in the polypoid and nonpolypoid mucosae of patients with Cronkhite-Canada syndrome is an important clue that distinguishes it from other polyposis disorders and sporadic lesions. Importantly, close clinicopathologic correlation in combination with careful evaluation for the presence of ectodermal manifestations is necessary to aid the distinction between different hamartomatous polyposis syndromes. Evaluation of patients with multiple juvenile or inflammatory-type polyps should include molecular testing for the possibility of any one of these hamartomatous polyposis syndromes.

## SUMMARY AND CONCLUSIONS

Nonadenomatous polyposis syndromes are increasingly classified based on underlying molecular abnormalities. However, not all patients with heritable disorders have detectable genetic alterations, and the clinical manifestations of disease are often variable. Thus, careful pathologic assessment of morphologic features and distribution of disease is vital to the evaluation of patients with multiple nonadenomatous polyps. In general, a single pathologist should review all relevant pathology materials in the event that a polyposis disorder is suspected. If those materials are not available, then clinicians should be alerted to the possibility of a heritable disorder by key diagnoses in the past medical history. Potential red flags include the presence of hyperplastic and inflammatory polyps of the gastrointestinal tract, particularly if they are seen in multiple samples, affect different organs, or develop in the proximal small bowel where such lesions are uncommon. Although isolated ganglioneuromas, lipomas, and perineurinomas may occur in otherwise healthy individuals, the presence of multiple diagnoses in a single patient should raise concern, particularly if they occur in combination with hyperplastic polyps or adenomas.

# References

1. Burkart AL, Sheridan T, Lewin M, et al. Do sporadic Peutz-Jeghers polyps exist? Experience of a large teaching hospital. *Am J Surg Pathol* 2007;31(8):1209–1214.
2. McGarrity TJ, Kulin HE, Zaino RJ. Peutz-Jeghers syndrome. *Am J Gastroenterol* 2000;95(3):596–604.
3. Offerhaus GJ, Billaud M, Gruber SB. Peutz-Jeghers syndrome. In: Bosman FT, Carneiro F, Hruban RH, et al., eds. *WHO Classification of Tumours of the Digestive System*. 4th ed. Lyon, France: International Agency for Research on Cancer; 2009:168–170.

4. Derici H, Peker Y, Tatar F, et al. Multiple malign gastrointestinal polyps and rectal carcinoma in a young patient with Peutz-Jeghers syndrome. *Int J Colorectal Dis* 2007;22(1):85–86.
5. Dong K, Li B. Peutz-Jeghers syndrome: case reports and update on diagnosis and treatment. *Chin J Dig Dis* 2004;5(4):160–164.
6. Perzin KH, Bridge MF. Adenomatous and carcinomatous changes in hamartomatous polyps of the small intestine (Peutz-Jeghers syndrome): report of a case and review of the literature. *Cancer* 1982;49(5):971–983.
7. van Lier MG, Westerman AM, Wagner A, et al. High cancer risk and increased mortality in patients with Peutz-Jeghers syndrome. *Gut* [Multicenter Study] 2011;60(2):141–147.
8. Lam-Himlin D, Park JY, Cornish TC, et al. Morphologic characterization of syndromic gastric polyps. *Am J Surg Pathol* [Comparative Study] 2010;34(11):1656–1662.
9. Petersen VC, Sheehan AL, Bryan RL, et al. Misplacement of dysplastic epithelium in Peutz-Jeghers Polyps: the ultimate diagnostic pitfall? *Am J Surg Pathol* 2000;24(1):34–39.
10. Xie X, Wang Z, Chen Y. Association of LKB1 with a WD-repeat protein WDR6 is implicated in cell growth arrest and p27(Kip1) induction. *Mol Cell Biochem* [Research Support, Non-U.S. Gov't] 2007;301(1–2):115–122.
11. Amos CI, Bali D, Thiel TJ, et al. Fine mapping of a genetic locus for Peutz-Jeghers syndrome on chromosome 19p. *Cancer Res* 1997;57(17):3653–3656.
12. Trojan J, Brieger A, Raedle J, et al. Peutz-Jeghers syndrome: molecular analysis of a three-generation kindred with a novel defect in the serine threonine kinase gene STK11. *Am J Gastroenterol* 1999;94(1): 257–261.
13. Trojan J, Raedle J, Zeuzem S. Mutated serine-threonine kinase gene (STK11) is the cause of Peutz-Jeghers syndrome. *Z Gastroenterol* 1998;36(9):871–873.
14. Schreibman IR, Baker M, Amos C, et al. The hamartomatous polyposis syndromes: a clinical and molecular review. *Am J Gastroenterol* [Review] 2005;100(2):476–490.
15. Chow E, Macrae F. A review of juvenile polyposis syndrome. *J Gastroenterol Hepatol* [Research Support, Non-U.S. Gov't Review] 2005;20(11):1634–1640.
16. Giardiello FM, Hamilton SR, Kern SE, et al. Colorectal neoplasia in juvenile polyposis or juvenile polyps. *Arch Dis Child* 1991;66(8):971–975.
17. Offerhaus GJ, Howe JR. Juvenile polyposis. In: Bosman FT, Carneiro F, Hruban RH, et al., eds. *WHO Classification of Tumours of the Digestive System*. 4th ed. Lyon, France: International Agency for Research on Cancer; 2009:166–167.
18. Gallione CJ, Repetto GM, Legius E, et al. A combined syndrome of juvenile polyposis and hereditary haemorrhagic telangiectasia associated with mutations in MADH4 (SMAD4). *Lancet* [Research Support, Non-U.S. Gov't Research Support, U.S. Gov't, P.H.S.] 2004;363(9412):852–859.
19. Baert AL, Casteels-Van Daele M, Broeckx J, et al. Generalized juvenile polyposis with pulmonary arteriovenous malformations and hypertrophic osteoarthropathy. *AJR Am J Roentgenol* [Case Reports] 1983;141(4):661–662.
20. Murday V, Slack J. Inherited disorders associated with colorectal cancer. *Cancer Surv* 1989;8(1):139-57.
21. Gupta SK, Fitzgerald JF, Croffie JM, et al. Experience with juvenile polyps in North American children: the need for pancolonoscopy. *Am J Gastroenterol* 2001;96(6):1695–1697.
22. Heiss KF, Schaffner D, Ricketts RR, et al. Malignant risk in juvenile polyposis coli: increasing documentation in the pediatric age group. *J Pediatr Surg* 1993;28(9):1188–1193.
23. Jarvinen H, Franssila KO. Familial juvenile polyposis coli: increased risk of colorectal cancer. *Gut* 1984;25(7):792–800.
24. Delnatte C, Sanlaville D, Mougenot JF, et al. Contiguous gene deletion within chromosome arm 10q is associated with juvenile polyposis of infancy, reflecting cooperation between the BMPR1A and PTEN tumor-suppressor genes. *Med Sci (Paris)* 2006;22(11):912–913.
25. Howe JR, Sayed MG, Ahmed AF, et al. The prevalence of MADH4 and BMPR1A mutations in juvenile polyposis and absence of BMPR2, BMPR1B, and ACVR1 mutations. *J Med Genet* [Multicenter Study Research Support, Non-U.S. Gov't] 2004;41(7):484–491.
26. Zhou XP, Woodford-Richens K, Lehtonen R, et al. Germline mutations in BMPR1A/ALK3 cause a subset of cases of juvenile polyposis syndrome and of Cowden and Bannayan-Riley-Ruvalcaba syndromes. *Am J Hum Genet* [Research Support, Non-U.S. Gov't Research Support, U.S. Gov't, Non-P.H.S. Research Support, U.S. Gov't, P.H.S.] 2001;69(4):704–711.
27. DiLiberti JH. Inherited macrocephaly-hamartoma syndromes. *Am J Med Genet* [Review] 1998;79(4): 284–290.

28. Nelen MR, Kremer H, Konings IB, et al. Novel PTEN mutations in patients with Cowden disease: absence of clear genotype-phenotype correlations. *Eur J Hum Genet* [Research Support, Non-U.S. Gov't] 1999;7(3):267–273.
29. Bannayan GA. Lipomatosis, angiomatosis, and macrencephalia. A previously undescribed congenital syndrome. *Arch Pathol* 1971;92(1):1–5.
30. Gorlin RJ, Cohen MM Jr, Condon LM, et al. Bannayan-Riley-Ruvalcaba syndrome. *Am J Med Genet* [Case Reports] 1992;44(3):307–314.
31. Ruvalcaba RH, Myhre S, Smith DW. Sotos syndrome with intestinal polyposis and pigmentary changes of the genitalia. *Clin Genet* [Case Reports] 1980;18(6):413–416.
32. Butler MG, Dasouki MJ, Zhou XP, et al. Subset of individuals with autism spectrum disorders and extreme macrocephaly associated with germline PTEN tumour suppressor gene mutations. *J Med Genet* [Case Reports Research Support, Non-U.S. Gov't] 2005;42(4):318–321.
33. Reardon W, Zhou XP, Eng C. A novel germline mutation of the PTEN gene in a patient with macrocephaly, ventricular dilatation, and features of VATER association. *J Med Genet* [Case Reports] 2001;38(12):820–823.
34. Zhou XP, Marsh DJ, Morrison CD, et al. Germline inactivation of PTEN and dysregulation of the phosphoinositol-3-kinase/Akt pathway cause human Lhermitte-Duclos disease in adults. *Am J Hum Genet* [Research Support, Non-U.S. Gov't Research Support, U.S. Gov't, P.H.S.] 2003;73(5):1191–1198.
35. Nelen MR, Padberg GW, Peeters EA, et al. Localization of the gene for Cowden disease to chromosome 10q22-23. *Nat Genet* 1996;13(1):114–116.
36. Zbuk KM, Eng C. Cancer phenomics: RET and PTEN as illustrative models. *Nat Rev Cancer* [Research Support, N.I.H., Extramural Research Support, Non-U.S. Gov't Review] 2007;7(1):35–45.
37. Starink TM, van der Veen JP, Arwert F, et al. The Cowden syndrome: a clinical and genetic study in 21 patients. *Clin Genet* 1986;29(3):222–233.
38. Pilarski R, Eng C. Will the real Cowden syndrome please stand up (again)? Expanding mutational and clinical spectra of the PTEN hamartoma tumour syndrome. *J Med Genet* [Review] 2004;41(5):323–326.
39. Wirtzfeld DA, Petrelli NJ, Rodriguez-Bigas MA. Hamartomatous polyposis syndromes: molecular genetics, neoplastic risk, and surveillance recommendations. *Ann Surg Oncol* [Review] 2001;8(4):319–327.
40. Perriard J, Saurat JH, Harms M. An overlap of Cowden's disease and Bannayan-Riley-Ruvalcaba syndrome in the same family. *J Am Acad Dermatol* [Case Reports Research Support, Non-U.S. Gov't Review] 2000;42(2 Pt 2):348–350.
41. Minaguchi T, Waite KA, Eng C. Nuclear localization of PTEN is regulated by Ca(2+) through a tyrosil phosphorylation-independent conformational modification in major vault protein. *Cancer Res* [Research Support, Non-U.S. Gov't] 2006;66(24):11677–11682.
42. Bayley JP. Succinate dehydrogenase gene variants and their role in Cowden syndrome. *Am J Hum Genet* [Comment Letter] 2011;88(5):674–675; author reply 6.
43. Cronkhite LW Jr, Canada WJ. Generalized gastrointestinal polyposis; an unusual syndrome of polyposis, pigmentation, alopecia and onychotrophia. *N Engl J Med* 1955;252(24):1011–1015.
44. Daniel ES, Ludwig SL, Lewin KJ, et al. The Cronkhite-Canada syndrome. An analysis of clinical and pathologic features and therapy in 55 patients. *Medicine (Baltimore)* 198261(5):293–309.
45. Blonski WC, Furth EE, Kinosian BP, Compher C, Metz DC. A case of Cronkhite-Canada syndrome with taste disturbance as a leading complaint. *Digestion* 2005;71(4):201–205.
46. Ward E, Wolfsen HC, Ng C. Medical management of Cronkhite-Canada syndrome. *South Med J* 2002;95(2):272–274.
47. Ward EM, Wolfsen HC. Pharmacological management of Cronkhite-Canada syndrome. *Expert Opin Pharmacother* 2003;4(3):385–389.
48. Nagata J, Kijima H, Hasumi K, et al. Adenocarcinoma and multiple adenomas of the large intestine, associated with Cronkhite-Canada syndrome. *Dig Liver Dis* 2003;35(6):434–438.
49. Watanabe T, Kudo M, Shirane H, et al. Cronkhite-Canada syndrome associated with triple gastric cancers: a case report. *Gastrointest Endosc* 1999;50(5):688–691.
50. Kaneko Y, Kato H, Tachimori Y, et al. Triple carcinomas in Cronkhite-Canada syndrome. *Jpn J Clin Oncol* 1991;21(3):194–202.
51. Egawa T, Kubota T, Otani Y, et al. Surgically treated Cronkhite-Canada syndrome associated with gastric cancer. *Gastric Cancer* 2000;3(3):156–160.
52. Yashiro M, Kobayashi H, Kubo N, et al. Cronkhite-Canada syndrome containing colon cancer and serrated adenoma lesions. *Digestion* 2004;69(1):57–62.

53. Malhotra R, Sheffield A. Cronkhite-Canada syndrome associated with colon carcinoma and adenomatous changes in C-C polyps. *Am J Gastroenterol* 1988;83(7):772–776.
54. Kao KT, Patel JK, Pampati V. Cronkhite-Canada syndrome: a case report and review of literature. *Gastroenterol Res Pract* 2009;2009:619378.
55. Takeuchi Y, Yoshikawa M, Tsukamoto N, et al. Cronkhite-Canada syndrome with colon cancer, portal thrombosis, high titer of antinuclear antibodies, and membranous glomerulonephritis. *J Gastroenterol* [Case Reports] 2003;38(8):791–795.
56. Burke AP, Sobin LH. The pathology of Cronkhite-Canada polyps. A comparison to juvenile polyposis. *Am J Surg Pathol* 1989;13(11):940–946.

SECTION

# III

# Pathologic Features of Colorectal Carcinoma

# Handling of Colorectal Cancer Resection Specimens

# 6

Rhonda K. Yantiss

Virtually all carcinomas of the colorectum develop from preexisting neoplasms, namely, adenomas, serrated polyps, and inflammatory bowel disease–related dysplasia. Improved endoscopic techniques and widely available colorectal cancer screening and surveillance programs enable clinicians to remove large, potentially malignant lesions with minimally invasive approaches. As a result, pathologists increasingly encounter invasive carcinomas in endoscopically obtained samples as well as colectomy specimens. Pathologists must perform several functions when assessing cancer specimens, namely, tumor staging, assessment of resection adequacy, and documentation of background disease, if present. Understanding the anatomy and features of colorectal cancer in resection specimens is necessary to accurately document extent of disease and judiciously submit an appropriate number of tissue blocks. The purpose of this chapter is to discuss the gross handling of colorectal cancer specimens.

## ENDOSCOPICALLY OBTAINED POLYPECTOMY SPECIMENS

Colorectal polyps are classified as epithelial, mesenchymal, and mixed polyps based on their primary components. The nature of a polyp may be suspected at the time of gross examination. Epithelial polyps, such as adenomas, are mostly composed of a proliferation of epithelial cells and, thus, display expansion of the mucosa that is readily apparent on cross section (Figure 6.1). Most polyps composed of mesenchymal elements are derived from the muscularis mucosae or submucosa and appear as sessile nodules with a rounded, smooth surface (Figure 6.2). Mixed polyps, including mucosal prolapse polyps and hamartomas, may contain splayed bundles of smooth muscle cells emanating from the hyperplastic muscularis mucosae, which produce a thick, dense stalk (Figure 6.3).

Colorectal adenomas are classified as pedunculated or sessile based on their endoscopic appearance. Pedunculated adenomas contain a stalk comprising normal mucosa and submucosa, presumably resulting from chronic trauma as the polyp is pulled in the direction of the fecal stream (Figure 6.4). Sessile polyps rest on the colonic mucosa without an apparent stalk (Figure 6.5). Pedunculated polyps typically display a tubular morphology, whereas sessile polyps are tubular, villous, or tubulovillous. Colorectal adenomas are entirely benign and cured by complete excision. Less than 5% harbor malignant foci, although approximately 20% of adenomas spanning more than 2 cm contain invasive adenocarcinoma. Other risk factors for cancer development in adenomas include the presence of high-grade dysplasia and/or a villous component that accounts for at least 25% of the polyp volume.[1,2] Early invasive adenocarcinomas limited to the submucosa may be amenable to endoscopic excision, particularly if associated with a pedunculated adenoma, as discussed in Chapter 8.[3]

### Gross Processing of Polypectomy Specimens

Pedunculated and sessile colorectal adenomas are amenable to snare polypectomy and endoscopic removal. Pedunculated polypectomy specimens often contain an identifiable base or stalk, the latter of which may appear slightly retracted. If the polyp base is identified, then a small amount of ink should be placed at the resection margin. Sessile polyps can be removed by injecting the polyp base with a combination of norepinephrine and saline to lift the lesion off the submucosa, although larger lesions may require piecemeal resection. Injection of a flat polyp creates a fluid-filled wheal at the base that simulates the appearance of a stalk in histologic sections. Thus, the gross appearance of a polyp is best determined at the time of endoscopic evaluation. Large sessile polyps of the distal rectum may also be excised with an attached disc of mucosa and submucosa. The underside and lateral aspects of these mucosal resection specimens represent surgical margins, which are commonly inked, pinned out (deep margin side down), and fixed for a few hours prior to sectioning. Intact and fragmented polyps are sectioned at 2 mm intervals and submitted entirely for histologic evaluation (Figure 6.6).

## Gross Evaluation of Colectomy Specimens

Systematic pathologic evaluation of colorectal cancer resection specimens plays a vital role in determining the patient's prognosis and facilitating decisions regarding use of adjuvant therapy. Awareness of the clinical history and nature of the surgical procedure ensures appropriate handling of the case. It is important to accurately document all components of a resection specimen, note the anatomic location of the tumor and its relationship to relevant surgical margins, and describe the presence, if any, of underlying conditions. Specific details about the tumor, including configuration (i.e., ulcerated, polypoid, fungating) and size, should be noted and documented with photography, if available. Although there are no universally

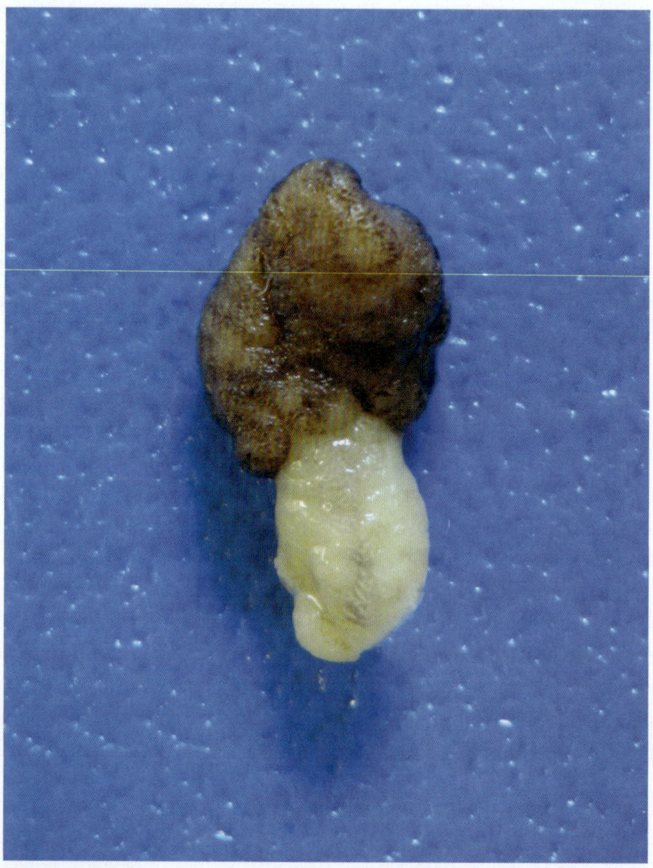

A

**FIGURE 6.1:** A large adenoma has a lobulated, slightly granular surface, reflecting expansion of its mucosa by neoplastic epithelium (**A**).

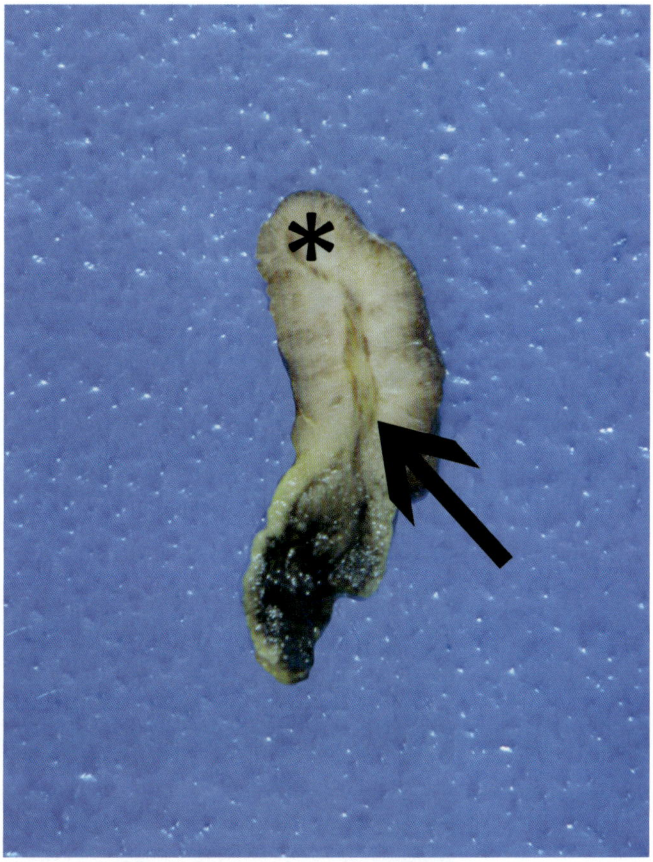

B

FIGURE 6.1: (*Continued*) A cross section through the adenoma demonstrates a thickened mucosa (*asterisk*), which is demarcated from the underlying submucosa (*arrow*). The base of the polyp is inked (**B**).

accepted guidelines regarding the appropriate number of sections obtained from colorectal cancer resection specimens, we advocate submission of at least four sections of the tumor, including a minimum of two sections documenting deepest invasion and one of the adjacent mucosa, all regional lymph nodes, margins as appropriate, any other findings (e.g., polyps, tattoo, inflammation), and sampling of other organs composing the specimen, such as the ileum or appendix.

Pathologists evaluate colorectal tumors in order to assign tumor stage, assess resection adequacy, and document background disease, if present. Colorectal surgery is the mainstay of therapy for most types of neoplasia, in which case the resection specimen usually contains an adenoma, carcinoma, or other tumor type. Surgery can also follow endoscopic manipulation or neoadjuvant therapy, both of which alter the appearance of the lesion. Early invasive adenocarcinomas in large polyps may produce ulcers or surface irregularities that prompt gastroenterologists to tattoo the mucosa with India ink (Figure 6.7). In other situations, the diagnosis of invasive adenocarcinoma is only made following polypectomy, so subsequent resections are performed for lymph node staging and contain only a polypectomy site with, or without, an associated tattoo. Finally, locally advanced rectal adenocarcinomas and anal squamous cell carcinomas are routinely treated with neoadjuvant therapy that induces variable tumor regression prior to surgery. Treated cancers form ulcers in the distal rectum with scarring of the wall and pericolic fat that should be extensively sampled to document residual disease, as described in Chapters 8 and 9 (Figure 6.8).

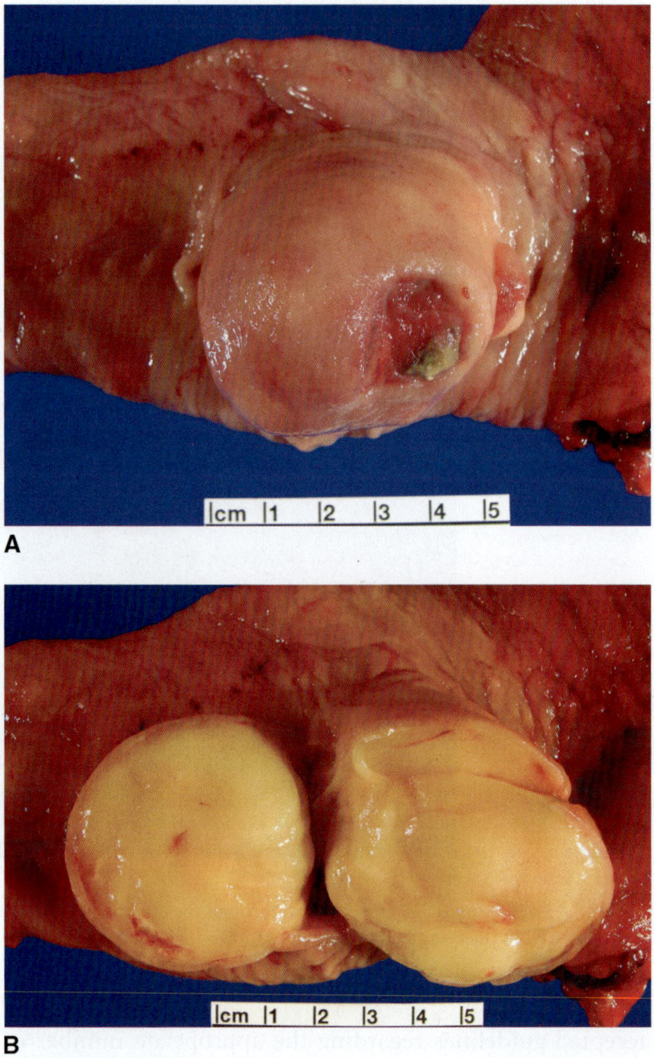


**FIGURE 6.2:** A submucosal lipoma has a smooth round appearance except in the area of an ulcer (**A**). This polyp displays a fatty *yellow* cut surface (**B**).

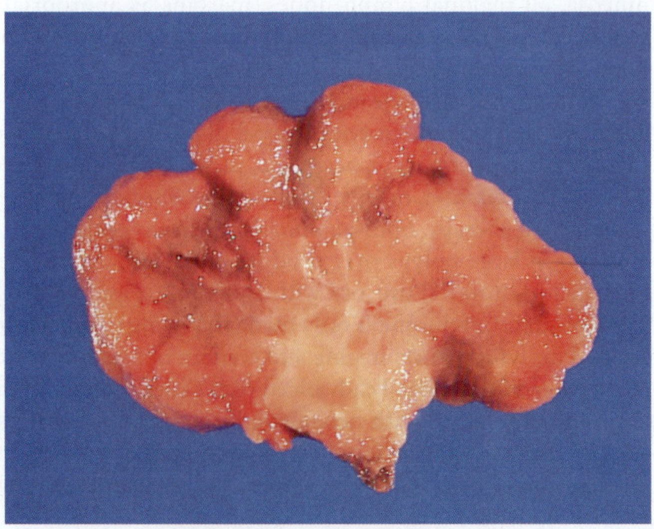

**FIGURE 6.3:** A Peutz-Jeghers polyp has a lobulated appearance owing to aggregates of mucosal elements at the surface. The stalk is pale and firm, reflecting the presence of smooth muscle fibers emanating from the muscularis mucosae at the polyp base.

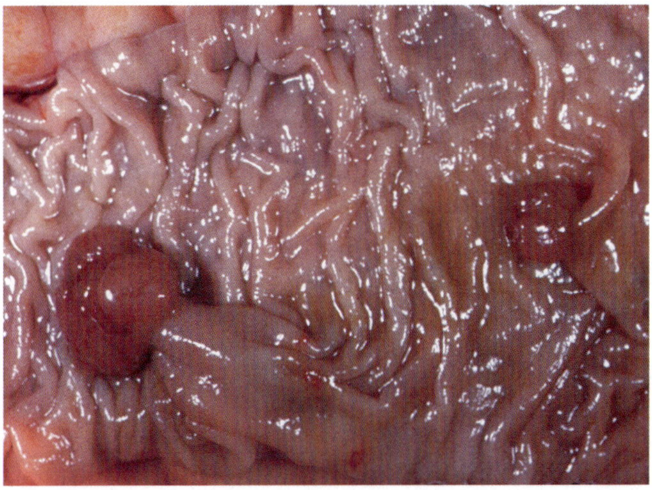

FIGURE 6.4: A pedunculated polyp in the sigmoid colon is erythematous and lobulated. The stalk comprises normal mucosa that is similar to the background mucosa. A second, smaller polyp is also present on a short stalk (**right**).

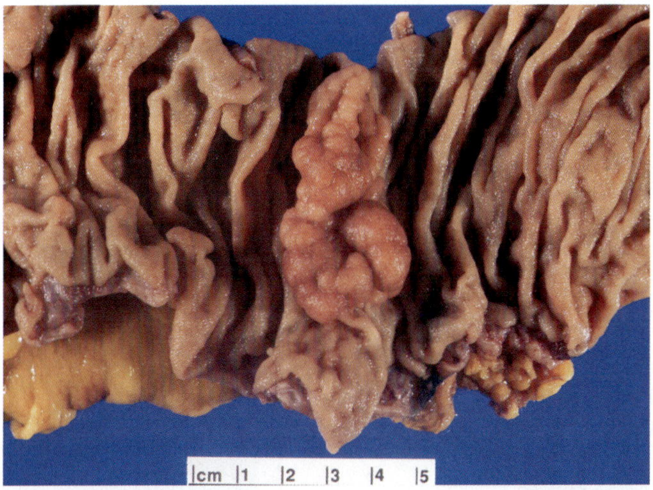


FIGURE 6.5: A sessile adenoma of the ascending colon forms a flat, irregular plaque on the mucosal surface.

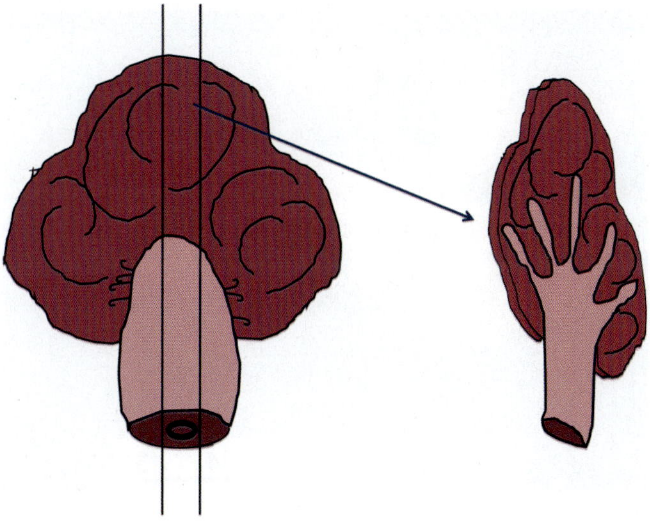

FIGURE 6.6: Colorectal polyps are always sectioned perpendicularly to the polyp base such that the relationship between the mucosa and submucosa is maintained. Most pedunculated polyps are bisected or trisected in the long axis of the polyp.

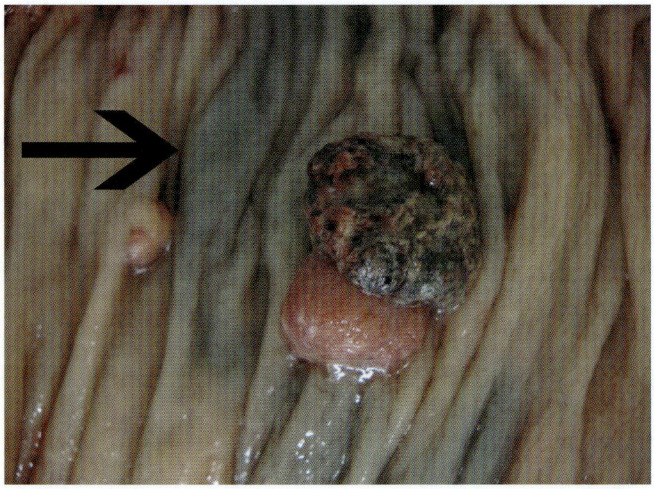

**FIGURE 6.7:** This polyp was identified during surveillance colonoscopy. Its large size and surface irregularity prompted the gastroenterologist to tattoo the site at the time of biopsy, thereby imparting *blue* discoloration to the background mucosa (*arrow*). A second, smaller polyp is present below the *arrow*.

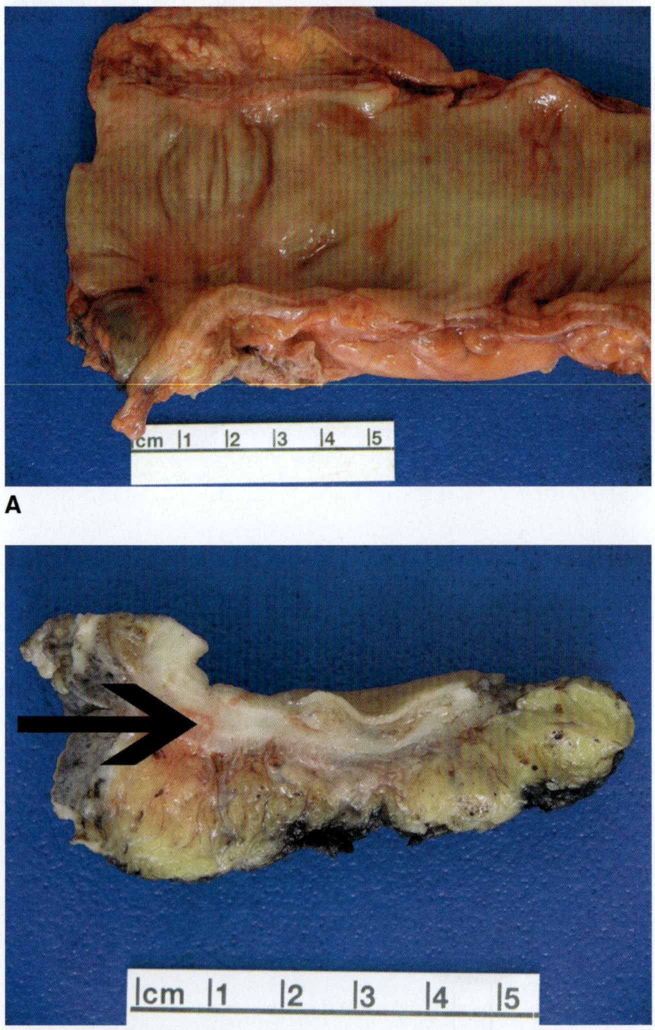


**FIGURE 6.8:** Neoadjuvant chemotherapy and radiation induced near complete regression of a rectal cancer. This tumor was a circumferential fungating mass at the time of diagnosis but now shows a substantial response to treatment. An ulcer is present near the distal margin (**A**). A cross section through the ulcerated area reveals residual carcinoma in the submucosa and superficial muscularis propria (*arrow*). Fibrosis in perirectal fat reflects tumor regression (**B**).

## Inking and Evaluating Resection Margins

A number of problems arise when assessing surgical resection margins on colectomy specimens, although most issues are resolved following close examination of the specimen, review of the radiology report, and direct conversation with the surgeon. Common problems include inadvertent inclusion of the serosa as a resection margin and failure to recognize the radial resection margin. All colorectal resection specimens have at least three margins: the proximal and distal visceral margins of the tubular gut and one, or more, soft tissue (radial) margins. The ileum always comprises the proximal margin of right colonic resection specimens. Tubular gut resection margins of abdominal colon cancers are usually distant from the tumor. Those that are greater than 3 cm from the advancing tumor edge are sufficiently evaluated by gross examination alone since primary colorectal carcinomas do not show extensive lateral or submucosal tumor spread in most cases.[4] Colonic resection margins located 1 to 3 cm from the tumor edge may be taken *en face*, but margins less than 1 cm from the tumor should be inked and sampled with perpendicular sections.

The radial margin is a soft tissue resection margin, and its nature varies depending on the anatomic location of the tumor and the type of surgical specimen obtained (Table 6.1). For example, the sigmoid colon lies within the peritoneal cavity and is supported by a mesentery transection of which represents the radial margin. The remaining pericolic fat on the sigmoid colon is surfaced by mesothelial cells (e.g., serosa) and does not constitute a surgical resection margin. Thus, a tumor that invades through the sigmoid colon wall and extends to the surface of peritonealized fat is assigned a pT4a pathologic stage with a negative margin, whereas a tumor extending to the mesenteric margin (usually designated with sutures at the vascular pedicle) is assigned a pT3 pathologic stage with a positive margin. Other parts of the colon that lie partially within the peritoneal cavity (i.e., ascending and descending colon) are surfaced anteriorly by peritoneum but lie on the posterior abdominal wall, which represents a margin. Tumors that occur in these areas have both mesenteric and posterior radial margins, although the latter are rarely of clinical significance. The serosa of the colon is not a surgical margin, although some pathologists may advocate inking it in order to document serosal penetration (pT4a) in some cases. Should one adopt this practice, a different color is used to denote the serosa in order to avoid potential confusion with the radial margin.

**Table 6.1** Radial Margins on Colorectal Resection Specimens

| Source of Specimen | Extent of Peritoneum | Radial Margin |
|---|---|---|
| Cecum | Entirely covered | Mesentery |
| Right colon | Covered anterolaterally | Mesentery<br>Posterior aspect of right colon |
| Transverse colon | Intraperitoneal with mesentery | Mesentery |
| Descending colon | Covered anterolaterally | Mesentery<br>Posterior aspect of left colon |
| Sigmoid colon | Intraperitoneal with mesentery | Mesentery |
| Rectosigmoid colon | Intraperitoneal proximally<br>Covered anterolaterally in upper rectum | Sigmoid colon mesentery<br>Mesorectum, posterior |
| Rectum | Covered anterolaterally in upper rectum<br>Covered anteriorly in middle rectum<br>No peritoneum in distal rectum | Mesorectum, posterior<br>Mesorectum, posterolateral<br>Mesorectum, circumferential |

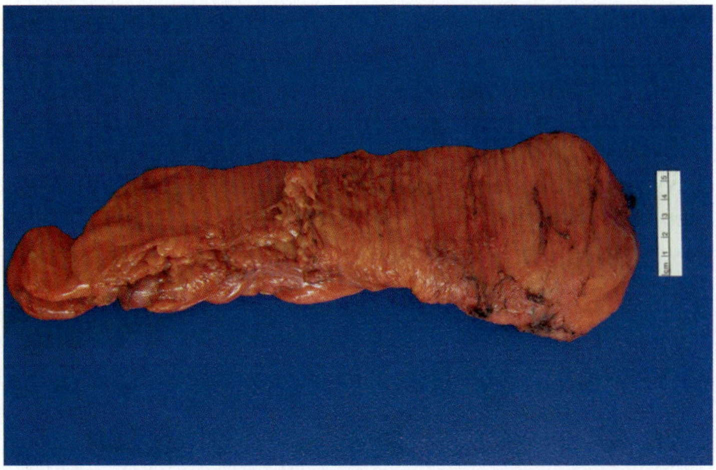

FIGURE 6.9: A total mesorectal excision specimen comprises the rectum and all regional lymph nodes within perirectal fat. The posterior aspect of the specimen is entirely ensheathed by the mesorectal envelope, which imparts a glistening appearance to the surface of the specimen. The mesorectum is contiguous with the mesentery of the sigmoid colon (**left**). The perirectal soft tissue is bulky and of largest diameter at the distal end of the resection specimen (**right**). This specimen would be considered to represent a complete mesorectal excision.

The rectum lies below the peritoneal reflection, which extends more distally on the anterior rectal surface. Adipose tissue on the posterior aspect of the upper and middle rectum and that surrounding the lower rectum is contained within fibroconnective areolar tissue, termed the mesorectum.[5] The rectal radial margin reflects sharp dissection from the soft tissues and adjacent structures within the pelvis. This margin comprises the posterior surface superiorly, the posterolateral surface in the middle, and the entire circumference distally on resection specimens that contain the entire rectum. The radial resection margin is the most important margin on rectal cancer resection specimens, and its status is a powerful predictor of local recurrence.[6] Rectal carcinomas are removed *via* total mesorectal excision, which is performed by dissecting along the areolar plane outside the mesorectal fascia and entirely removing the rectum, mesorectum, and all regional lymph nodes (Figure 6.9).[7] This surgical technique decreases the risk of local recurrence and improves overall survival, so comments regarding adequacy of mesorectal excision are incorporated into the surgical pathology report.[6,8,9] Criteria used in determining the adequacy of resection include smoothness of mesorectal surface, presence or absence of defects in the mesorectal envelope, and bulk of mesorectal connective tissue, particularly near the distal margin (Table 6.2).[10] Disruptions in the mesorectal envelope may be superficial or small, in which case they impart slight irregularity to the mesorectal surface (Figure 6.10). More substantial disruptions appear as large ragged defects that extend into the muscularis propria (Figure 6.11).

## Assessing Depth of Tumor Invasion

Understanding of colorectal anatomy and careful examination of resection specimens are vitally important during gross handling of colorectal cancer specimens. Skilled assessment of depth of invasion at gross examination accurately predicts pathologic tumor stage. Tubular adenomas have a smooth, erythematous surface, whereas villous adenomas tend to be sessile lesions with soft, frond-like projections. Adenomas are composed of neoplastic epithelium limited to the mucosa and, thus, are clearly demarcated from the underlying submucosa on cross section (Figure 6.12). Invasive adenocarcinomas induce mucosal irregularities and/or ulcers when associated with preexisting adenomas (Figure 6.13). More deeply invasive cancers obliterate normal tissue planes as they infiltrate the bowel wall and can be best appreciated on cross section (Figure 6.14). Serosal involvement induces grossly apparent alterations at the peritoneal surface, including a scar-like

**Table 6.2 Assessment for Resection Adequacy for Rectal Cancer Specimens**

| Status of Mesorectum | Gross Features |
|---|---|
| Incomplete | Little bulk to mesorectal tissue<br>Coning of connective tissue at distal margin<br>Large defects in mesorectal fat<br>Defects extending into muscularis propria<br>Sectioning reveals irregular circumferential margin |
| Nearly complete | Slightly irregular mesorectal fascia<br>Moderate bulk with occasional defects greater than 5 mm, no defects that extend to muscularis propria<br>No areas of muscularis propria visibility |
| Complete | Intact, bulky mesorectum with smooth surface<br>Minor irregularities in mesorectal surface (<5 mm)<br>No coning at distal margin |

pucker or nodular irregularity on the peritoneal surface, as well as rough, shaggy adhesions on the colon or in pericolic fat (Figure 6.15). Detecting serosal penetration is facilitated by cytology preparations obtained from the outer aspect of the colon subjacent to the tumor, as described in Chapter 8.

## Documentation of Background Disease

Some colorectal carcinomas arise in association with adenomas, serrated polyps, or chronic inflammatory disorders. The extent to which pathologists document background disease in these situations is somewhat discretionary since further sampling will, at best, identify an occult tumor that is unlikely to substantially impact management decisions. Documentation of background disease is important for other reasons. For example, a minimum number of adenomas must be reported to qualify patients for germline testing when a polyposis disorder is clinically suspected. Documentation of background disease is also useful when subclassifying types of inflammatory bowel disease and has clinical implications with respect to surveillance practices among patients with ulcerative colitis and Crohn disease.

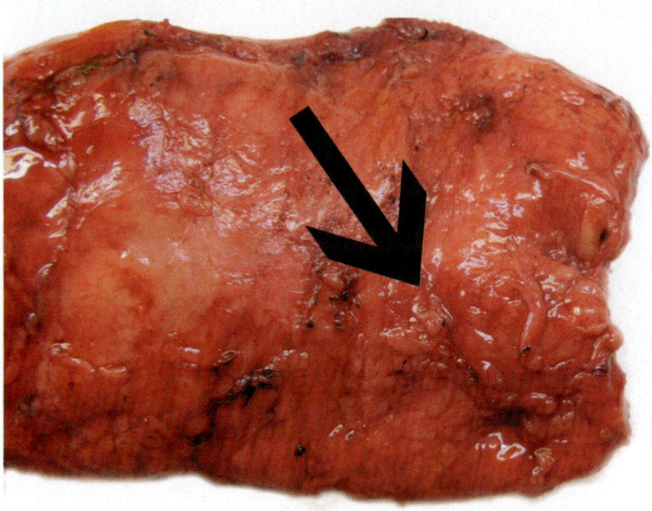

**FIGURE 6.10:** Superficial disruptions of the mesorectal envelope impart a slight irregularity to the resection margin (*arrow*). This specimen is classified as a nearly complete mesorectal excision. (Photograph courtesy of Dr. Nicholas West, Leeds Institute of Molecular Medicine, St. James's University Hospital, Leeds, UK.)

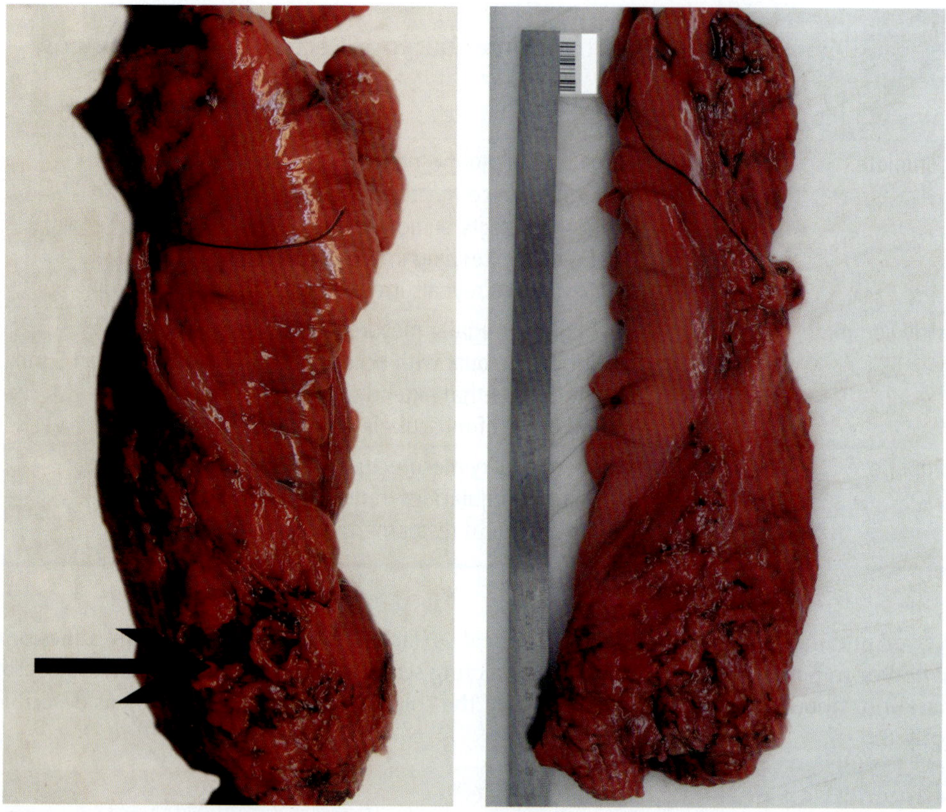


**FIGURE 6.11:** An incomplete mesorectal excision shows large disruptions in the mesorectal envelope (*arrow*) and a defect in the perirectal fat (**A**). This specimen shows disruption of at least 50% of the mesorectal envelope inferiorly (**B**). Muscularis propria is clearly visible through the fat at the distal end of the specimen where the mesorectal fat is not bulky. Lack of soft tissue bulk at the distal end of the specimen has been termed "coning" and is evidence of an inadequate resection. (Photograph courtesy of Dr. Nicholas West, Leeds Institute of Molecular Medicine, St. James's University Hospital, Leeds, UK.)

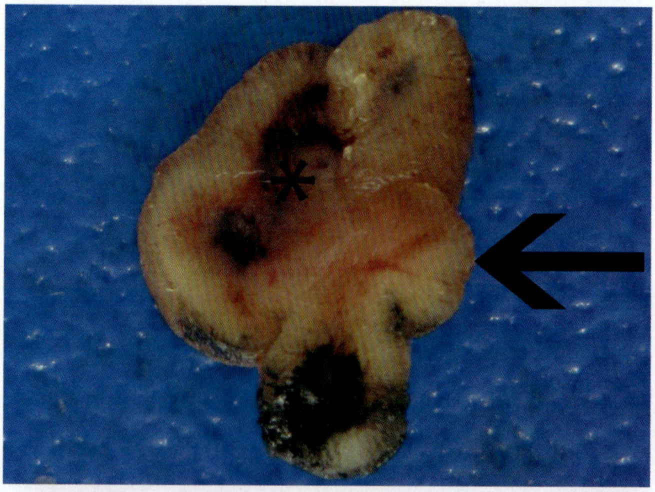

**FIGURE 6.12:** The cross section of a pedunculated adenoma reveals expansion of the mucosa (*arrow*) overlying the soft and gelatinous submucosa (*asterisk*). The cauterized polyp base is inked black.

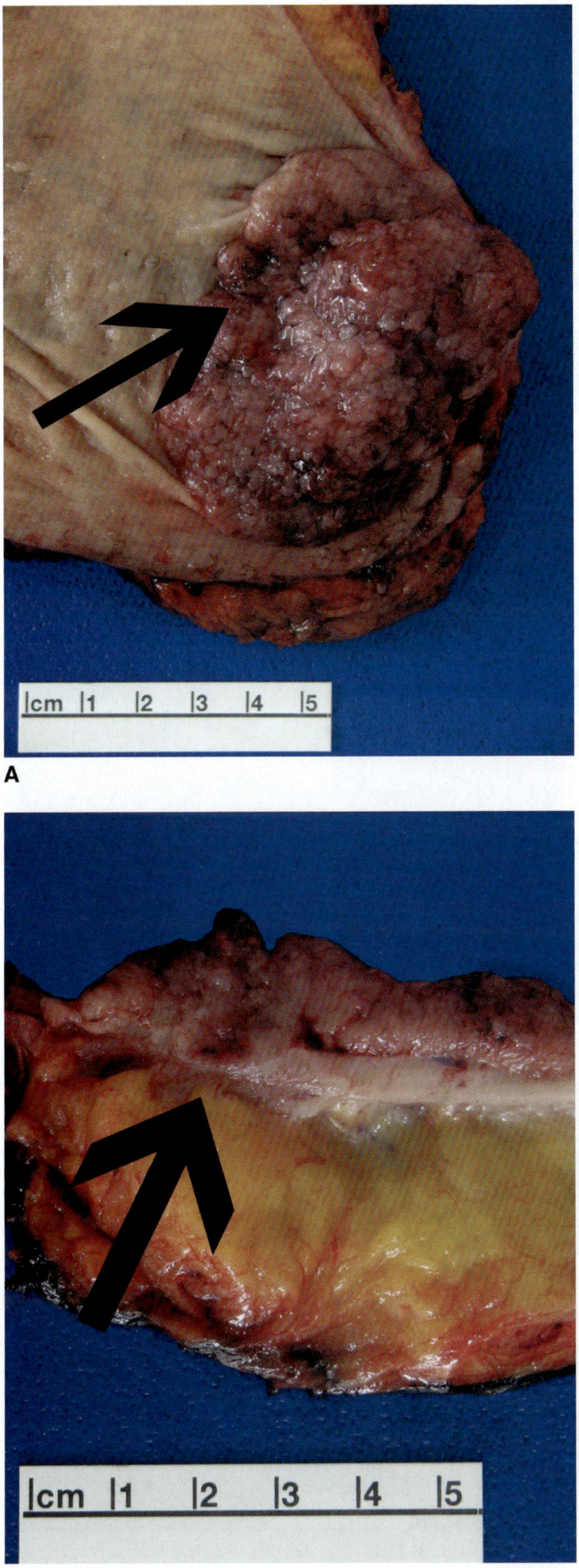


A

B

FIGURE 6.13: A large villous adenoma of the rectum contains a focus of early invasive adenocarcinoma (**A**). The sessile polyp is composed of erythematous frond-like projections that correspond to villous adenoma (**right**). However, there is an area of surface irregularity corresponding to invasive carcinoma (*arrow*). A cross section through this area reveals invasive carcinoma extending into the muscularis propria (*arrow*), whereas the rest of the tumor is limited to the mucosa (**B**).

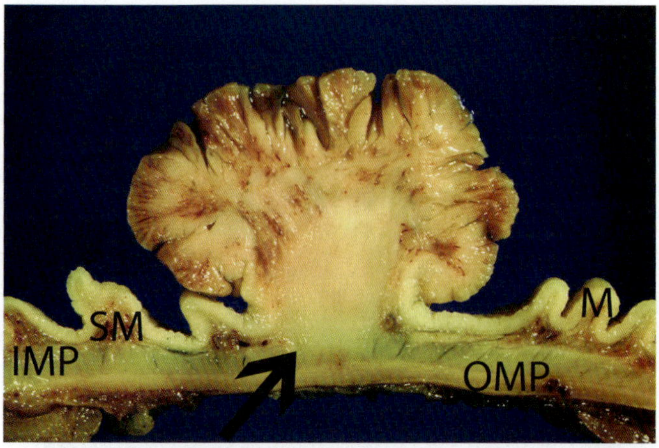


**FIGURE 6.14:** A polypoid invasive cancer obliterates the submucosa and invades the superficial muscularis propria (*arrow*). The layers of the colonic wall are clearly demonstrated distant from the tumor. (M, mucosa; SM, submucosa; IMP, inner layer, muscularis propria; OMP, outer layer, muscularis propria.) (Reprinted from Panarelli N, Yantiss R. *Frozen Section Laboratory: Appendix, Colon, and Anus*. New York, NY: Springer; 2010, with permission.)

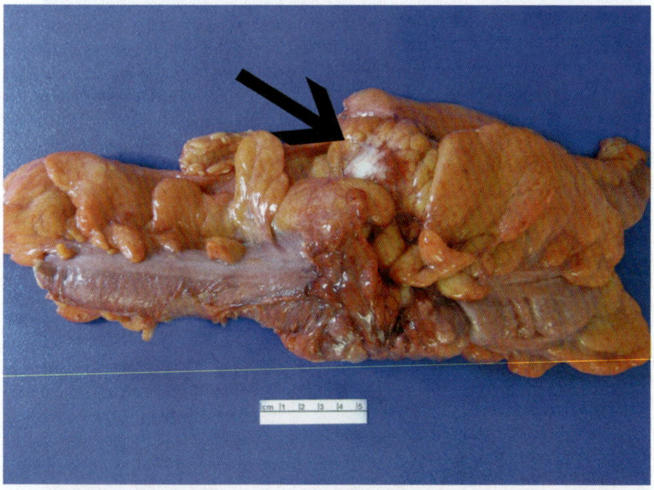

A

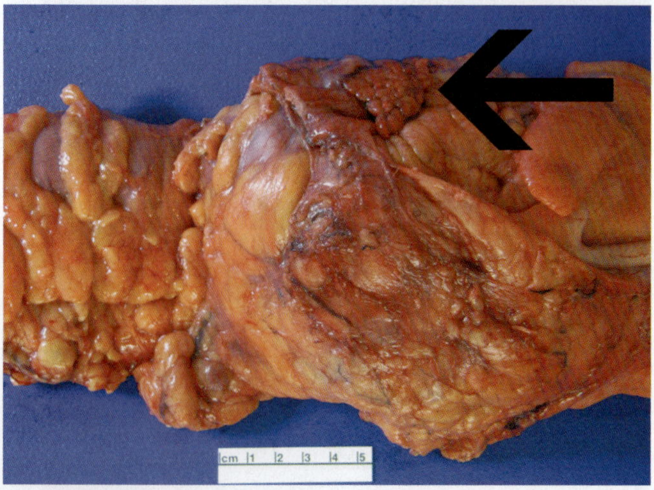

B

**FIGURE 6.15:** A locally advanced sigmoid colon cancer penetrates the serosa, producing a white scar in the subserosal fat (*arrow*) and tumor nodules on the antimesenteric aspect of the colon (**A**). There are serosal adhesions and a piece of attached omentum (*arrow*) overlying the tumor (**B**).

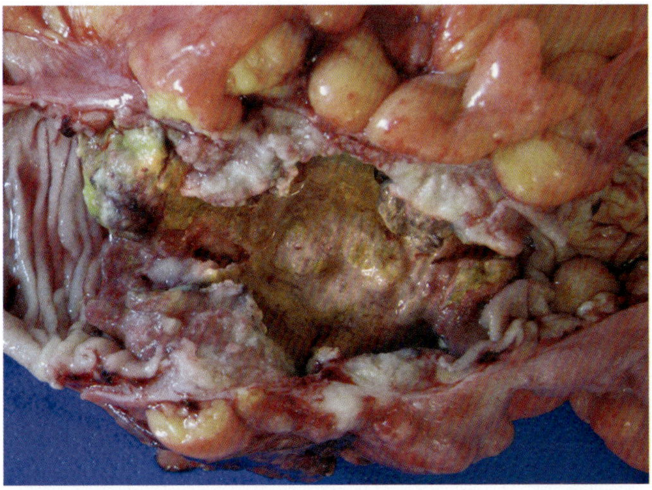

C

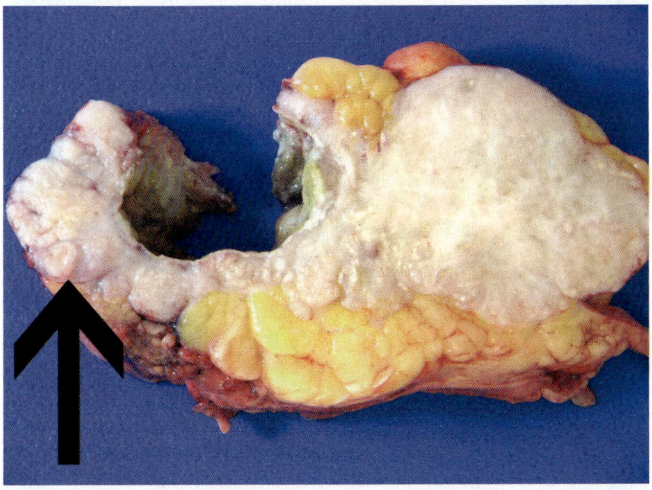

D

FIGURE 6.15: (*Continued*) Opening the colon reveals tumor infiltration through the wall (**C**). Cross sections through the cancer demonstrate extensive serosal penetration on the antimesenteric aspect of the colon (*arrow*) as well as bulky tumor in mesenteric fat that extends to the peritoneal surface (**D**).

Most patients with familial adenomatous polyposis undergo prophylactic colectomy to prevent colorectal cancer. Adequate evaluation of these specimens includes gross photography, palpation of the colonic wall for firm areas, documentation of the site and approximate number of polyps in the gross description, and sampling of the mucosa for histologic evaluation. Although there are no established guidelines for handling these cases, we suggest that all polyps larger than 1 cm in diameter and those that show any unusual features, such as depressed or ulcerated areas, be submitted entirely with full-thickness sections of the colonic wall. Recording the location of any suspicious polyps facilitates complete regional lymph node dissection in the event of an occult malignancy. We also obtain additional representative sections of smaller polyps and mucosa at a rate of approximately one section per 5 cm of affected colon. These representative sections may consist solely of amputated polyps, mucosa, and submucosa, provided that the subjacent wall is of normal pliancy. Occasional patients with familial adenomatous polyposis already have an overt cancer at the time of colectomy. In this situation, the location and size of the tumor and other polyps are recorded. Tissue samples are obtained to pathologically stage the tumor and regional lymph nodes, similar to sporadic cancers, and all large (≥1 cm) or unusual polyps are submitted to detect occult malignancies. Representative sections documenting at least 10 additional polyps are probably adequate provided they are accompanied by a gross photograph and comprehensive description (Figure 6.16).

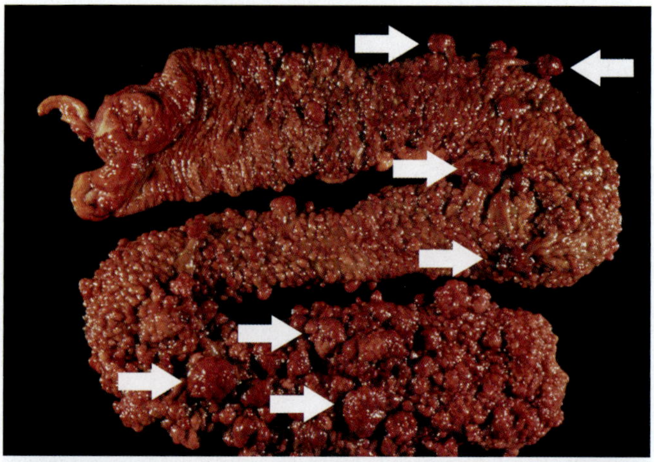

**FIGURE 6.16:** A colectomy specimen from a patient with familial adenomatous polyposis contains innumerable polyps carpeting the mucosa. Some of the polyps are quite large and require complete sampling (*arrows*), whereas representative sections of smaller lesions are probably adequate.

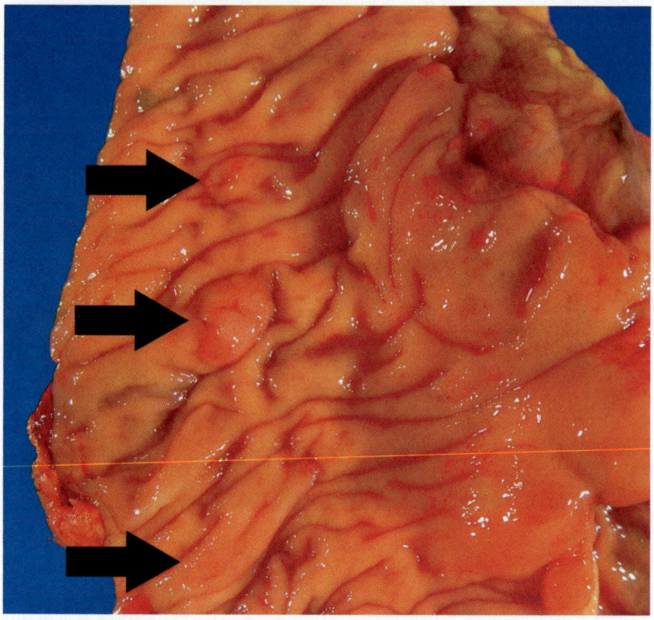

**FIGURE 6.17:** A colon affected by serrated polyposis contains multiple sessile serrated polyps that are difficult to discern from the nonpolypoid mucosa. The polyps are slightly erythematous raised plaques or thickened folds (*arrows*).

Serrated (hyperplastic) polyposis is a disorder characterized by numerous nondysplastic and dysplastic polyps that is clearly associated with increased cancer risk, as discussed in Chapter 4. The disorder is defined by the presence of any one of the following: (i) 20 or more nondysplastic serrated (hyperplastic) polyps anywhere in the colon; (ii) ≥5 nondysplastic serrated polyps in the abdominal colon, at least 2 of which span ≥1 cm; or (iii) any number of nondysplastic serrated polyps in a first-degree relative of a patient who carries the diagnosis.[11] Patients usually have other types of polyp, including serrated, tubular, and villous adenomas, which tend to be more numerous among older patients with the disorder. Serrated polyps show a predilection for the proximal colon and appear as plaque-like excrescences or thickened mucosal folds (Figure 6.17). These lesions may contain foci of high-grade dysplasia or invasive carcinoma despite their relatively small size. We recommend that colectomy specimens be photographed to document the site and approximate number of polyps. Careful palpation of the colonic wall to exclude an early cancer is followed by complete submission of all lesions spanning ≥1 cm and representative sections of polyps and mucosa at a rate of approximately one section per 5 cm of affected colon. Smaller polyps may be better appreciated if the mucosa is evaluated in the fixed state.

Chronic inflammatory bowel disease causes variable mucosal injury ranging from mild mucosal inflammation to severe, extensive ulceration, transmural inflammation, necrosis, and perforation. The disease distribution and extent in the bowel wall are clues to the diagnosis of ulcerative colitis or Crohn disease and, thus, should be carefully evaluated in light of available clinical information. Although some individuals with inflammatory bowel disease undergo colectomy for medically refractory disease, neoplastic complications of chronic injury still account for a large number of surgeries among these patients. Unlike sporadic colorectal cancers and adenomas, chronic colitis–related neoplasia is often multifocal and may be difficult to discern based on visual inspection alone. Gross photography and palpation of the wall are best performed in the fresh state, but areas of dysplasia and early carcinoma may be better appreciated after fixation. Full-thickness sections that include all layers of the bowel wall are obtained at a rate of approximately one section per 5 cm of affected colon in order to document severity of inflammation and facilitate disease classification (Crohn disease versus ulcerative colitis). Extensive sampling of any abnormalities (e.g., mucosal irregularities, polyps, plaques, firm areas, ulcers) is often required to detect areas of neoplasia and evaluate for depth of invasion among early carcinomas (Figure 6.18). Documenting the anatomic location and size of these abnormalities is also important, in the event that carcinoma is detected and a subsequent lymph node dissection is necessary.

## Gross Photography

Examination of resection specimens in the fresh state allows one to best determine which anatomic structures are present and, in the case of a low anterior resection, whether the mesorectum is intact or disrupted. Gross photographs are most demonstrative when obtained of organs in the fresh state. Photographs of the outer surface of a resection specimen document extent of the surgical procedure and are obtained before opening or inking it. Probing the specimen prior to opening allows one to locate the lesion and open along the opposing side or on the antimesenteric side for circumferential lesions. Photographs of the luminal aspect of the specimen and a tumor cross section are also necessary in order to document depth of invasion. Specimens are fixed only after all measurements and photography have been performed.

## Detection of Regional Lymph Nodes

Regional lymph nodes include all lymph nodes in a segmental resection or those within approximately 15 to 20 cm of the tumor in more extensive surgical resections, such as total colectomy specimens. All grossly negative regional lymph nodes are to be submitted entirely, whereas representative sections of positive lymph nodes adequately document extent of disease. Ill-defined nodules in pericolic fat are also sampled in order to document soft tissue tumor deposits, which are

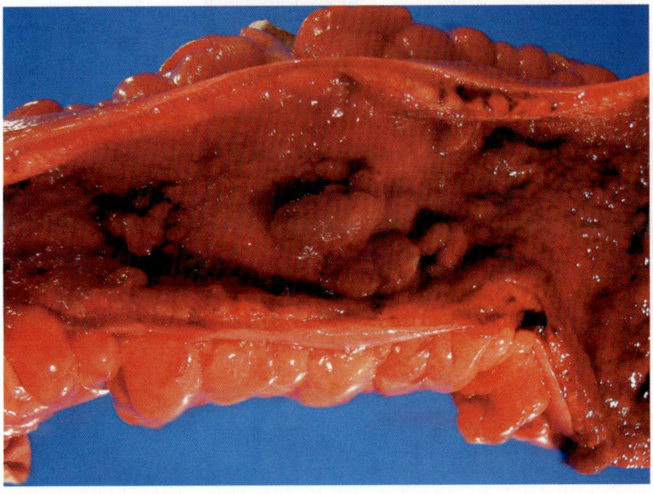

**FIGURE 6.18:** An invasive adenocarcinoma forms a multinodular mass in the colon of a patient with long-standing ulcerative colitis. The background mucosa is atrophic. Foci of polypoid dysplasia are present at the periphery.

prognostically important. Examination of at least 12 negative regional lymph nodes is generally considered adequate for staging purposes, and thus, a minimum of 12 to 15 regional lymph nodes should be examined for every colorectal cancer resection specimen, including those from patients who have been neoadjuvantly treated.[12,13] Pathology reports that describe inadequate lymph node counts may preclude patients from study protocols or be used as a quality assurance measure for surgeons in some institutions. Thus, failure to identify adequate numbers of lymph nodes in initial tissue sections warrants submission of additional soft tissue and/or use of clarifying solutions, such as graded alcohol solutions followed by xylene.[14] Treatment of specimens with these solutions should be performed only after the radial resection margin has been adequately assessed.

Some centers advocate identification of sentinel lymph nodes in patients with colorectal carcinoma. Sentinel lymph nodes are detected by circumferentially injecting blue dye into the colonic wall subjacent to the primary tumor and isolating the first few lymph nodes that display a color change.[1–4] Techniques to evaluate these lymph nodes include complete histologic evaluation, obtaining multiple tissue levels, and immunohistochemical stains to detect cancer cells. However, there are no data to suggest that exhaustive evaluation of sentinel lymph nodes reliably predicts prognosis among colorectal cancer patients or are these methods superior to complete evaluation of regional lymph nodes in assigning tumor stage to colorectal cancers.[15,16] Similarly, detection of tumor cells in histologically negative lymph nodes by molecular techniques has not been shown to predict clinical outcome better than pathologic stage assessment.

## Assessment of Distant Metastatic Disease

Distant metastases include nonregional lymph node deposits, tumor nodules in the peritoneum, and parenchymal metastases in other organs, particularly the liver. Up to 25% of colorectal cancer patients have tumor deposits in the liver at diagnosis, and another 20% develop hepatic metastases following treatment of the primary tumor.[17] Patients with hepatic metastases are increasingly managed with a combination of chemotherapy, ablative techniques, and surgical resection, the latter of which is performed with the goal of complete resection and maximal preservation of hepatic function, as discussed in Chapter 17.[18] The extent of hepatic resection depends on the anatomic location of the tumor deposit, and thus, knowledge of the radiographic findings and surgical procedure is helpful when evaluating resection specimens (Figure 6.19). The status of the resection margin is an important prognostic indicator among patients undergoing hepatic

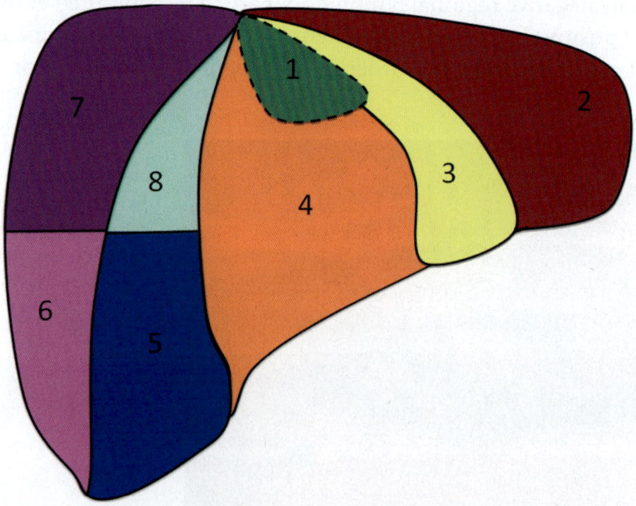


**FIGURE 6.19:** The Couinaud classification scheme divides the liver into eight segments, reflecting the hepatic biliary drainage and vascular supply. Each segment has its own vascular inflow, vascular outflow, and biliary drainage. The caudate lobe is considered segment 1 and is located posteriorly, as indicated by the *dashed line*. The remaining segments are numbered in a clockwise fashion in the frontal plane.

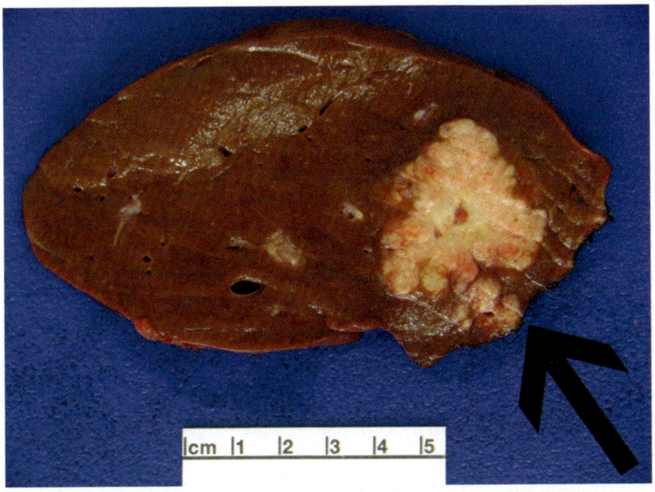


**FIGURE 6.20:** A deposit of metastatic colonic adenocarcinoma closely approximates the hepatic resection margin (*arrow*). The tumor is a multinodular mass with a slightly depressed center owing to areas of necrosis and fibrosis.

resection for metastatic disease: Patients with positive resection margins do not enjoy improved survival compared to those that do not undergo surgery, and resection margins less than 1 cm are associated with decreased survival.[19,20] Sections are obtained perpendicular to the cauterized resection margin to demonstrate its relationship to the tumor deposit (Figure 6.20).

## SUMMARY AND CONCLUSIONS

Pathologic evaluation of resection specimens plays a crucial role in planning management of colorectal cancer patients. Careful gross assessment and submission of appropriate tissue sections impact our ability to document depth of invasion and status of the margin in polypectomy specimens that contain cancer. Not only are these features predictive of prognosis, they are taken into account when determining whether additional surgery is warranted. Judicious grossing practices and cytology preparations facilitate pathologic stage assessment of surgical resection specimens, particularly when documenting extent of local disease. Correlations between gross observations and microscopic findings improve documentation of underlying conditions that predispose to cancer development in some patients and raise awareness of potential risk among family members.

# References


1. Morson B. President's address. The polyp-cancer sequence in the large bowel. *Proc R Soc Med* 1974; 67(6 Pt 1):451–457.
2. Muto T, Bussey HJ, Morson BC. The evolution of cancer of the colon and rectum. *Cancer* 1975; 36(6):2251–2270.
3. Haggitt RC, Glotzbach RE, Soffer EE, et al. Prognostic factors in colorectal carcinomas arising in adenomas: implications for lesions removed by endoscopic polypectomy. *Gastroenterology* 1985;89(2): 328–336.
4. Hughes TG, Jenevein EP, Poulos E. Intramural spread of colon carcinoma. A pathologic study. *Am J Surg* 1983;146(6):697–699.
5. Salerno G, Daniels IR, Moran BJ, et al. Clarifying margins in the multidisciplinary management of rectal cancer: the MERCURY experience. *Clin Radiol* 2006;61(11):916–923.
6. Kapiteijn E, Marijnen CA, Nagtegaal ID, et al. Preoperative radiotherapy combined with total mesorectal excision for resectable rectal cancer. *New Engl J Med* 200130;345(9):638–646.

7. Wasserberg N, Gutman H. Resection margins in modern rectal cancer surgery. *J Surg Oncol* 2008;98(8):611–615.
8. Arbman G, Nilsson E, Storgren-Fordell V, et al. A short diagnostic delay is more important for rectal cancer than for colonic cancer. *Eur J Surg* 1996;162(11):899–904.
9. Nagtegaal ID, van de Velde CJ, van der Worp E, et al. Macroscopic evaluation of rectal cancer resection specimen: clinical significance of the pathologist in quality control. *J Clin Oncol* 2002;20(7):1729–1734.
10. Hermanek P, Junginger T. The circumferential resection margin in rectal carcinoma surgery. *Tech Coloproctol* 2005;9(3):193–199; discussion 199–200.
11. Rosty C, Buchanan DD, Walsh MD, et al. Phenotype and polyp landscape in serrated polyposis syndrome: a series of 100 patients from genetics clinics. *Am J Surg Pathol* [Research Support, N.I.H., Extramural Research Support, Non-U.S. Gov't] 2012;36(6):876–882.
12. Swanson RS, Compton CC, Stewart AK, et al. The prognosis of T3N0 colon cancer is dependent on the number of lymph nodes examined. *Ann Surg Oncol* 2003;10(1):65–71.
13. Prandi M, Lionetto R, Bini A, et al. Prognostic evaluation of stage B colon cancer patients is improved by an adequate lymphadenectomy: results of a secondary analysis of a large scale adjuvant trial. *Ann Surg* 2002;235(4):458–463.
14. Scott KW, Grace RH. Detection of lymph node metastases in colorectal carcinoma before and after fat clearance. *Br J Surg* 1989;76(11):1165–1167.
15. Bertagnolli M, Miedema B, Redston M, et al. Sentinel node staging of resectable colon cancer: results of a multicenter study. *Ann Surg* 2004;240(4):624–628; discussion 628–630.
16. Redston M, Compton CC, Miedema BW, et al. Analysis of micrometastatic disease in sentinel lymph nodes from resectable colon cancer: results of Cancer and Leukemia Group B Trial 80001. *J Clin Oncol* 2006;24(6):878–883.
17. Scheele J, Stangl R, Altendorf-Hofmann A. Hepatic metastases from colorectal carcinoma: impact of surgical resection on the natural history. *Br J Surg* 1990;77(11):1241–1246.
18. Chua TC, Liauw W, Chu F, et al. Summary outcomes of two-stage resection for advanced colorectal liver metastases. *J Surg Oncol* 2012;107(2):211–216.
19. Ruers T, Bleichrodt RP. Treatment of liver metastases, an update on the possibilities and results. *Eur J Cancer* 2002;38(7):1023–1033.
20. Elias D, Cavalcanti A, Sabourin JC, et al. Resection of liver metastases from colorectal cancer: the real impact of the surgical margin. *Eur J Surg Oncol* 1998;24(3):174–179.

# Morphologic Classification of Colorectal Epithelial Tumors

# 7

Rhonda K. Yantiss

Malignant colorectal epithelial neoplasms are broadly classified as carcinomas and (neuro)endocrine tumors. Invasive colorectal carcinomas are defined by infiltration through the muscularis mucosae into the submucosa and/or deeper soft tissues. More than 90% are gland-forming adenocarcinomas with an intestinal phenotype, although several other histopathologic subtypes exist (Table 7.1). These variants are important to recognize because some are associated with specific molecular characteristics, such as microsatellite instability (MSI-H), whereas others are defined as high-grade neoplasms at risk for biologically aggressive behavior. (Neuro)endocrine neoplasms are classified as well-differentiated and poorly differentiated tumors and included in the *AJCC Cancer Staging Manual*, seventh edition.[1] The purpose of this chapter is to discuss the types of malignant colorectal epithelial tumors, their clinical features, morphologic characteristics, and molecular associations.

## COLORECTAL CARCINOMA

### Clinical Features

Colorectal carcinoma is largely a disease of older adults and is slightly more common among men than women. Higher rates are observed in industrialized countries of Europe and North America, as well as Australia and New Zealand, relative to less well-developed countries. Cancer rates increase among immigrants and their descendants from low-incidence regions to match those of their adoptive countries. Obesity, meat consumption, smoking, and alcohol are all considered modifiable colorectal cancer risk factors, whereas decreased risk is associated with increased fiber intake; diets rich in fruits, vegetables, and grains; and chronic nonsteroidal anti-inflammatory drug use. The epidemiologic features of colorectal carcinoma are further discussed in Chapter 2.

Most carcinomas are located in the distal colorectum, although cancers of the proximal colon become more common with advancing age. Many tumors are asymptomatic, early stage lesions that are detected during screening or surveillance colonoscopy. Proximal colonic cancers rarely cause obstructive symptoms because the right colon is quite distensible and contains mostly liquid stool. Tumors of the abdominal colon tend to be quite large and bleed intermittently, producing positive fecal occult blood tests and iron deficiency anemia (Figure 7.1). Carcinomas of the distal colorectum are more likely to cause changing bowel habits. Annular tumors partially obstruct the lumen, resulting in narrow caliber stools and sensations of incomplete evacuation, constipation, bloating, and distention (Figure 7.2). Some patients with obstructing cancers have diarrheal symptoms due to leakage of liquid stool around impacted solid feces. Bleeding distal tumors also cause hematochezia, especially when they develop in the rectum.

### Intestinal-Type Adenocarcinoma

More than 90% of colorectal adenocarcinomas are composed of glands with an intestinal phenotype. Malignant glands harbor columnar epithelial cells, some of which contain cytoplasmic mucin vacuoles. The tumor cell nuclei are round or ovoid with irregular membranes, heterogeneous

**Table 7.1 Morphologic Variants of Epithelial Cell Neoplasms of the Colorectum**

| Morphologic Subtype |
| --- |
| Intestinal-type adenocarcinoma |
| Micropapillary carcinoma |
| Cribriform comedo–type adenocarcinoma |
| Serrated adenocarcinoma |
| Mucinous adenocarcinoma |
| Signet ring cell carcinoma |
| Medullary carcinoma |
| Rare variants<br>Adenosquamous carcinoma<br>Spindle cell carcinoma<br>Undifferentiated carcinoma<br>Choriocarcinoma<br>Villous cdenocarcinoma<br>Clear cell adenocarcinoma |
| (Neuro)endocrine tumors<br>Well-differentiated (neuro)endocrine tumor<br>Low-grade (neuro)endocrine tumor<br>High-grade (neuro)endocrine tumor<br>Poorly-differentiated (neuro)endocrine tumor<br>(Neuro)endocrine carcinoma, non–small cell type<br>(Neuro)endocrine carcinoma, small cell type<br>Mixed adenoneuroendocrine carcinoma |

chromatin, prominent nucleoli, and numerous mitotic figures. Single cell and luminal necrosis are often prominent (Figure 7.3). Some tumors contain cells with abundant clear cytoplasm and subnuclear vacuoles that simulate the appearance of secretory endometrium or other müllerian-type malignancies, particularly when they present in extraintestinal sites (Figure 7.4). Well-differentiated tumors may show a predominantly villous architecture that closely simulates the appearance of an adenoma. Intestinal-type adenocarcinomas of the colorectum show a characteristic immunophenotype. They are negative for cytokeratin 7 and display positivity for cytokeratin 20, CDX-2, and CDH17.[2]

## Micropapillary Carcinoma

Approximately 10% of colorectal carcinomas contain a micropapillary component, but fewer than 1% of tumors are classified as micropapillary carcinomas. This tumor type is more aggressive than conventional adenocarcinoma, and the presence of a micropapillary component is an adverse prognostic factor among stage I and stage II colorectal carcinomas.[3,4] More than half of cases are locally advanced with lymphovascular invasion and multiple (>4) regional lymph node metastases.[4,5] Micropapillary tumors contain solid cell clusters within lacunar spaces that simulate vascular invasion (Figure 7.5). They show peripheral staining for MUC1, a glycoprotein necessary for maintenance of cell lumina, which may inhibit tumor cell/stromal interactions and contribute to the morphologic appearance of this tumor type.[6] Micropapillary carcinomas show cytokeratin 20 positivity and negativity for cytokeratin 7 and are usually microsatellite stable (MSS).

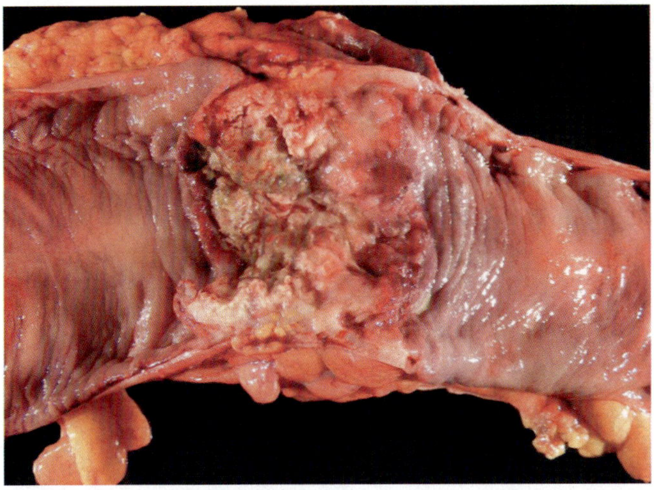

FIGURE 7.1: This transverse colectomy specimen contains a large fungating adenocarcinoma with necrosis and hemorrhage. The tumor was discovered during evaluation for microcytic anemia.

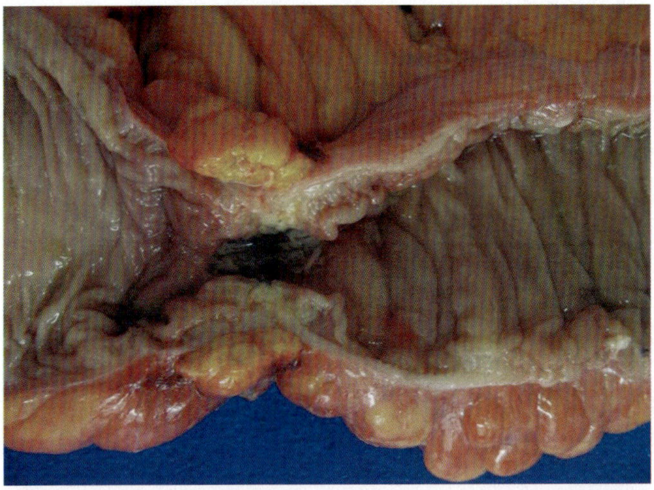

FIGURE 7.2: An annular adenocarcinoma of the sigmoid colon produces an area of luminal narrowing. The proximal end of the specimen shows mild dilation (**left**).

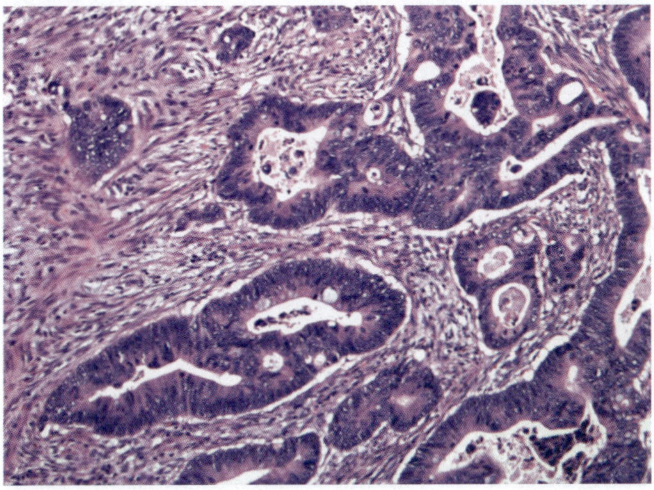

FIGURE 7.3: Low-grade intestinal-type colorectal carcinomas consist of infiltrating glands enmeshed in desmoplastic stroma. The tumor cells contain eosinophilic cytoplasm and occasional mucin vacuoles. The nuclei are polarized at the base of each cell and display heterogeneous chromatin. Luminal necrotic debris is evident.

## Cribriform–Comedo–Type Adenocarcinoma

Cribriform–comedo–type adenocarcinoma is recognized by the WHO as a colorectal cancer subtype with morphologic features reminiscent of ductal carcinoma in situ of the breast.[7] Tumors with this morphology account for less than 1% of all colorectal carcinomas and tend to occur in the proximal colon of older adults.[8] Cribriform–comedo–type adenocarcinomas are composed of expansile sheets of malignant glands with a fused growth pattern. Luminal necrotic material is prominent (Figure 7.6). The tumor cells show high-grade cytologic features with enlarged nuclei

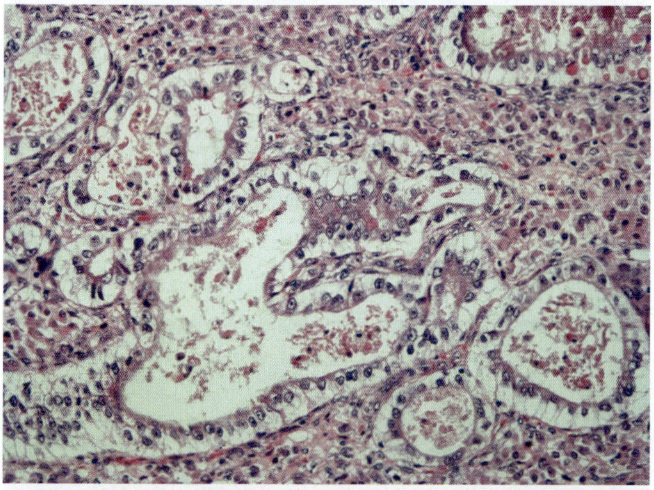

**FIGURE 7.4:** Metastatic clear cell colonic carcinoma in the ovary consists of malignant glands lined by cells with abundant clear cytoplasm. Subnuclear vacuoles are reminiscent of secretory endometrium. However, the nuclei are quite atypical with open chromatin and prominent nucleoli. Luminal necrotic material characteristic of intestinal-type carcinoma is present. The background stromal cells are luteinized.

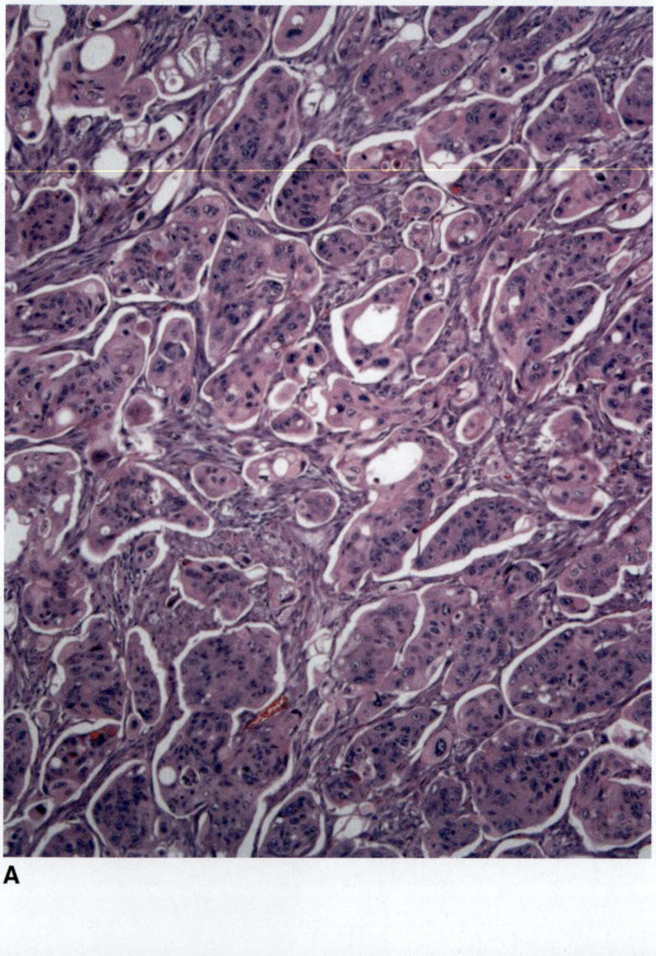

A

**FIGURE 7.5:** Micropapillary carcinoma contains sheets of tumor cells without apparent gland formation (**A**).

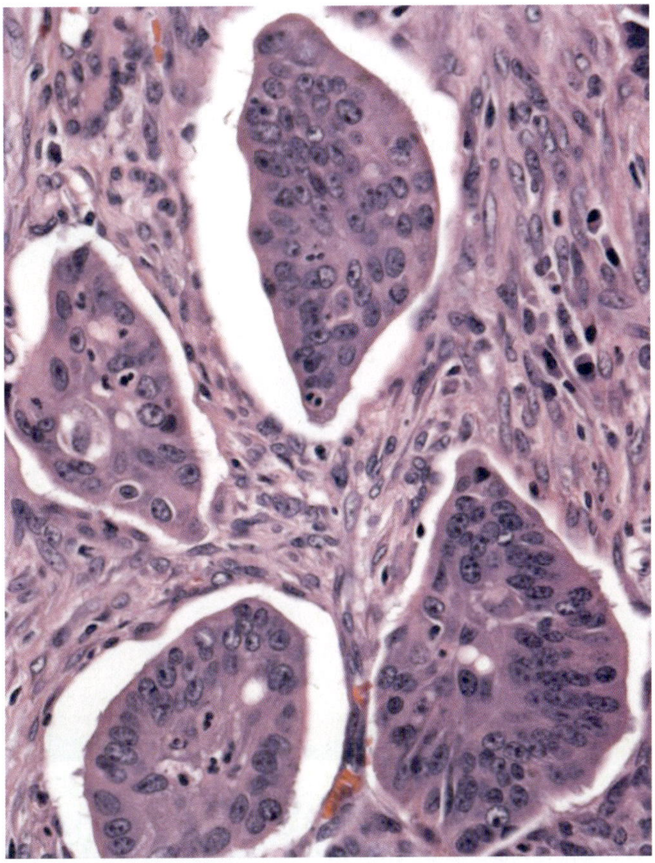

B

FIGURE 7.5: (*Continued*) The tumor cell clusters are associated with retraction artifact that simulates lymphovascular invasion. Tumor cells are arranged in clusters, some of which display central fibrovascular cores (**B**).

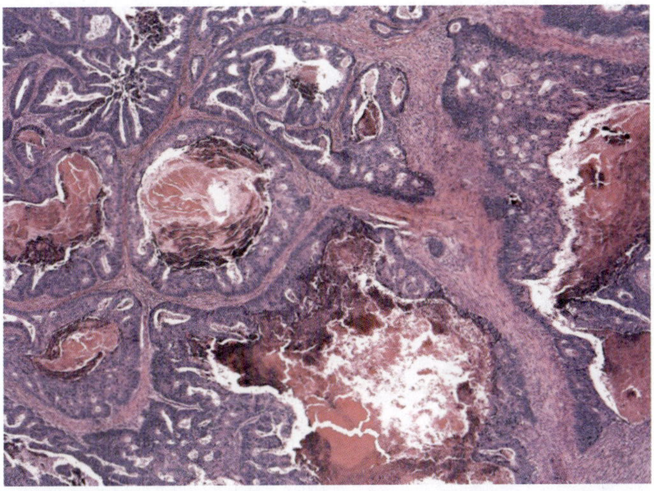

FIGURE 7.6: Cribriform–comedo–type adenocarcinoma contains cystically dilated glands with abundant luminal necrotic debris. The dilated glands harbor malignant cells with a fused, cribriform growth pattern.

and prominent nucleoli. Cribriform–comedo–type carcinomas are usually MSS, but show CpG island hypermethylation.[8]

## Serrated Adenocarcinoma

Serrated adenocarcinomas typically arise in the abdominal colon and are more common among older female adults.[7] They represent one putative endpoint of the serrated neoplastic pathway, as discussed in Chapter 4, although most colonic carcinomas derived from serrated polyps do not have a serrated appearance. In fact, serrated polyps may be seen in combination with 17% of proximal colonic carcinomas, but less than 20% of these tumors have morphologic features that warrant classification as serrated adenocarcinoma.[9] Serrated adenocarcinomas are often small, plaque-like nodules that may be associated with sessile polyps (Figure 7.7). They contain neoplastic glands with a serrated architecture and abundant, often eosinophilic, cytoplasm; large nuclei; and prominent nucleoli (Figure 7.8).

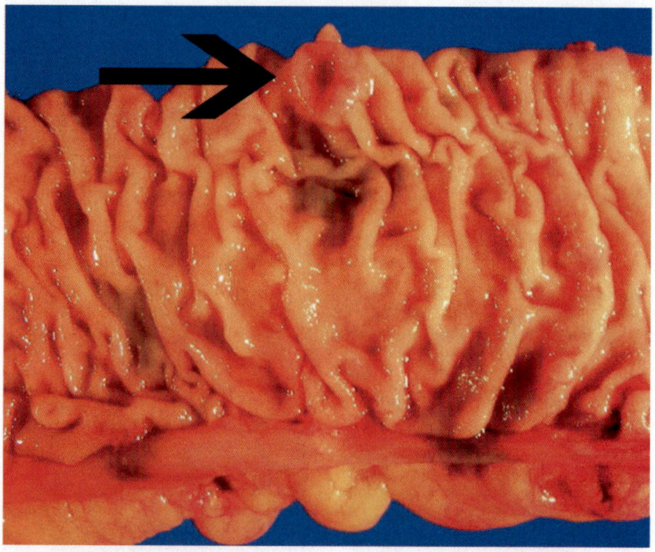

**FIGURE 7.7:** A serrated adenocarcinoma forms a small plaque-like nodule with central umbilication (*arrow*).

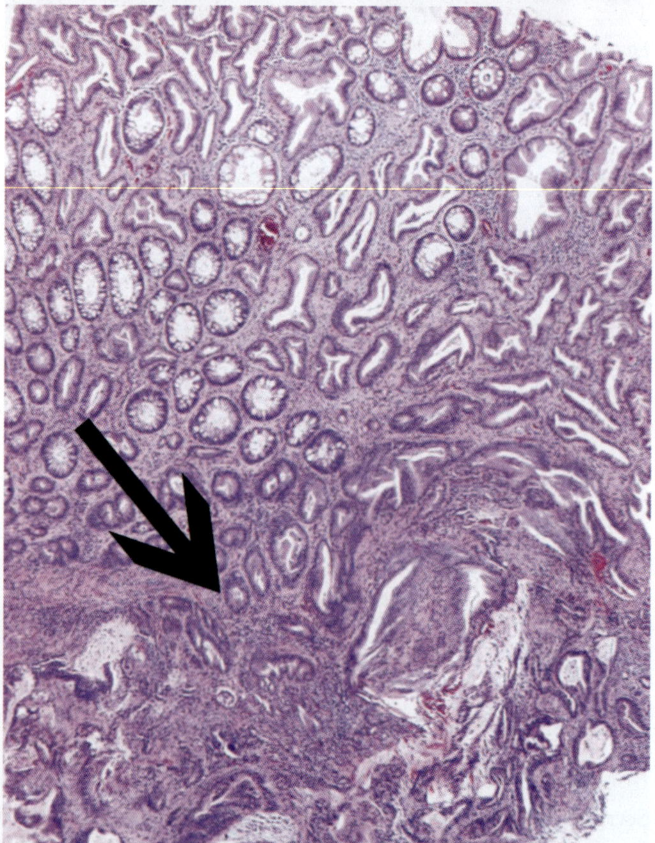

A

**FIGURE 7.8:** An early invasive serrated adenocarcinoma is associated with a serrated polyp in the mucosa (**A**).

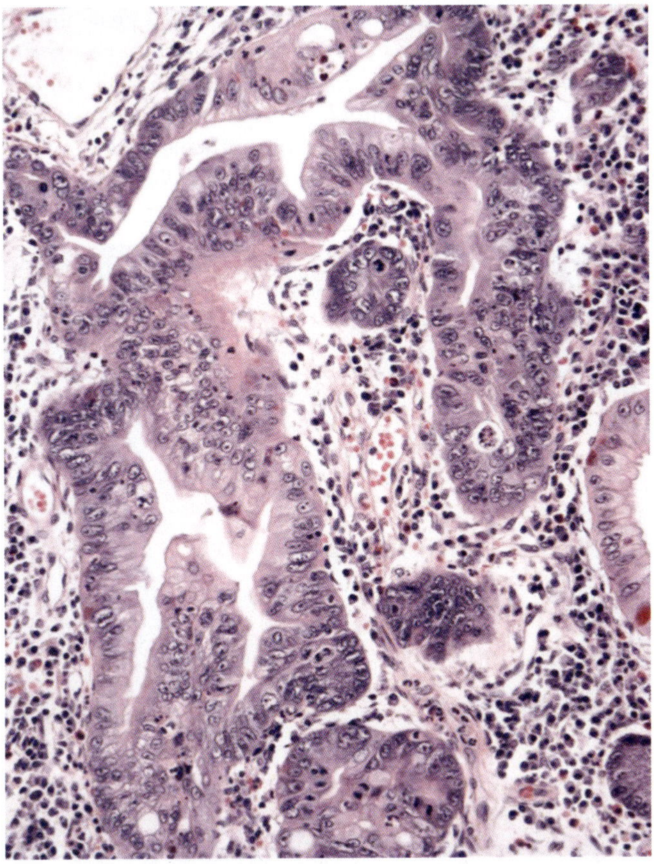

B

FIGURE 7.8: (*Continued*) The tumor is composed of irregular, infiltrative glands with a serrated contour (*arrow*). The tumor cells contain abundant eosinophilic cytoplasm and large nuclei with open chromatin, prominent nucleoli, and numerous mitotic figures (**B**).

These tumors frequently contain other elements, including cribriform glands, mucin pools, and signet ring cells. The molecular features of serrated adenocarcinoma are variable. Fewer than 20% of tumors show molecular features typical of the serrated neoplastic pathway, namely, *BRAF* mutations, CpG island hypermethylation, and MSI-H. They may be MSS, harbor *KRAS* mutations, or display relatively little DNA hypermethylation.[9]

# COLORECTAL CARCINOMAS WITH SPECIFIC CLINICOPATHOLOGIC CHARACTERISTICS

## Mucinous Adenocarcinoma

Up to 10% of all colorectal adenocarcinomas are classified as mucinous carcinomas, as defined by the presence of extracellular mucin pools comprising more than 50% of the tumor volume. Carcinomas that show less than 50% mucinous differentiation are classified as adenocarcinomas with a mucinous component. Mucinous adenocarcinomas occur in two specific situations. They are the most common adenocarcinomas to complicate chronic anal sinuses and fistulae in patients with, or without, Crohn disease.[10] In addition, 20% to 60% of mucinous adenocarcinomas show underlying MSI-H, and thus, their clinical features and biologic behavior mirror those of sporadic MSI-H cancers in older adults and heritable tumors affecting patients with Lynch syndrome.[11,12] Mucinous tumors with MSI-H are associated with a better prognosis than MSS mucinous adenocarcinomas.[13] The WHO classifies MSI-H carcinomas as low-grade carcinomas, regardless of their morphologic features, but does not recommend grading criteria for MSS mucinous adenocarcinomas.[7]

Mucinous carcinomas are often bulky tumors of the abdominal colon with a glistening or gelatinous cut surface (Figure 7.9). Freely floating strips or clusters of tumor cells are present within mucin pools or adherent to their peripheries (Figure 7.10A). The tumor cells contain abundant cytoplasmic mucin and display nuclear features comparable to those of intestinal-type adenocarcinomas (Figure 7.10B). Some mucinous carcinomas harbor epithelial cells arranged singly or in cords within mucin pools (Figure 7.11). Mucinous carcinomas that contain cohesive

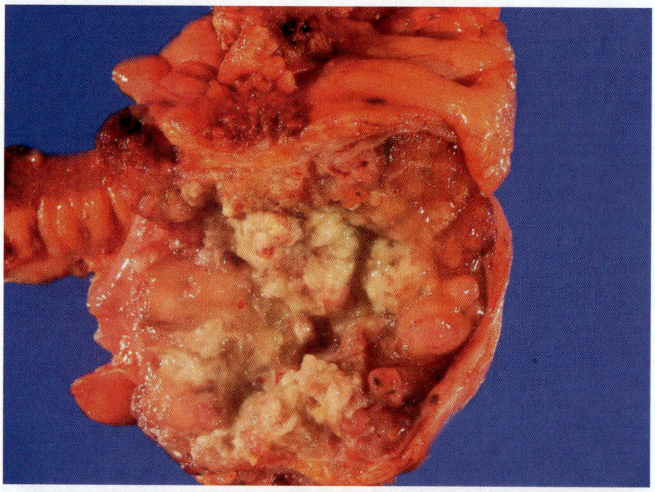

**FIGURE 7.9:** This mucinous adenocarcinoma of the splenic flexure is a large, bulky tumor with a gelatinous cut surface.

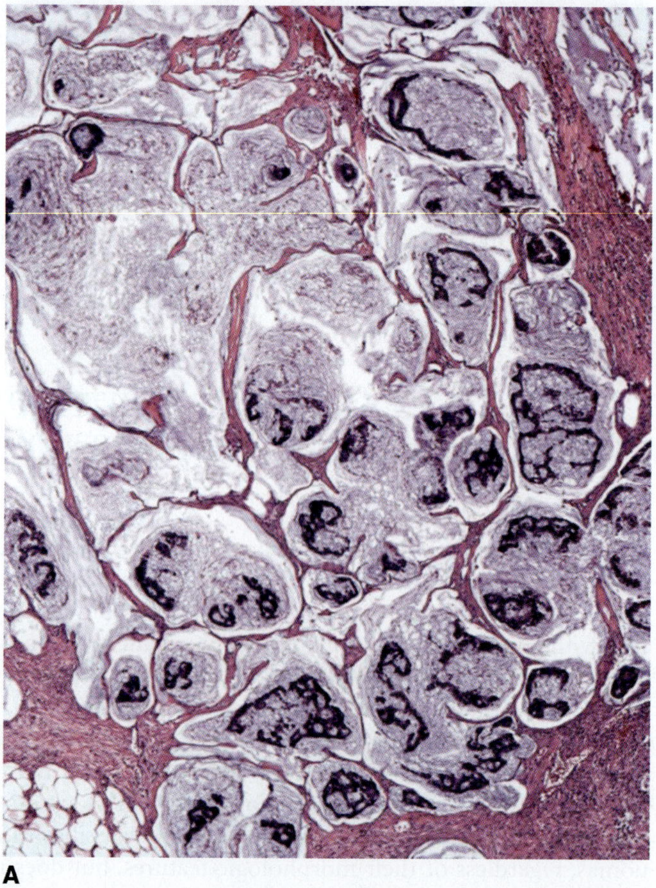

**FIGURE 7.10:** Mucinous adenocarcinomas contain strips and clusters of tumor cells floating in extracellular pools of mucin (**A**).

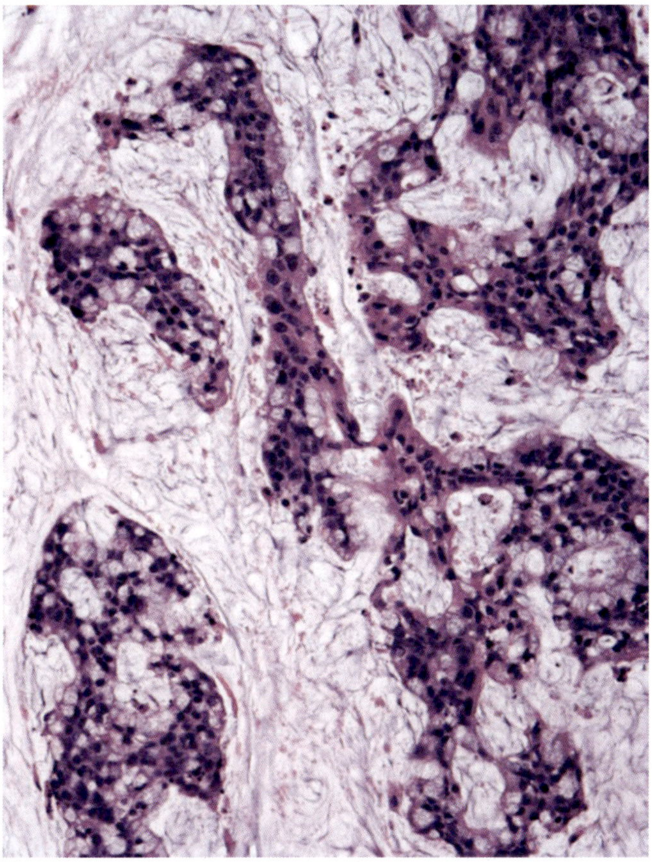

B

FIGURE 7.10: (*Continued*) The tumor cells are arranged in fused glands and contain abundant cytoplasmic mucin with enlarged, hyperchromatic nuclei and prominent nucleoli (**B**).

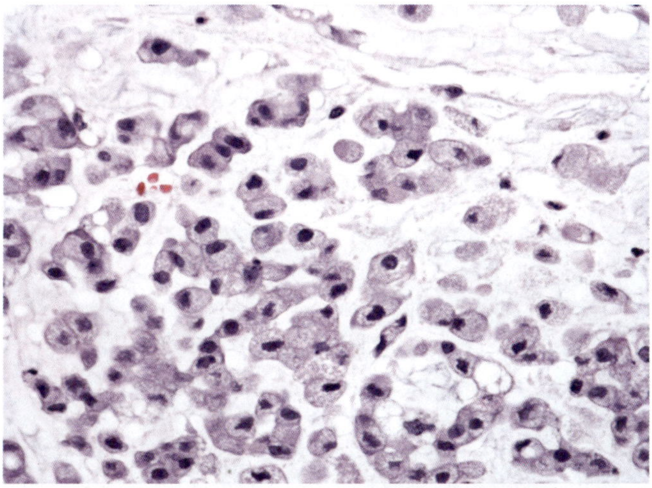

FIGURE 7.11: Some high-grade mucinous adenocarcinomas contain clusters of single floating cells within mucin pools. This growth pattern reflects aggressive behavior in some cases and, thus, is variably classified as high-grade mucinous adenocarcinoma and signet ring cell carcinoma.

strips of cells distended with mucin have a better prognosis than those that contain floating signet ring cells. For this reason, the former are classified as low-grade mucinous carcinomas, and the latter are considered high-grade mucinous carcinomas.[14] High-grade mucinous carcinoma may be associated with infiltrating signet ring cell carcinoma, and thus, its detection should prompt a careful search for a more aggressive lesion.[11]

## Signet Ring Cell Carcinoma

Only 2% of colorectal cancers are classified as signet ring cell carcinoma, which is defined by the presence of signet ring cells accounting for at least 50% of the tumor volume. Signet ring cell carcinoma is overrepresented among cancer patients with inflammatory bowel disease. Up to 35% of Crohn disease–related intestinal cancers have a signet ring cell component.[15] The clinical features of signet ring cell carcinomas that develop in this situation mirror those of inflammatory bowel disease–related neoplasia, occurring in younger patients who have long-standing disease. Signet ring cell carcinoma may also be seen in association with mucinous carcinoma. Approximately 20% to 30% show MSI-H, in which case they occur more commonly in the proximal colon and tend to affect older women.[11] MSS signet ring cell carcinomas that are unassociated with inflammatory bowel disease show a predilection to affect young patients (<40 years of age) and present at advanced stage.[16,17] More than one-third of patients have peritoneal carcinomatosis at the time of diagnosis, although parenchymal metastases to the liver are uncommon.[18,19] The WHO considers MSI-H signet ring cell carcinomas to be low grade, but most data have failed to demonstrate an improved prognosis among patients with MSI-H signet ring cell carcinomas compared to those that are MSS, the latter of which generally pursue an aggressive clinical course.[20]

Three patterns of signet ring cell carcinoma have been described. The first consists of cords and singly arranged signet ring cells floating in pools of mucin, although such tumors are more appropriately classified as high-grade mucinous adenocarcinomas, as described above (Figure 7.12).[7,14] The second pattern displays tumor cells arranged in cords and nests that do not elicit a desmoplastic stromal response. The cells contain globoid mucin vacuoles and peripherally compressed nuclei reminiscent of "crypt cell carcinoma/goblet cell carcinoid" tumors of the appendix (Figure 7.13). Both of these variants may be MSI-H and are often present in combination with other morphologic variants, such as mucinous carcinoma.[21] Finally, some signet ring cell carcinomas are composed of single infiltrating tumor cells that dissect through reactive stroma, similar to invasive signet ring cell carcinomas of the stomach (Figure 7.14). Tumors with this appearance are usually MSS and biologically aggressive.

## Medullary Carcinoma

Medullary carcinoma accounts for approximately 1% of all colorectal cancers. Virtually all medullary carcinomas show underlying MSI-H, and thus, their clinical features mirror those of Lynch-related (HNPCC) and sporadic colonic carcinomas with MSI-H. These tumors are more common among older women and are extremely uncommon among African Americans.[22] They typically occur in the proximal colon where they attain a large size and have not been

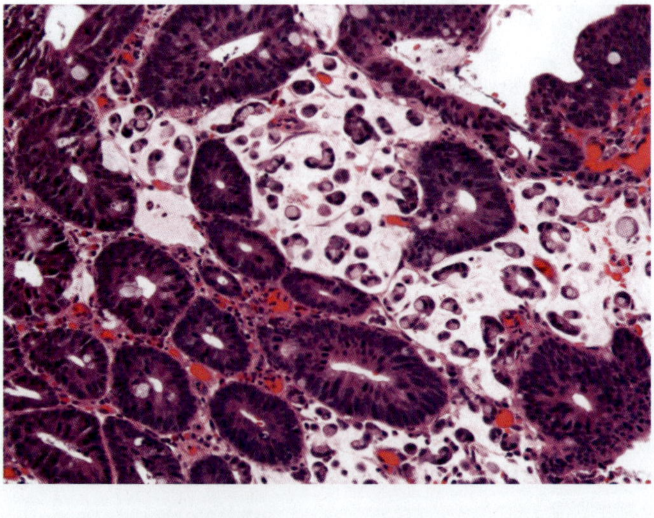

**FIGURE 7.12:** High-grade mucinous adenocarcinomas contain infiltrating mucin pools with freely floating signet ring cells. Classification of these lesions may be confusing, since they have been considered to represent invasive signet ring cell carcinoma by some authors.

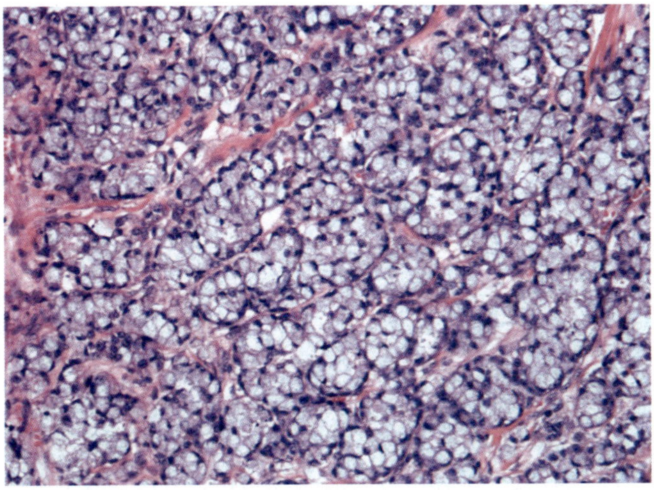

FIGURE 7.13: Invasive signet ring cell carcinomas may grow as sheets, cords, and nests of tumor cells that elicit very little stromal reaction and contain large mucin vacuoles with crescentic peripheral nuclei. This pattern of growth is usually associated with areas of mucinous adenocarcinoma.

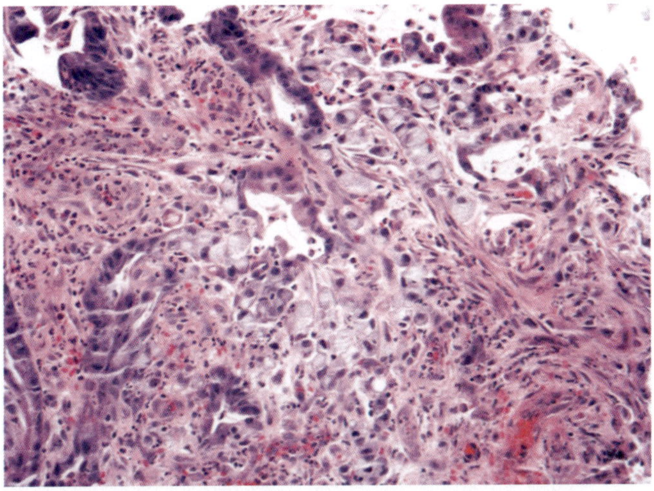

FIGURE 7.14: This signet ring cell carcinoma developed in a young patient with long-standing Crohn disease and chronic anorectal disease. The tumor is composed of single infiltrating cells that destroy the lamina propria and are associated with desmoplastic stroma. The tumor cells contain large mucin vacuoles and display considerable cytologic atypia.

convincingly demonstrated in the rectum. Less than half of cases are associated with elevated serum carcinoembryonic antigen levels. Most medullary carcinomas are stage II at the time of diagnosis, although approximately 10% of cases metastasize to regional lymph nodes. This tumor type is associated with a better clinical outcome than gland-forming colonic adenocarcinomas of comparable stage.[23,24]

Medullary carcinomas are large, bulky tumors that display an expansile growth pattern and contain syncytial nests and sheets of tumor cells with minimal gland formation (Figure 7.15A). The tumor cells are polygonal with abundant eosinophilic cytoplasm, large nuclei with open chromatin, and prominent nucleoli. Lymphocytes are abundant within tumor stroma and interdigitate between neoplastic epithelial cells (Figure 7.15B). Medullary carcinomas also elicit a Crohn-like lymphoid reaction, as discussed in Chapter 9. They are typically diploid by flow cytometry and display MSI-H, but lack *KRAS* and *TP53* mutations.[23]

## Other Rare Colorectal Cancer Variants

A variety of uncommon colorectal cancer subtypes exist, accounting for less than 1% of all colorectal carcinomas. Although these variants probably show similar clinical features with intestinal-type tumors, their rarity precludes comprehensive analysis of their epidemiologic

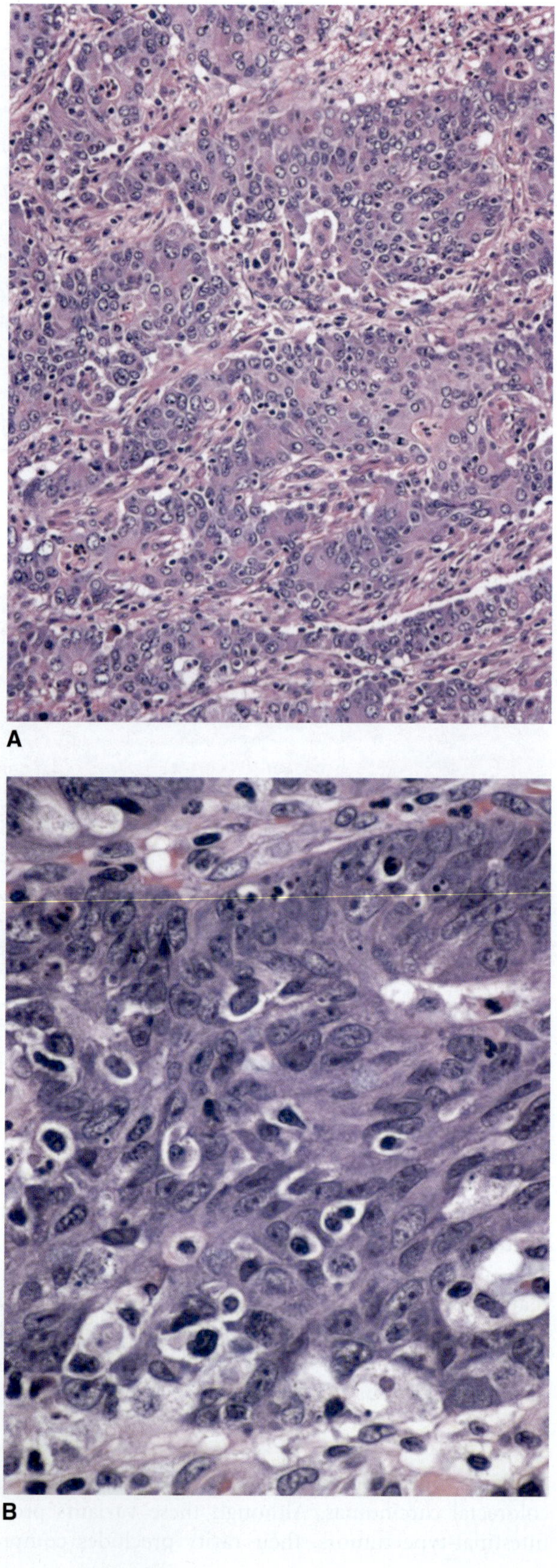

A

B

FIGURE 7.15: Medullary carcinoma contains syncytia of tumor cells with abundant eosinophilic cytoplasm that are intimately associated with tumor-infiltrating lymphocytes as well as inflammatory stroma (**A**). The tumor cells contain large nuclei with irregular contours, coarse chromatin, and prominent nucleoli (**B**).

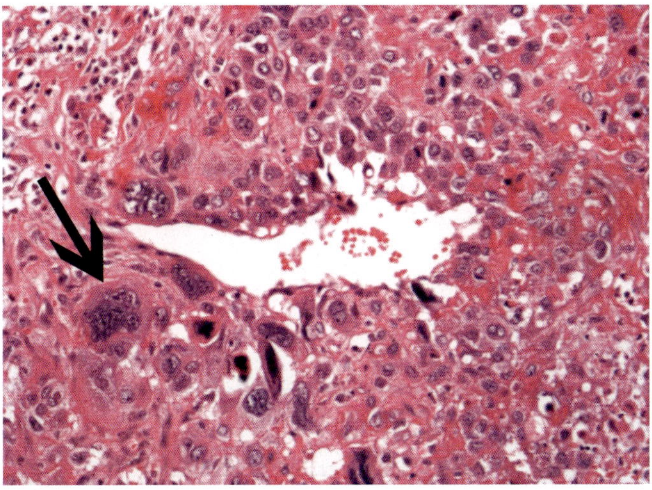

FIGURE 7.16: Colonic choriocarcinoma is usually seen as a component of adenocarcinoma. It consists of sheets of highly atypical mononuclear cells with abundant cytoplasm, hemorrhage, and necrosis. The tumor cells are associated with fibrin and invade blood vessels. Mitotic figures are numerous and syncytiotrophoblast-type cells are readily apparent (*arrow*).

characteristics. Adenosquamous, spindle cell (sarcomatoid), and undifferentiated carcinomas have all been described in both the colon and rectum. Choriocarcinoma may occur in pure form, although it is usually seen in combination with intestinal-type adenocarcinoma (Figure 7.16).

# (NEURO)ENDOCRINE TUMORS OF THE COLORECTUM

## History

Early investigators postulated that small cell carcinomas and "carcinoid" tumors were derived from the neural crest and, thus, considered these lesions to be "neuroendocrine" in nature.[25] Even today, authors contend that morphologically related tumors of the gastrointestinal (GI) tract that stain for chromogranin, synaptophysin, or both contain neurosecretory granules, although they provide no compelling evidence that distinguishes a "neurosecretory" granule from a "secretory" one. Recent studies confirm that there is no normal "neuroendocrine" cell in the GI tract nor are endocrine cells of this organ system derived from the neural crest. Epithelial stem cells with potential for divergent differentiation give rise to endocrine cells, Paneth cells, goblet cells, and absorptive cells. Endocrine cells of the diffuse endocrine system express a variety of peptide markers, such as chromogranin A, synaptophysin, and neuron-specific enolase that are incorrectly considered to be "neuroendocrine" markers. Chromogranin A is the precursor to secreted functional peptides, namely, pancreastatin, parastatin, and vasostatins I and II, and is best classified as a marker of endocrine differentiation. It follows that cells (and tumors) expressing peptide hormones are appropriately classified as endocrine cells (and neoplasms), whereas the term "neuroendocrine" should be reserved for situations in which unequivocal neural and endocrine differentiation are observed. True neuroendocrine cells are observed in the pituitary gland, sympathetic chain, and adrenal gland, and examples of neuroendocrine tumors include paragangliomas and pheochromocytomas. "Neuroendocrine" is inaccurate when applied to the islets of Langerhans and tubular gut endocrine cells and is misleading when used to describe tumors that recapitulate the phenotype of GI endocrine cells. Nonetheless, the current WHO and AJCC classification schemes utilize the term "neuroendocrine," rather than "endocrine," to denote colorectal epithelial tumors with characteristic morphologic and immunohistochemical features, as described below.

## Classification and Grading of (Neuro)Endocrine Tumors

The classification of endocrine tumors is based on degree of differentiation and tumor grade. Differentiation describes the extent to which tumor cells resemble normal endocrine cells of the tubular gut, whereas grade refers to severity of cytologic atypia reflected by nuclear size

Table 7.2 Grading Scheme for (Neuro)Endocrine Tumors of the Colorectum

| Tumor Classification | Grade | Mitotic Rate | | Ki-67 Labeling |
|---|---|---|---|---|
| Well differentiated | | | | |
| Low grade | G1 | <2/10 high-power fields | AND | <3% |
| Intermediate grade | G2 | 2–20/10 high-power fields | OR | 3%–20% |
| Poorly differentiated | | | | |
| High grade | G3 | >20/10 high-power fields | OR | >20% |

and contour, chromatin pattern, nucleolar prominence, mitotic activity, and the presence, or absence, of necrosis. Endocrine neoplasms of the colorectum are classified as well-differentiated and poorly differentiated tumors based on a combination of mitotic activity and immunohistochemical labeling with Ki-67 (Table 7.2). Well-differentiated tumors contain neoplastic cells that bear a close resemblance to normal endocrine cells and encompass low- and intermediate-grade tumors. As a group, they show relatively little mitotic activity and a low proliferation rate with no or minimal necrosis. Poorly differentiated tumors show high-grade cytologic features, including irregular nuclei with coarse or vesicular chromatin, numerous mitotic figures, high proliferation rates, and frequent necrosis. They show high Ki-67 labeling indices, often in excess of 50%.

## Well-Differentiated (Neuro)Endocrine Tumors of the Colorectum

Well-differentiated endocrine tumors of the abdominal colon are rare, accounting for less than 1% of all colonic tumors and less than 10% of GI endocrine tumors. Most are considered to be biologically aggressive. Approximately 5% are associated with the carcinoid syndrome, and two-thirds are metastatic at the time of diagnosis. Five-year survival rates range from 70% for localized disease to 25% for disease associated with distant spread. Rectal endocrine tumors account for approximately 17% of GI endocrine tumors and show a low propensity for lymph node metastases and distant spread. The overall 5-year survival is approximately 72%. Superficial small tumors are usually treated adequately by polypectomy alone, but adverse prognostic factors, including size greater than 2 cm, necrosis, and invasion of the muscularis propria, should prompt more extensive resection. Pathologic stage of endocrine tumors is assigned using the *AJCC Cancer Staging Manual*, seventh edition.[1]

Well-differentiated endocrine tumors of the colorectum tend to appear as yellow, or tan, submucosal nodules, although those that produce serotonin may be associated with dense fibrosis in the bowel wall and/or mesentery, resulting in luminal narrowing. Endocrine tumors of the GI tract show a variety of histologic growth patterns that reflect, in part, their derivation from the embryologic foregut, midgut, and hindgut. Foregut tumors commonly contain well-formed glands or acini, whereas midgut tumors display a nested growth pattern, and hindgut tumors are composed of nests and ribbon-like cords of neoplastic cells. Although these growth patterns formed the basis for early classification schemes, they are not entirely specific and one may frequently observe multiple growth patterns within the same tumor, or in different tumors of the same anatomic region. Tumor morphology is less important than tumor grade in predicting biologic potential.

Colonic endocrine tumors are considered to be of midgut origin and display a nested growth pattern. Rectal endocrine tumors are derived from the hindgut and often composed of L cells. They contain small nests and ribbon-like cords of neoplastic cells. Both low- and intermediate-grade tumors typically contain cells with abundant cytoplasm, stippled nuclear chromatin, and small but conspicuous nucleoli. Some tumor cells may contain abundant clear, or eosinophilic, cytoplasm or show degenerative cytologic atypia with multinucleated tumor cells and intranuclear inclusions, but none of these features is predictive of biologic behavior. Low-grade tumors show minimal cytologic atypia without appreciable mitotic activity and no necrosis. Tumor cells have round, smooth nuclei with stippled chromatin and inconspicuous nucleoli (Figure 7.17A). Intermediate-grade tumors contain crowded cells with slight nuclear enlargement and hyperchromasia, as well as scattered mitotic figures (Figure 7.17B). Immunohistochemical stains directed against Ki-67 are used to distinguish between low- and intermediate-grade tumors. Low-grade lesions display a Ki-67 labeling index of less than 2%, whereas intermediate-grade lesions show nuclear staining in 2% to 20% of tumor cells. Labeling indices between 2% and 20% may be associated with biologically aggressive behavior, even if the cytologic features within the tumor are low-grade.

## (Poorly Differentiated) High-Grade (Neuro)Endocrine Carcinoma

High-grade endocrine carcinomas of the colorectum account for less than 1% of all colorectal carcinomas and are classified as small cell and non–small cell carcinomas. Small cell carcinomas tend to be more common in sites normally surfaced by squamous mucosa, namely, the esophagus and anus, whereas non–small cell variants arise from sites with glandular mucosa. Both tumor types pursue an aggressive course with a mean survival of approximately 10 months and 2-year survival of 25%.[26,27] High-grade endocrine carcinomas may be treated using a small cell carcinoma protocol in some institutions, and thus, their recognition is clinically important. These lesions were largely considered to be MSS in the past; however, recent data suggest that up to

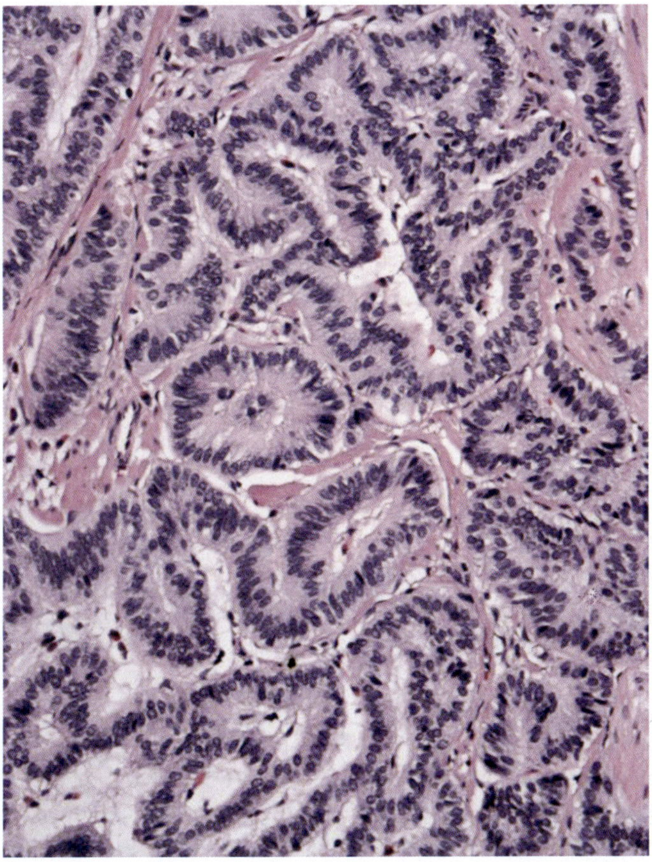

A

FIGURE 7.17: Low-grade well-differentiated rectal endocrine tumors contain ribbons and cords of tumor cells with variably hyalinized stroma. The tumor cells are monotonous with round, or ovoid, nuclei; inconspicuous nucleoli; and negligible mitotic activity (A).

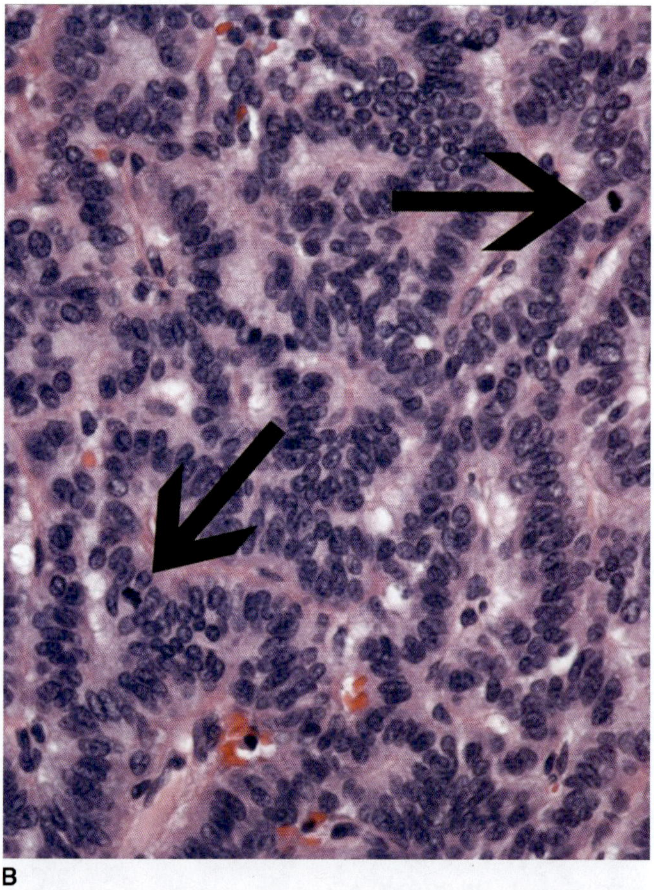


**FIGURE 7.17:** (*Continued*) Intermediate-grade well-differentiated tumors show a similar growth pattern, but the nuclei are larger and crowded (**B**). They contain coarse chromatin with irregular membranes, occasional nucleoli, and readily identifiable mitotic figures (*arrows*).

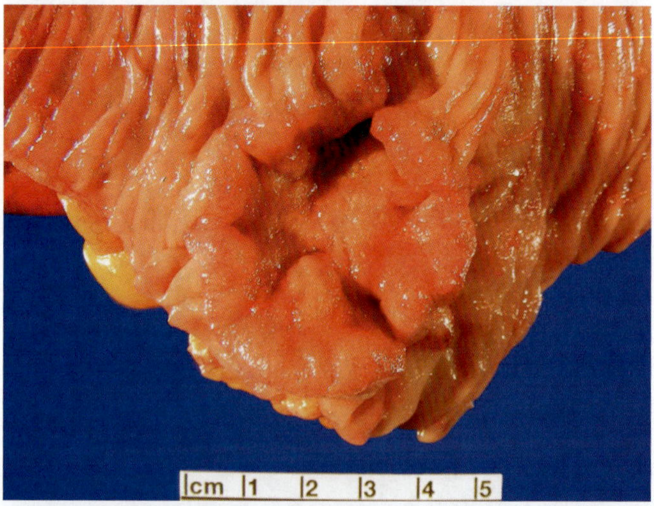


**FIGURE 7.18:** A high-grade (neuro) endocrine carcinoma of the proximal colon forms an ulcerated mass with rolled borders that is grossly similar to conventional adenocarcinoma. This tumor was associated with numerous metastatic deposits in regional lymph nodes at the time of surgery, and the patient developed hepatic metastases within 6 months of presentation.

15% show MSI-H and DNA hypermethylation.[28,29] High-grade endocrine carcinomas have not been reported in association with Lynch syndrome.

High-grade endocrine tumors are often large, bulky tumors that are advanced at the time of diagnosis (Figure 7.18). Small cell carcinomas share considerable morphologic overlap with their pulmonary counterparts and comprise small to medium-sized cells with scant cytoplasm and brisk mitotic activity. The tumor cell nuclei are angulated with coarse chromatin, inconspicuous

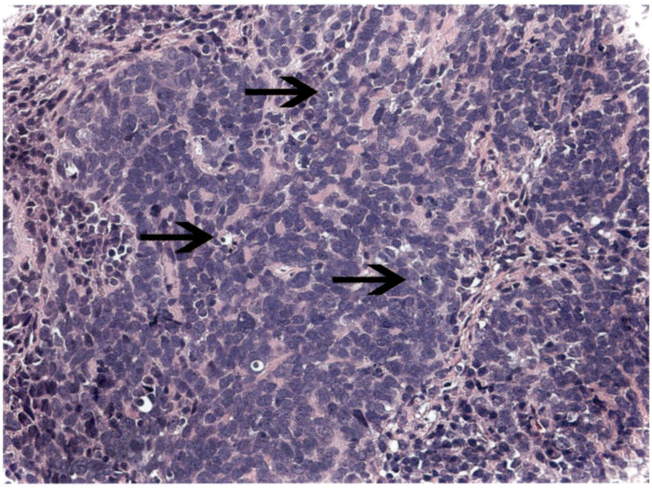

FIGURE 7.19: High-grade (neuro)endocrine carcinoma of the anorectum resembles pulmonary small cell carcinoma. The tumor is composed of sheets of cells with large, irregular nuclei and scant cytoplasm. The nuclei contain coarse chromatic with inconspicuous nucleoli. Apoptotic debris is readily apparent (*arrows*).

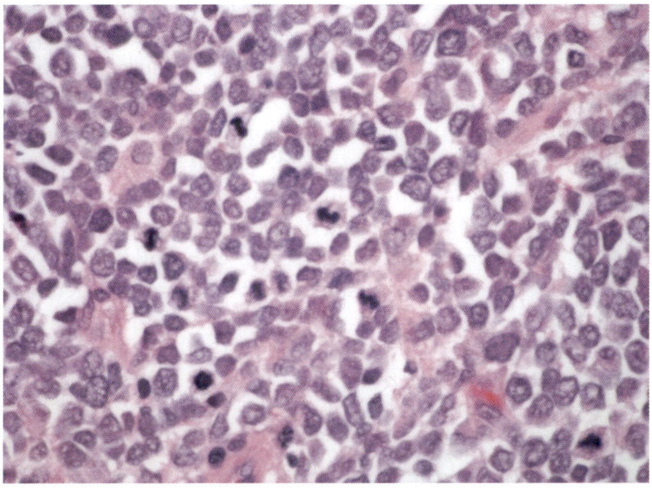

FIGURE 7.20: High-grade (neuro)endocrine carcinomas of the colorectum usually contain intermediate-to-large cells with eosinophilic cytoplasm. The nuclei display open chromatin and prominent nucleoli. Numerous mitotic figures are present.

nucleoli, and readily apparent apoptotic debris (Figure 7.19). Approximately 25% of cases are associated with an adenocarcinoma when occurring in the colorectum, whereas tumors of the anal canal may contain areas of squamous cell carcinoma. Similar to small cell carcinomas that arise elsewhere, most tumors of the colorectum express at least one endocrine marker (e.g., synaptophysin, CD56, and chromogranin) as well as dot-like staining for keratin. Approximately 20% of tumors show nuclear CDX-2 staining. Small cell carcinomas of the colorectum may also display strong nuclear staining for TTF-1, so positivity for this marker should not lead one to conclude that an endocrine carcinoma in the colorectum represents a metastasis.[30]

Non–small cell endocrine carcinomas contain appreciable eosinophilic cytoplasm with brisk mitotic activity and are subclassified as large and intermediate cell types based on tumor cell size. Tumor cells are arranged in a diffuse growth pattern, organoid nests, trabeculae, and rosettes and commonly display areas of squamous and/or glandular differentiation.[26] Most arise de novo or contain areas of adenocarcinoma, but are not derived from preexisting well-differentiated endocrine tumors. Tumor cells harbor intermediate-to-large nuclei with open chromatin and prominent nuclei (Figure 7.20). They express endocrine markers and show variable staining for other colorectal cancer markers, such as cytokeratin 20 and CDX-2. Coexpression of cytokeratins 7 and 20 occurs in a minority of cases.[29]

### Mixed Adenoneuroendocrine Carcinoma

Some colorectal carcinomas contain substantial amounts of high-grade endocrine and glandular elements. Carcinomas that display overtly malignant endocrine and glandular differentiation, each of which account for at least 30% of the tumor volume, are classified as mixed adenoneuroendocrine carcinomas by the WHO.[30] However, this designation should only be applied to carcinomas that show morphologically evident endocrine differentiation that is confirmed by immunohistochemical stains. It should not be used to denote conventional adenocarcinomas with immunopositivity for endocrine markers, since immunopositivity for chromogranin, synaptophysin, or neuron-specific enolase occurs in approximately 40% of colorectal adenocarcinomas without morphologic evidence of endocrine differentiation.[31] Mixed adenoneuroendocrine should not be applied to early adenocarcinomas that contain occasional nests of low-grade–appearing endocrine cells.[32]

## SUMMARY

More than 90% of colorectal carcinomas are gland-forming adenocarcinomas with an intestinal phenotype. However, several other morphologic variants exist, and these are important to recognize for a variety of reasons. Some tumor types are frequently associated with underlying MSI-H, which may imply the presence of a cancer syndrome in some cases or influence decisions regarding adjuvant therapy in other instances. Other variants, such as micropapillary carcinoma and signet ring cell carcinoma, are defined as high-grade neoplasms at risk for biologically aggressive behavior. GI endocrine tumors represent a morphologically and biologically heterogeneous group of tumors that have, until recently, been poorly characterized. Recent advances in our understanding of their pathogenesis have led to recommendations regarding pathology reporting of these lesions. Required information for pathology reporting of endocrine tumors includes tumor site and type of procedure, tumor stage and grade, adequacy of resection, and Ki-67 labeling indices. Other variables, such as tumor stage and prognostically important stage-independent factors, are discussed in Chapters 8 and 9.

# References


1. Neuroendocrine tumors. In: Edge S, Byrd D, Compton CC, et al., eds. *AJCC Cancer Staging Manual*. 7th ed. New York, NY: Springer; 2009:181–189.
2. Su MC, Yuan RH, Lin CY, et al. Cadherin-17 is a useful diagnostic marker for adenocarcinomas of the digestive system. *Mod Pathol* 2008;21(11):1379–1386.
3. Xu F, Xu J, Lou Z, et al. Micropapillary component in colorectal carcinoma is associated with lymph node metastasis in T1 and T2 stages and decreased survival time in TNM stages I and II. *Am J Surg Pathol* 2009;33(9):1287–1292.
4. Lino-Silva LS, Hernandez RA, Caro-Sanchez CH. Colonic micropapillary carcinoma, a recently recognized subtype associated with histologic adverse factors. Clinicopathologic analysis of 15 cases. *Colorectal Dis* 2012;14(9):e567–e572.
5. Verdu M, Roman R, Calvo M, et al. Clinicopathological and molecular characterization of colorectal micropapillary carcinoma. *Mod Pathol* 2011;24(5):729–738.
6. Ohtsuki Y, Kuroda N, Umeoka T, et al. KL-6 is another useful marker in assessing a micropapillary pattern in carcinomas of the breast and urinary bladder, but not the colon. *Med Mol Morphol* 2009;42(2):123–127.
7. Hamilton SR, Bosman FT, Boffetta P, et al. Tumors of the colon and rectum. In: Bosman FT, Carneiro F, Hruban RH, et al., eds. *WHO Classification of Tumours of the Digestive System*. 4th ed. Lyon, France: International Agency for Research on Cancer; 2010:134–146.

8. Chirieac LR, Shen L, Catalano PJ, et al. Phenotype of microsatellite-stable colorectal carcinomas with CpG island methylation. *Am J Surg Pathol* 2005;29(4):429–436.
9. Tuppurainen K, Makinen JM, Junttila O, et al. Morphology and microsatellite instability in sporadic serrated and non-serrated colorectal cancer. *J Pathol* 2005;207(3):285–294.
10. Schaffzin DM, Stahl TJ, Smith LE. Perianal mucinous adenocarcinoma: unusual case presentations and review of the literature. *Am Surg* 2003;69(2):166–169.
11. Sung CO, Seo JW, Kim KM, et al. Clinical significance of signet-ring cells in colorectal mucinous adenocarcinoma. *Mod Pathol* 2008;21(12):1533–1541.
12. Yantiss RK, Goodarzi M, Zhou XK, et al. Clinical, pathologic, and molecular features of early-onset colorectal carcinoma. *Am J Surg Pathol* 2009;33(4):572–582.
13. Leopoldo S, Lorena B, Cinzia A, et al. Two subtypes of mucinous adenocarcinoma of the colorectum: clinicopathological and genetic features. *Ann Surg Oncol* 2008;15(5):1429–1439.
14. Vakiani E, Shia J, Dhall J, et al. Prognostic significance of morphologic features in mucinous colorectal carcinomas. *Lab Invest* 2008;88:138A.
15. Palascak-Juif V, Bouvier AM, Cosnes J, et al. Small bowel adenocarcinoma in patients with Crohn's disease compared with small bowel adenocarcinoma de novo. *Inflamm Bowel Dis* 2005;11(9):828–832.
16. Wachtel MS, Haynes AL III, Griswold JA. Signet ring, high grade, and undifferentiated colorectal adenocarcinomas differ. *J Surg Res* 2010;163(2):250–256.
17. Chang DT, Pai RK, Rybicki LA, et al. Clinicopathologic and molecular features of sporadic early-onset colorectal adenocarcinoma: an adenocarcinoma with frequent signet ring cell differentiation, rectal and sigmoid involvement, and adverse morphologic features. *Mod Pathol* 2012;25(8):1128–1139.
18. Tung SY, Wu CS, Chen PC. Primary signet ring cell carcinoma of colorectum: an age- and sex-matched controlled study. *Am J Gastroenterol* 1996;91(10):2195–2199.
19. Makino T, Tsujinaka T, Mishima H, et al. Primary signet-ring cell carcinoma of the colon and rectum: report of eight cases and review of 154 Japanese cases. *Hepatogastroenterology* 2006;53(72):845–849.
20. Kakar S, Smyrk TC. Signet ring cell carcinoma of the colorectum: correlations between microsatellite instability, clinicopathologic features and survival. *Mod Pathol* 2005;18(2):244–249.
21. Alexander J, Watanabe T, Wu TT, et al. Histopathological identification of colon cancer with microsatellite instability. *Am J Pathol* 2001;158(2):527–535.
22. Thirunavukarasu P, Sathaiah M, Singla S, et al. Medullary carcinoma of the large intestine: a population based analysis. *Int J Oncol* 2010;37(4):901–907.
23. Lanza G, Gafa R, Matteuzzi M, et al. Medullary-type poorly differentiated adenocarcinoma of the large bowel: a distinct clinicopathologic entity characterized by microsatellite instability and improved survival. *J Clin Oncol* 1999;17(8):2429–2438.
24. Ruschoff J, Dietmaier W, Luttges J, et al. Poorly differentiated colonic adenocarcinoma, medullary type: clinical, phenotypic, and molecular characteristics. *Am J Pathol* 1997;150(5):1815–1825.
25. Pearse AG, Polak JM. Neural crest origin of the endocrine polypeptide (APUD) cells of the gastrointestinal tract and pancreas. *Gut* 1971;12(10):783–788.
26. Shia J, Tang LH, Weiser MR, et al. Is non-small cell type high-grade neuroendocrine carcinoma of the tubular gastrointestinal tract a distinct disease entity? *Am J Surg Pathol* 2008;32(5):719–731.
27. Bernick PE, Klimstra DS, Shia J, et al. Neuroendocrine carcinomas of the colon and rectum. *Dis Colon Rectum* 2004;47(2):163–169.
28. Stelow EB, Moskaluk CA, Mills SE. The mismatch repair protein status of colorectal small cell neuroendocrine carcinomas. *Am J Surg Pathol* 2006;30(11):1401–1404.
29. La Rosa S, Marando A, Furlan D, et al. Colorectal poorly differentiated neuroendocrine carcinomas and mixed adenoneuroendocrine carcinomas: insights into the diagnostic immunophenotype, assessment of methylation profile, and search for prognostic markers. *Am J Surg Pathol* 2012;36(4):601–611.
30. Klimstra DS, Arnold R, Capella C, et al. Neuroendocrine neoplasms of the colon and rectum. In: Bosman FT, Carneiro F, Hruban RH, et al., eds. *WHO Classification of Tumours of the Digestive System*. 4th ed. Lyon, France: International Agency for Research on Cancer; 2010:174–177.
31. Yao GY, Zhou JL, Lai MD, et al. Neuroendocrine markers in adenocarcinomas: an investigation of 356 cases. *World J Gastroenterol* 2003;9(4):858–861.
32. Pulitzer M, Xu R, Suriawinata AA, et al. Microcarcinoids in large intestinal adenomas. *Am J Surg Pathol* 2006;30(12):1531–1536.

# 8 Pathologic Staging Issues: Implementation of the TNM Staging System

Rhonda K. Yantiss

Tumor stage is the single most powerful predictor of outcome among colorectal cancer patients and is determined by assessment of three parameters: local extent of the primary tumor, regional lymph node metastases, and distant metastases.[1] The TNM (*t*umor, lymph *n*odes, *m*etastasis) staging system for colorectal carcinoma is endorsed by the American Joint Committee on Cancer (AJCC) and Union for International Cancer Control and routinely used in the United States and Europe.[2] Unlike prior staging systems, this classification scheme provides pathologists, clinicians, and radiologists with a common language for uniform reporting of cancer stage and is continually updated as new elements prove to be of prognostic and/or therapeutic importance. Recent changes to pathologic stage assessment of colorectal carcinoma have been incorporated into the AJCC/TNM seventh edition *Cancer Staging Manual* and embraced by the College of American Pathologists (CAP), although definitional criteria for many elements are poorly reproducible and pathologists apply them in inconsistently.[3] The purpose of this chapter is to discuss some of the diagnostic problems encountered when applying staging criteria enumerated in the AJCC/TNM seventh edition *Cancer Staging Manual* to surgical pathology specimens.

## TNM DESCRIPTORS

Patients with colorectal carcinoma routinely undergo clinical staging prior to definitive surgical therapy. Clinical stage assignment is based on a combination of parameters including physical examination, endoscopic findings, and results of imaging studies. The clinical classification (cTNM) may differ from the final pathologic classification (pTNM) due to a variety of factors. Clinical stage is higher among patients in whom complete pathologic classification is not possible, such as individuals who have nonsurgical metastatic disease. Patients who receive neoadjuvant therapy for advanced cancers are assigned a clinical stage prior to initiation of treatment that is generally higher than the pathologic stage, which is assigned following surgical resection of a cancer that frequently shows some degree of regression. Alternatively, some patients are assigned a higher pathologic than clinical stage because their resection specimens contain more extensive disease than is clinically suspected prior to surgery. In these situations, the highest stage classification is used for final stage grouping.

The TNM stage assignment is subject to additional prefixes and suffixes in special situations. Stage is qualified by a "y" prefix (ypTNM) to denote cases in which classification is performed following neoadjuvant chemotherapy, radiotherapy, or both. This is particularly common among individuals with rectal tumors because most patients with advanced rectal cancer receive some form of therapy prior to definitive surgical resection. The "r" prefix (rpTNM) is used less frequently but identifies tumors that recur following a disease-free interval. Recurrent carcinomas that develop at a surgical anastomosis are, by convention, assigned to the proximal colonic segment and restaged. If the proximal segment is the small intestine, then the tumor is designated based upon the colonic or rectal portion of the anastomosis, as appropriate. Cancers that are classified at the time of autopsy are denoted with an "a" prefix (apTNM). The "m" suffix indicates the presence of multiple primary tumors at a single site (pTmNM). Pathologic stage is assigned based on extent of the most advanced carcinoma when multiple tumors are present.

## LOCAL EXTENT OF DISEASE (TUMOR STAGE)

The designation for pathologic tumor stage (pT) describes the deepest point of tumor penetration in the colonic wall. Colorectal epithelial neoplasms are assigned pathologic stages pTis, pT1, pT2, pT3, and pT4, as described below.

### Tumor Limited to the Muscularis Mucosae (pTis)

Cytologically malignant epithelial cell proliferations that are limited to the colorectal mucosa are classified as carcinomas in situ and assigned the pTis designation. However, both "carcinoma in situ" and pTis are generally avoided in routine practice because these terms apply to two different situations, are potentially confusing to treating clinicians, and may result in overly aggressive management. The pTis grouping includes intraepithelial carcinoma, as defined by an architecturally complex proliferation of neoplastic epithelial cells with malignant cytologic features (e.g., loss of polarization, nucleomegaly, macronucleoli, cellular necrosis, typical and atypical mitotic figures) that does not transgress the basement membrane (Figure 8.1). Carcinoma in situ (pTis) is also used to describe intramucosal carcinomas that breach the basement membrane

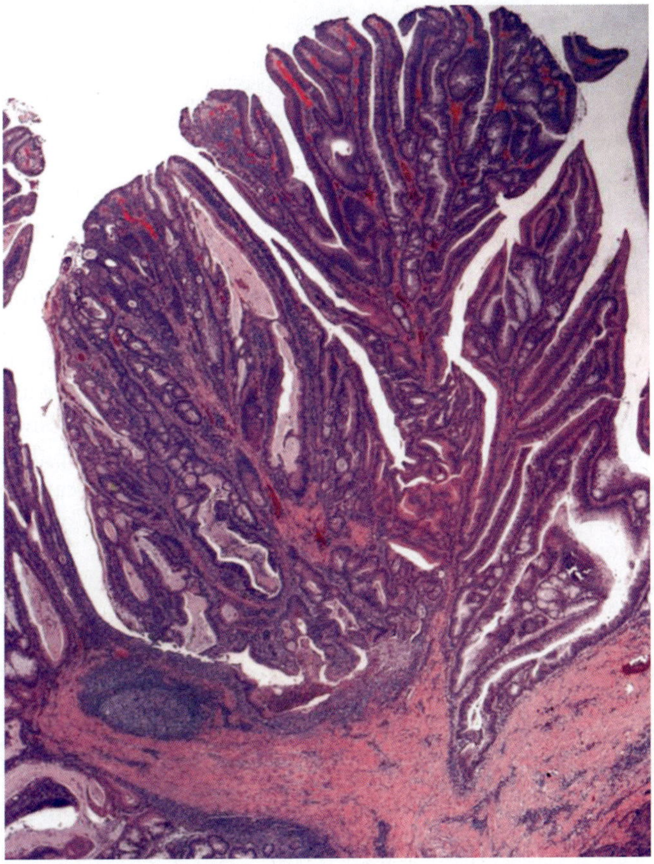

A

FIGURE 8.1: High-grade dysplasia (intraepithelial carcinoma) displays both architectural and cytologic atypia. Neoplastic epithelial cells are arranged in expansile aggregates of fused, cribriform glands (**A**).

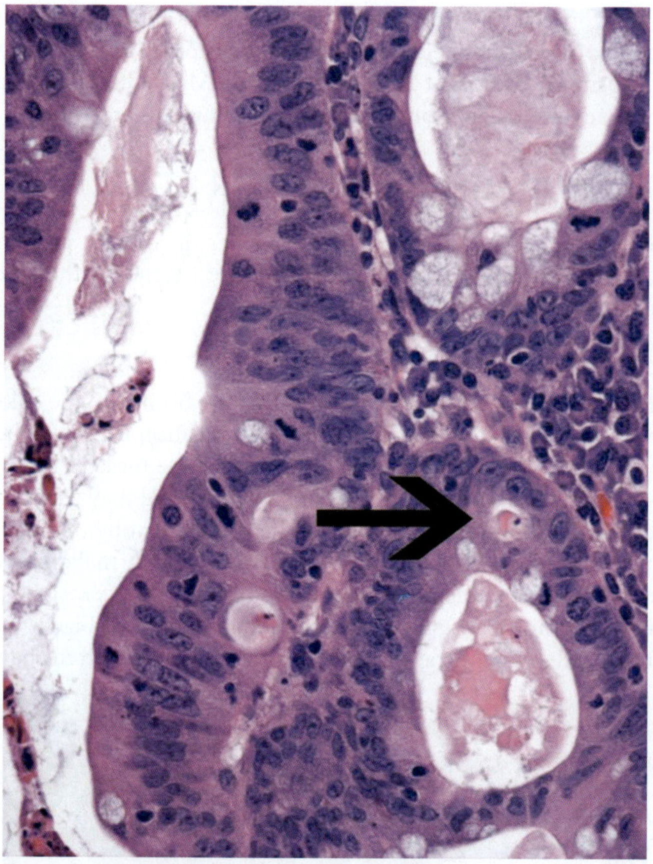
B

FIGURE 8.1: (*Continued*) The cells show loss of polarity and necrosis (*arrow*) but are limited by the basement membrane. They contain enlarged, hyperchromatic nuclei with easily identifiable mitotic figures (**B**).

and extend into the lamina propria or muscularis mucosae but do not invade the submucosa (Figure 8.2A). Intramucosal carcinomas consist of irregular clusters and nests of tumor cells that do not evoke a desmoplastic stromal response (Figure 8.2B). Neither intraepithelial nor intramucosal carcinoma has potential to metastasize, yet some clinicians may be alarmed by usage of the "carcinoma" terminology and be tempted to treat such lesions aggressively. For this reason, the World Health Organization has proposed alternative terms "intraepithelial neoplasia" and "intramucosal neoplasia" to denote intraepithelial and intramucosal carcinoma, respectively.[4] This suggestion has met with limited success. "Intraepithelial neoplasia" and "intramucosal neoplasia" are not commonly used as diagnostic terms in the United States. "High-grade dysplasia" is a more widely accepted term than either "intraepithelial carcinoma" or "intraepithelial neoplasia," and "intramucosal carcinoma" seems to be preferred over "intramucosal neoplasia."

## Tumor Invasive of, but Limited to, the Submucosa (pT1)

Most invasive colorectal adenocarcinomas limited to the submucosa (pT1) are detected in polypectomy specimens since these tumors are typically asymptomatic and identified during screening or surveillance colonoscopy. Invasive adenocarcinomas grow in an expansile, infiltrative pattern and are not accompanied by lamina propria tissue (Figure 8.3A). Invasion of the submucosa incites a desmoplastic stromal response in close proximity to malignant-appearing epithelial cells that display nuclear pleomorphism, nuclear membrane irregularities, and clumped chromatin (Figure 8.3B). Prior studies have shown that carcinomas arising in pedunculated adenomas may be adequately treated with polypectomy alone, provided the invasive carcinoma is low grade, lacks vascular invasion, and is

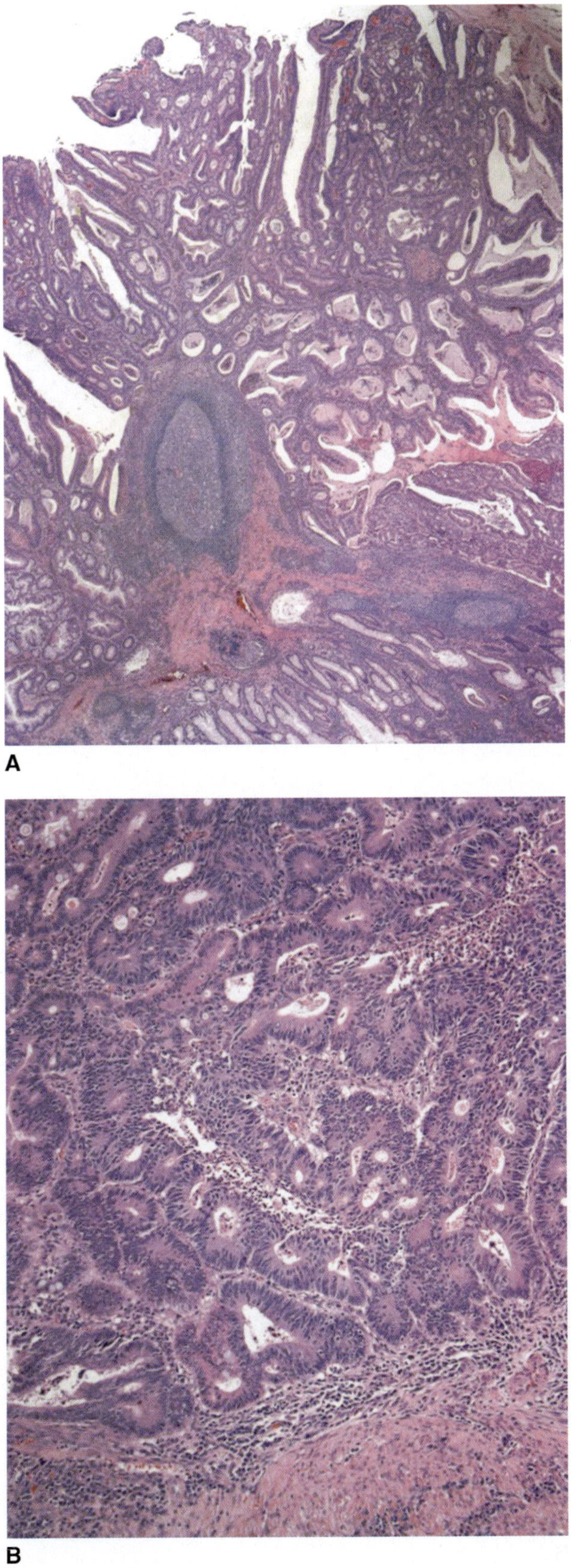

FIGURE 8.2: Intramucosal carcinomas show expansile growth in the lamina propria (**A**). The cytologic features are overtly malignant and include loss of cell polarity, increased nuclear size, hyperchromasia, mitotic activity, necrosis, and nucleolar prominence (**B**). The tumor cells do not elicit desmoplasia and are clearly limited by the muscularis mucosae (**bottom**).

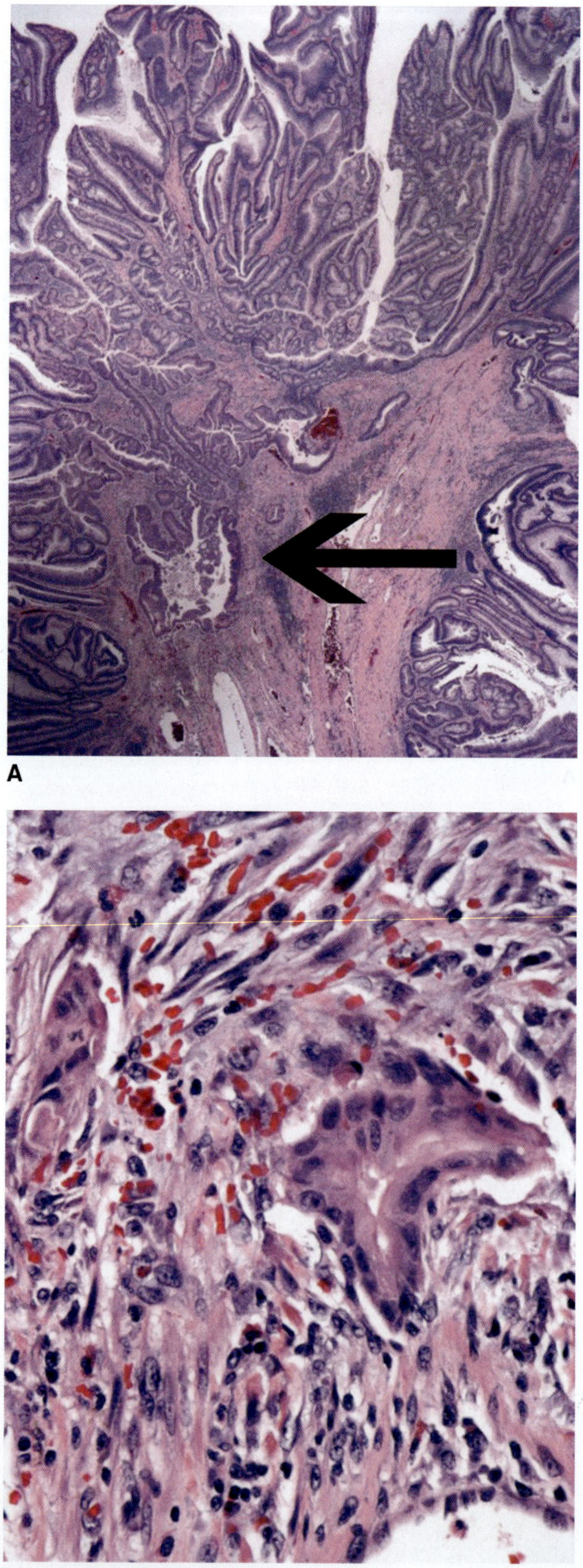

**FIGURE 8.3:** Invasive adenocarcinomas (*arrow*) are expansile tumors composed of irregularly distributed glands with an ill-defined advancing edge in the submucosa (**A**). Malignant glands are associated with desmoplastic stroma (**B**).

present at least 1 mm from the cauterized base of the polyp.[5–7] At a minimum, these three criteria should be incorporated in the final pathology report for all carcinomas present in polypectomy specimens. Other key components of the pathology report include anatomic location of the tumor, tumor size (invasive component), tumor budding, and distance of the tumor to the resection margin.

## Tumor Invasive of, but Limited to, the Muscularis Propria (pT2)

Colorectal carcinomas that invade into, but are limited to, the muscularis propria are assigned a pT2 pathologic stage, even if they are separated from the pericolic fat by as little as a single layer of smooth muscle cells (Figure 8.4). Recognition of muscularis propria invasion is generally straightforward, although problems may arise when assessing tumors that develop in colonic segments affected by diverticulosis. In this situation, herniations of mucosa through the colonic wall can be colonized by cancer cells (pT1) and simulate the appearance of a more advanced tumor in the muscularis propria or pericolic fat.

## Tumor Invasive of Pericolic or Perirectal Soft Tissue (pT3)

The absence of muscularis propria smooth muscle cells between the leading edge of the tumor and the pericolic fat represents the minimum criterion for pT3 classification (Figure 8.5). Some investigators suggest that cancers in the pericolic fat should be subclassified based upon their depth of invasion beyond the muscularis propria. Proposed schemes separate carcinomas invasive of pericolorectal soft tissue into four categories: pT3a (<1 mm beyond muscularis propria), pT3b (1 to 5 mm beyond muscularis propria), pT3c (>5 to 15 mm beyond muscularis propria), and pT3d (>15 mm beyond muscularis propria).[8] Although the AJCC/TNM seventh edition *Cancer Staging Manual* does not subdivide the pT3 category, tumors that extend less than 5 mm beyond

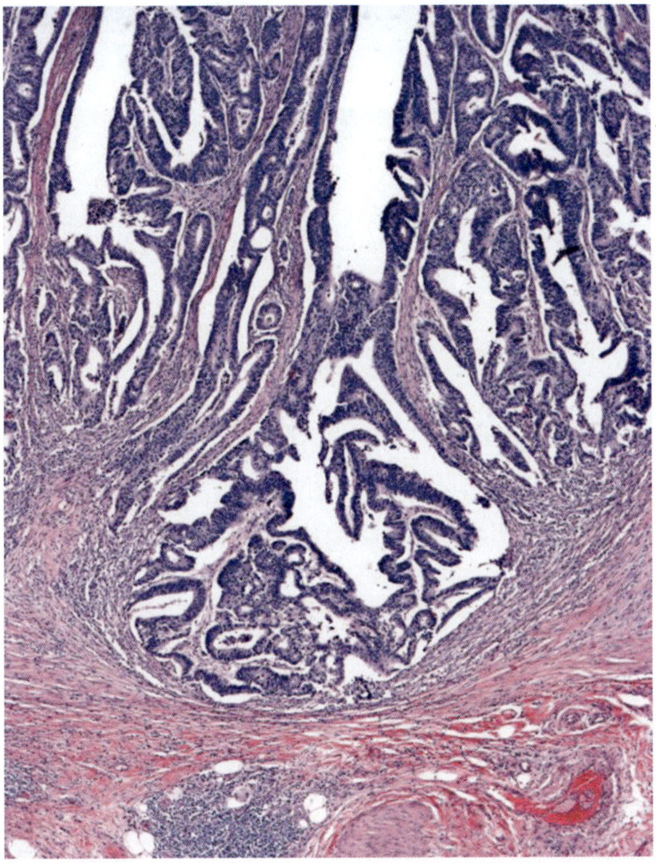

A

**FIGURE 8.4:** Tumors that invade the muscularis propria are staged as pT2 cancers (**A**).

**FIGURE 8.4:** (*Continued*) Carcinomas limited by a single layer of smooth muscle cells (*arrow*) are still staged in this category (**B**).

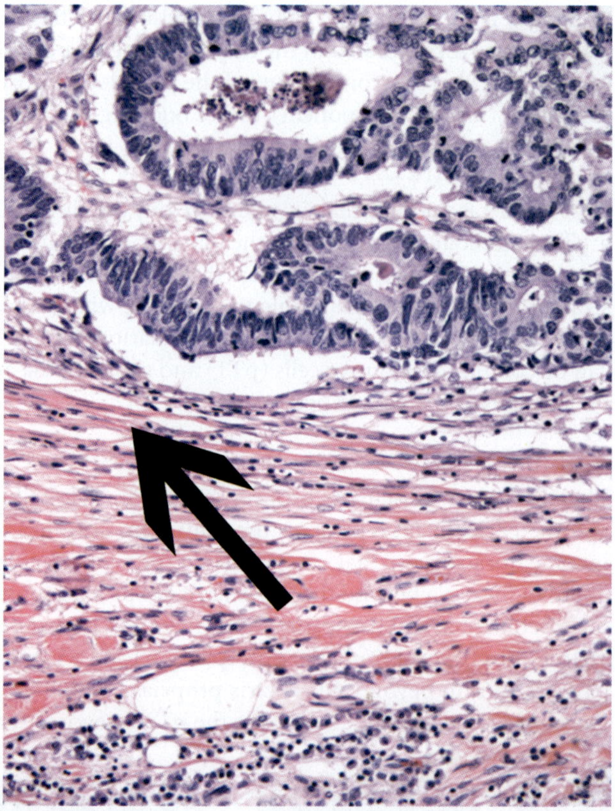

B

**FIGURE 8.5:** Colon cancers that extend through the muscularis propria into pericolic fact are designated as pT3 tumors.

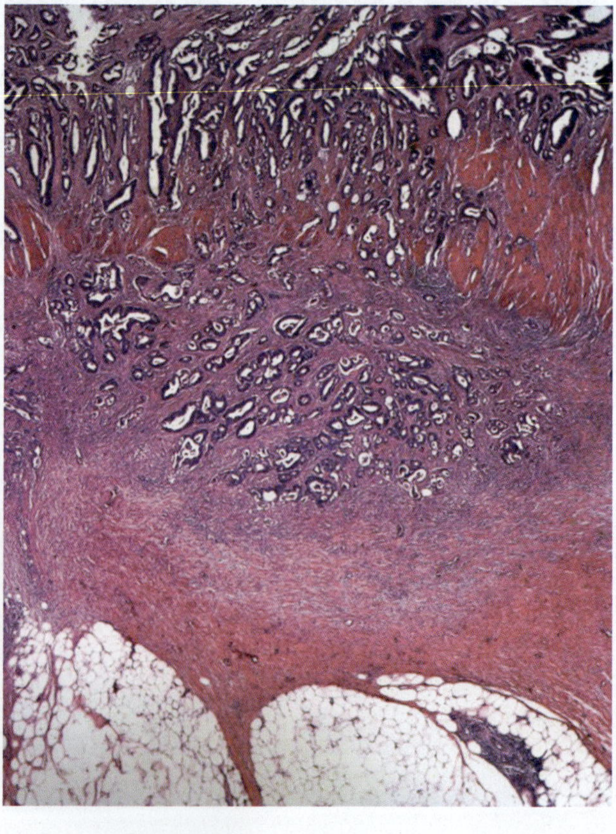

the muscularis propria are associated with a better prognosis than those that penetrate more deeply into the pericolic fat.[9] Thus, pathologists should assess extent of tumor beyond the muscularis propria and incorporate depth of invasion into the pathology report if possible.

## Tumor Penetrates the Peritoneum (pT4a) or Directly Invades Adjacent, Noncontiguous Structures (pT4b)

The most problematic aspect of pathologic tumor stage assignment is recognition of pT4 lesions. This group is subdivided in two categories: pT4a is defined as serosal penetration, whereas pT4b is defined as tumor that directly invades, or is adherent to, other organs or structures. The definitions for pT4a and pT4b in the AJCC/TNM seventh edition *Cancer Staging Manual* are different from those of prior AJCC/TNM staging systems, which defined pT4a as direct tumor extension into another organ and pT4b as serosal penetration.[10] Serosal penetration (pT4a) should be suspected upon gross examination of surgical resection specimens and appears as puckered sclerotic area that may be associated with fibrinous adhesions (Figure 8.6). Its presence can be documented at the time of gross examination by scraping the serosal surface of the unopened colon with the edge of a glass slide and preparing a cytology smear from the resultant material (Figure 8.7). The AJCC/TNM seventh edition *Cancer Staging Manual* and the CAP define serosal penetration as

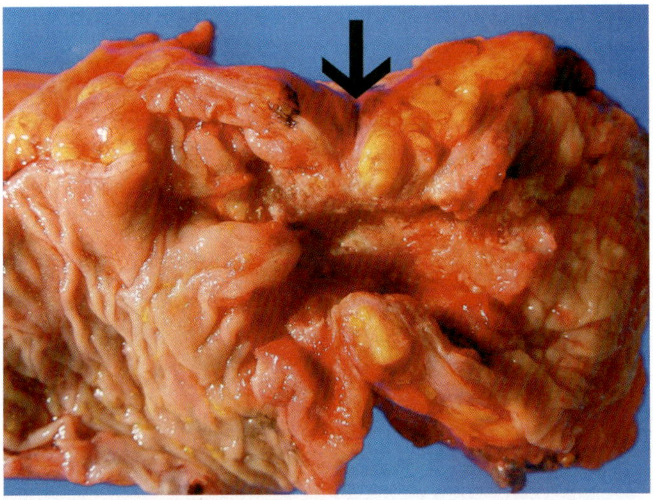

**FIGURE 8.6:** This cancer penetrates the serosa causing induration and a serosal "pucker" that appears as a *pale white* scar (*arrow*).

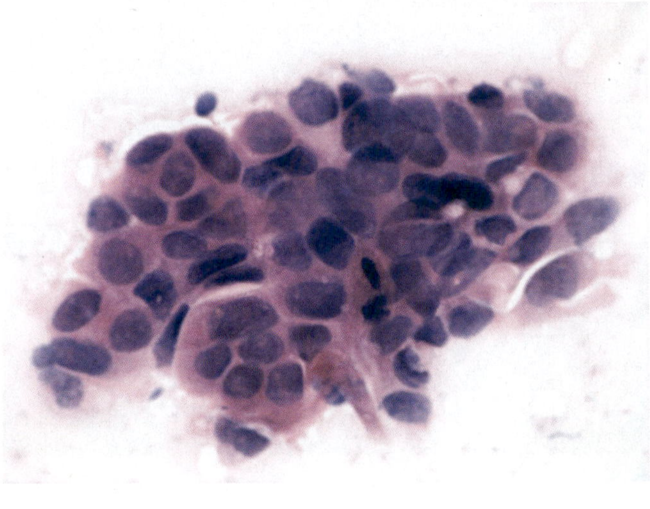

**FIGURE 8.7:** Pathologic stage assessment is augmented by cytologic evaluation. This cytology sample was prepared by scraping the serosal surface with a glass slide. It contains clusters of tumor cells with large, hyperchromatic nuclei; nuclear irregularities; prominent nucleoli; and mitotic figures.

either tumor cells present on the peritonealized surface of the abdominal colon or tumor cells present at the serosal surface in combination with mesothelial cell hyperplasia and/or an inflammatory reaction (Figures 8.8 and 8.9). However, many cancers that penetrate the peritoneal surface lack histologic criteria for definitive pT4a classification, even when there is ample evidence of a serosal perforation, such as a hole in the colon or free air under the diaphragm. Indeed, tumor cells less than 1 mm from a mesothelial reaction predict a similarly poor outcome to that associated with tumor cells on the serosal surface.[1,3,11] For this reason, many pathologists consider any one of the following three findings sufficient to categorize a tumor as pT4a: free tumor cells on the serosal surface, tumor cells present at the serosal surface accompanied by a mesothelial cell reaction, and tumor cells within 1 mm of the serosal surface associated with fibroinflammatory changes and mesothelial hyperplasia (Figure 8.10). Serosal penetration by colonic carcinoma should also be suspected when an exuberant fibroinflammatory response in the pericolic soft tissue surrounds cancers that have penetrated the muscularis propria. Neutrophil-rich peritumoral abscesses do not represent a host immune–mediated response to the cancer and typically imply the presence of tumor perforation (Figure 8.11). Their detection should prompt a careful search for other evidence of serosal penetration, including correlation with clinical findings and submission of additional sections, as necessary. Elastin stains may aid detection of peritoneal penetration by tumor cells in some cases. The normal abdominal colon contains a subserosal elastic lamina, but this layer of connective tissue is disrupted by deeply invasive colonic carcinomas.[12] Destruction of elastic fibers near the serosa is associated with increased risk of liver and peritoneal metastases as well as decreased overall survival.[13]

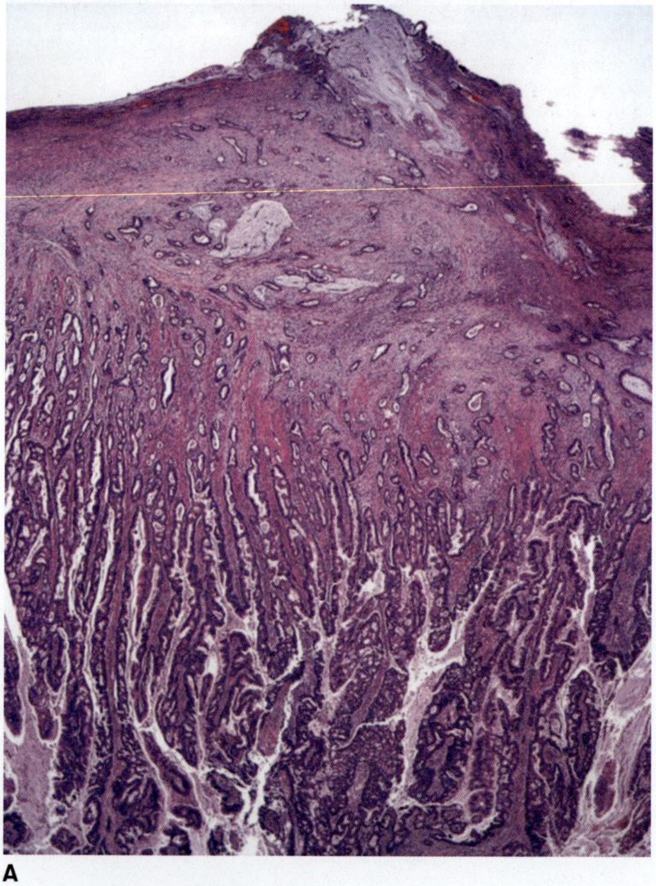

A

**FIGURE 8.8:** Peritoneal penetration (pT4a) is readily identified when tumor cells are present on the peritoneal surface (**A**),

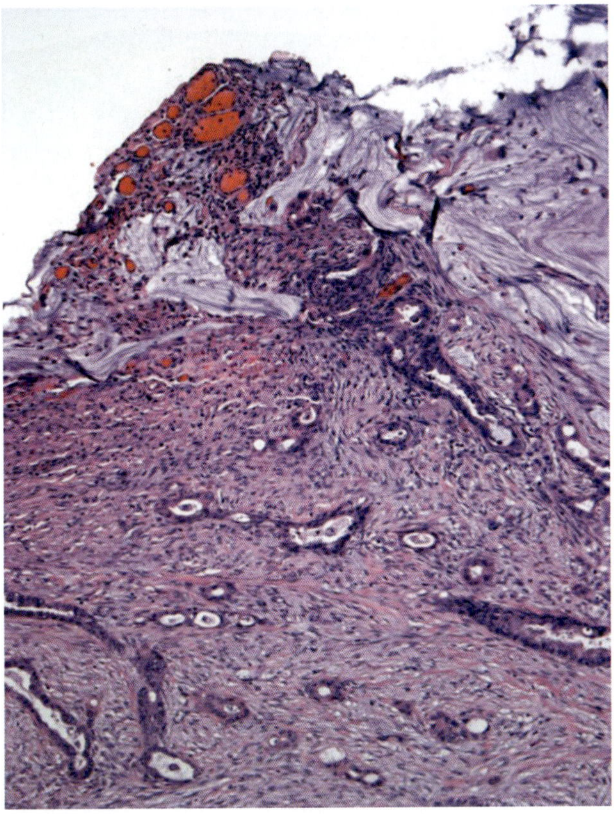

B

FIGURE 8.8: (*Continued*) although this is the least commonly observed finding among cancers that have transgressed the visceral peritoneum. Organizing mucus and tumor cells are associated with mesothelial cells and a fibroinflammatory tissue reaction (**B**).

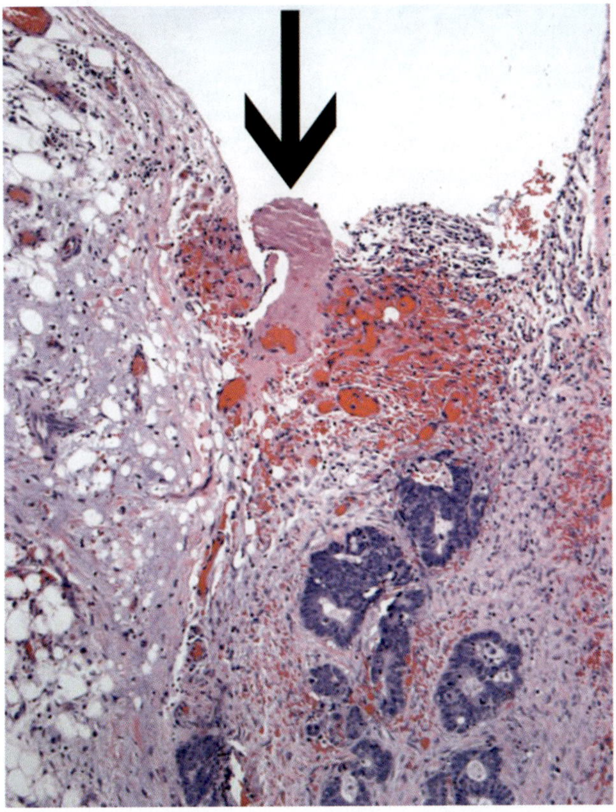

FIGURE 8.9: Tumors that penetrate the serosa elicit mesothelial hyperplasia and a fibroinflammatory response. Fibrin is present on the peritoneal surface (*arrow*).

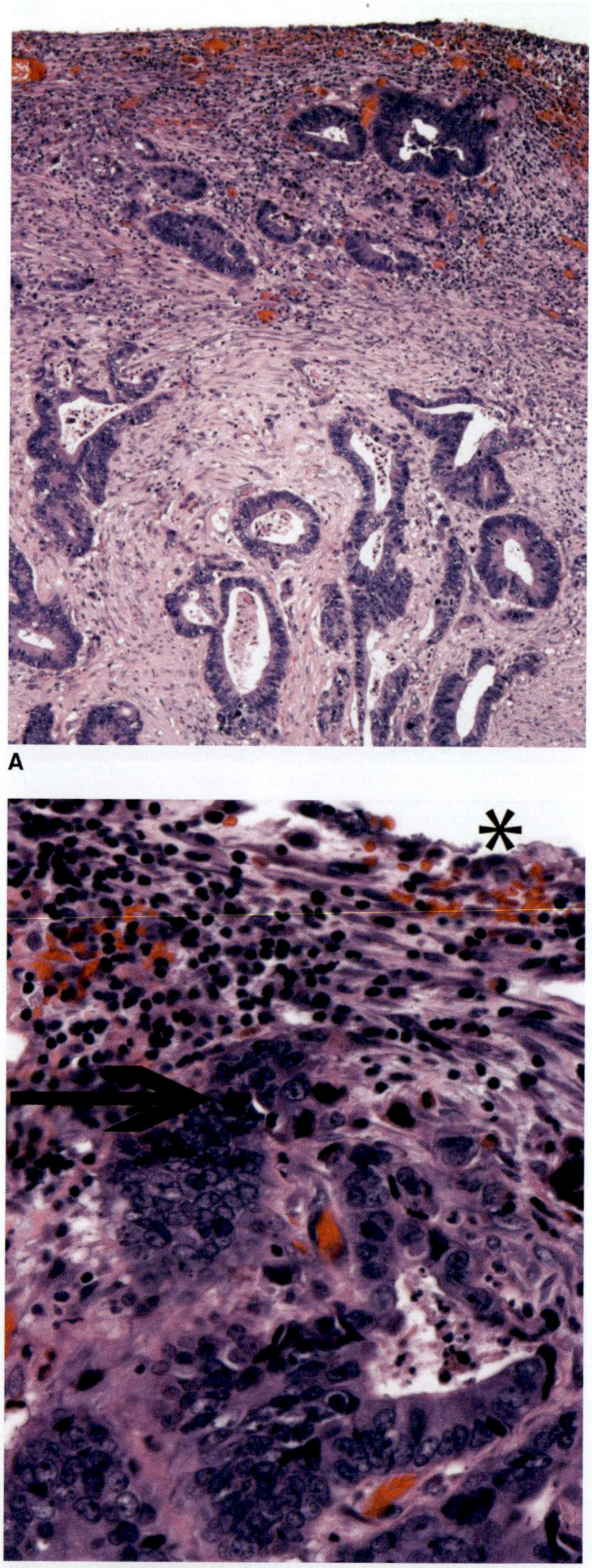

**FIGURE 8.10:** Cancers that penetrate the serosa commonly induce a granulation tissue–type reaction at the serosal surface (**A**). Mesothelial hyperplasia is present (*asterisk*) in close proximity to the tumor (*arrow*), although cancer is not identified on the serosa (**B**). The cytology smear prepared from a serosal scraping confirmed the presence of tumor cells on the serosa in this case.

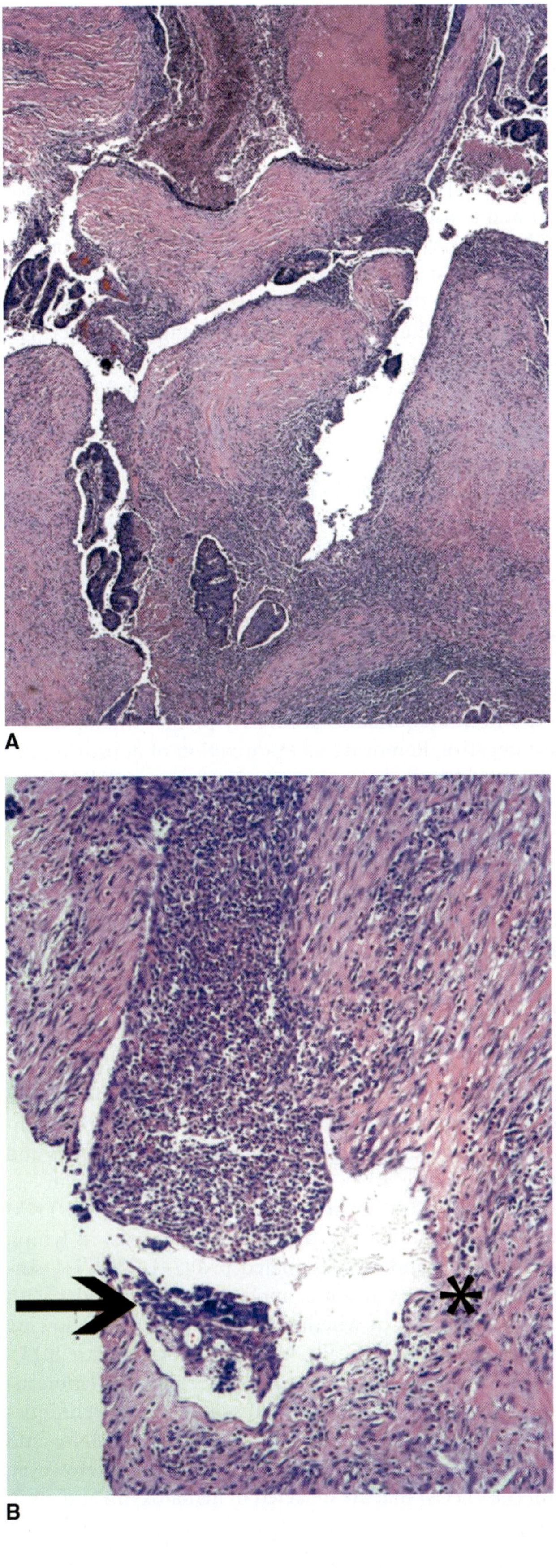


**FIGURE 8.11:** This perforated tumor was removed from a young woman who presented with an acute abdomen and feculent material in the peritoneal cavity. The tumor contained neutrophil-rich abscesses in pericolic fat (**A**). Careful examination of pericolic soft tissue revealed mesothelial cells (*asterisk*) associated with cancer (*arrow*) and an abscess (**B**).

Direct extension of colonic carcinoma into other organs is predicated by serosal penetration, so the AJCC/TNM seventh edition *Cancer Staging Manual* has designated the former with a higher pathologic stage (pT4b) than that of serosal involvement. The pT4b category should be assigned to colonic cancers that transgress the peritoneal surface and invade adjacent, noncontiguous organs or structures. Notably, tumor spread from the abdominal colon to a contiguous organ without serosal penetration (e.g., a cecal cancer that extends into the terminal ileum *via* the ileocecal valve) should not be designated as pT4b. Colon cancers that penetrate the serosa can induce adhesions between the tumor and a noncontiguous organ, such as another segment of the gastrointestinal tract, urinary bladder, or ovaries. In this situation, detection of tumor cells within the adhesion also results in a pT4b stage assignment, even if cancer is not detected in the adherent organ. Colonic carcinomas that penetrate the serosa and adhere to another organ, but do not show tumor cells in either the adhesion or the adherent organ, are staged as pT4a. The pT4a category does not apply to rectal carcinomas that lie entirely below the peritoneal reflection, although direct extension of these tumors into adjacent organs of the gynecologic and/or genitourinary tracts (pT4b) occurs in some cases.

## REGIONAL LYMPH NODE STAGING ISSUES

### Defining Regional Lymph Node Stage

Regional lymph nodes are staged as pN0, pN1, or pN2 and further subclassified depending upon the number involved by metastatic carcinoma, whereas nonregional lymph nodes that contain tumor deposits are staged as pM1 disease. All grossly negative, or equivocal, regional lymph nodes should be submitted entirely for pathologic evaluation, but representative sections of grossly positive lymph nodes are sufficient to document extent of disease. There is no universal agreement regarding the minimum number of lymph nodes required to accurately predict the likelihood that any unsampled lymph nodes are also negative. Removal and examination of approximately 12 to 15 negative lymph nodes is generally considered adequate for staging purposes.[14,15] If fewer than 12 lymph nodes are identified, additional sections of pericolorectal soft tissue should be submitted and visualizing techniques, such as use of clarifying solutions, may be considered.[16] Preoperatively treated rectal cancer resection specimens tend to contain smaller lymph nodes, but they still number between 30 and 60 in total mesorectal excision specimens.

The AJCC/TNM seventh edition *Cancer Staging Manual* subdivides regional lymph node status. Tumors without regional lymph node metastases are staged as pN0. Cases with regional lymph node metastases (pN1 and pN2) are further subclassified, such that N1a disease is defined as metastases present in one lymph node and pN1b denotes metastases in two to three lymph nodes. Higher stage nodal disease is also subdivided: pN2a denotes metastases in four to six lymph nodes and pN2b disease implies the presence of metastases in seven or more lymph nodes. The CAP recommends that tumor deposits spanning less than 2 mm in diameter be specifically designated. Metastatic tumor deposits measuring 0.2 to 2 mm are considered to represent micrometastases and staged as pN1(mic) or pN2(mic) for regional lymph node metastases and pM1(mic) for micrometastases at distant sites (Figure 8.12). Metastatic deposits that span less than 0.2 mm are regarded as isolated tumor cells (ITCs) by both the CAP and the AJCC/TNM seventh edition *Cancer Staging Manual*. These small clusters, or single tumor cells, in lymph nodes are not classified as lymph node metastases and are designated pN0(i+). The "i+" suffix is used to denote ITCs, not immunohistochemistry, and it is applied to lymph nodes with tumor deposits spanning less than 0.2 mm, regardless of whether they are detected following evaluation of hematoxylin and eosin or immunohistochemically stained sections (Figure 8.13). The pN0(mol+) designation is used when ITCs are identified using nonmorphologic (molecular) assays. There are no prospective data supporting the clinical utility of ancillary techniques to detect rare tumor cells in lymph nodes, and thus, use of immunohistochemical stains and molecular tests to enhance tumor cell detection is not recommended at this time.[2] However, tumor deposits spanning less than 0.2 mm (i.e., ITCs) that are detected in hematoxylin and eosin

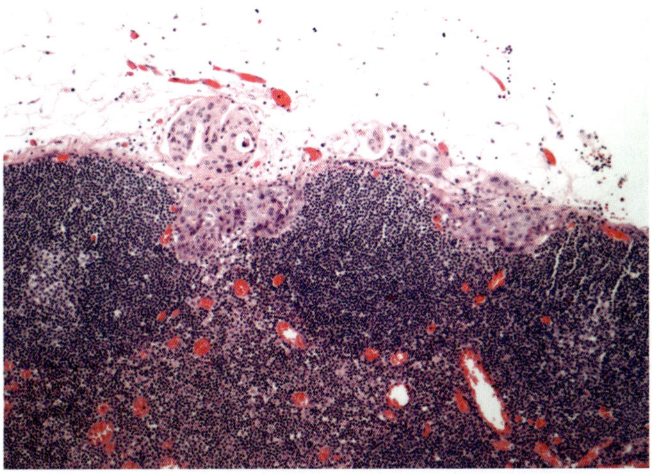

FIGURE 8.12: The CAP considers tumor deposits that span 0.2 to 2 mm in diameter to represent micrometastases and designates these lesions as pN1(mic) or pN2(mic). The AJCC/TNM seventh edition *Cancer Staging Manual* does not designate micrometastases separately from other tumor deposits in lymph nodes. (Courtesy of Dr. Alexandros Polydorides, Mount Sinai Medical School, New York, NY.)

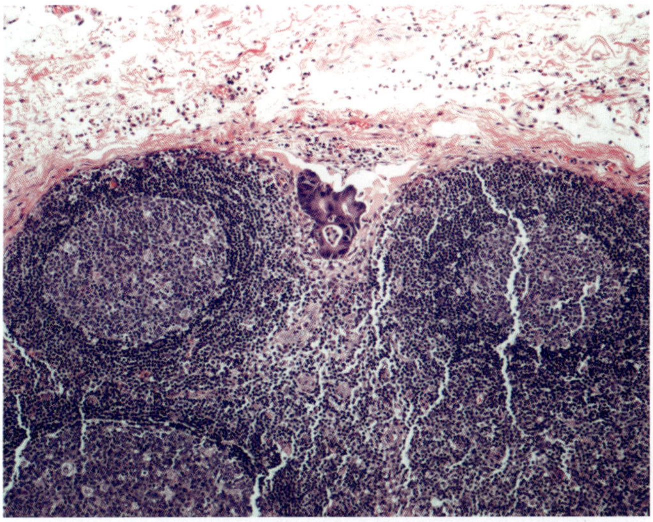

FIGURE 8.13: Tumor deposits that span less than 0.2 mm are classified as pN0(i+), regardless of whether they are detected upon examination of hematoxylin stained slides or following use of ancillary immunostains. (Courtesy of Dr. Alexandros Polydorides, Mount Sinai Medical School, New York, NY.)

stained sections should be evaluated with caution. Their biologic significance is not known and may not be negligible despite the pN0(i+) designation. Multiple tissue levels should always be examined since deeper tissue levels often reveal more substantial tumor deposits that alter stage assignment and directly impact patient care.

## Satellite Tumor Deposits in Pericolorectal Soft Tissue

The AJCC/TNM seventh edition *Cancer Staging Manual* introduced a novel classification scheme for satellite tumor deposits that is substantially different from prior staging guidelines. For example, the AJCC/TNM fifth edition *Cancer Staging Manual* (1997) classified tumor nodules with no underlying lymph node architecture based on their size.[17] Tumor nodules spanning at least 3 mm were considered to represent completely effaced lymph nodes, regardless of their morphology, and classified in the N category. Smaller tumor nodules were staged in the T (pT3) category because they presumably reflected vascular and/or perineural invasion extending into surrounding soft tissue or projections emanating from the primary tumor. The "3-mm rule" was replaced by the "contour rule" in the AJCC/TNM sixth edition *Cancer Staging Manual* (2002).[10] Round tumor nodules that were discontinuous with the main tumor were classified as positive lymph nodes and staged as pN1 or pN2, accordingly, even if no residual nodal tissue was identified

(Figure 8.14A). Ill-defined tumor nodules were considered to represent perineural or venous invasion with extension into soft tissue and staged in the T category (Figure 8.14B).

The AJCC/TNM seventh edition *Cancer Staging Manual* (2010) adopted a different approach to extramural tumor nodules because they are associated with poor clinical outcome.[18] Extramural satellite tumor deposits presumably reflect discontinuous extension from the primary tumor, extravascular spread of venous invasion, extension of perineural invasion into soft tissue, or completely replaced lymph nodes. Tumor nodules interpreted to represent completely effaced lymph nodes are classified as pN1a, pN1b, pN2a, or pN2b, depending upon the overall number of positive lymph nodes. Extramural satellite tumor deposits that are not believed to represent lymph nodes are counted, and their number is documented in the body of the pathology report. In addition, cancers associated with satellite tumor deposits are staged as pN1c, provided that other lymph node metastases are lacking. The AJCC/TNM seventh edition *Cancer Staging Manual (2010)* also states

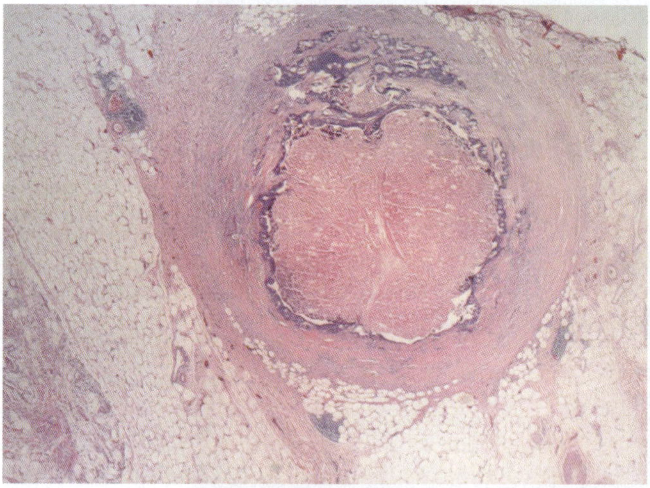

A

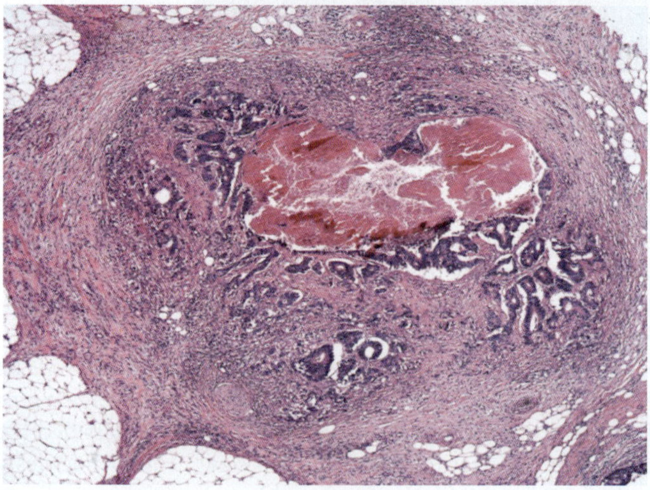

B

**FIGURE 8.14:** Tumor deposits with a smooth contour were staged as completely effaced lymph nodes (pN) in the AJCC/TNM sixth edition *Cancer Staging Manual* (**A**), whereas ill-defined nodules were considered to represent soft tissue extension of the primary tumor, perineural invasion, or vascular invasion and assigned a pT3 stage (**B**). Tumor deposits that are not considered to represent lymph nodes are evaluated differently in the AJCC/TNM seventh edition *Cancer Staging Manual.* Their number is specifically recorded and they are denoted pN1c, provided all other regional lymph nodes are negative for carcinoma.

that the pN1c category should only be used when satellite tumor nodules are found in pericolorectal tissues of cancers that extend no further than the muscularis propria (pT1 or pT2), although many pathologists use it to denote tumor deposits regardless of pathologic tumor (pT) stage. The number of tumor deposits should be recorded for all cases, even if the pN1c category is not used (i.e., tumor deposits are present in association with other regional lymph node metastases).

Unfortunately, distinction between completely replaced lymph nodes and satellite tumor deposits is subjective, and thus, reproducibility of the pN1c category is poor.[19] Features that suggest a tumor nodule represents an effaced lymph node include a round contour, fibrous capsule, lymph node sinuses, presence of a peripheral rim of lymphocytes, and lymphoid aggregates around, or in close proximity to, the tumor deposit. Anatomic structures, such as nerves, ganglia, and vascular bundles containing veins and arteries, are not normally present in lymph nodes. Their detection in a tumor nodule should lead one to classify it as a satellite tumor deposit, rather than an effaced lymph node. Ill-defined, stellate nodules without underlying nodal architecture should not be considered to represent effaced lymph nodes for staging purposes.

Some extramural tumor nodules should not be considered in the N category at all. Large vein invasion appears as rounded, or serpiginous, aggregates of malignant cells. Its presence should be suspected when tumor nodules are surrounded by smooth muscle cell bundles in pericolorectal fat or when they are located adjacent to arteries, reflecting the normal anatomy of a vascular bundle (Figure 8.15). Rounded nodules that reflect vascular invasion are designated as satellite tumor nodules, and the presence of large vein invasion recorded. Tumor nodules that involve the peritoneal surface distant from the primary mass likely represent peritoneal seeding (peritoneal carcinomatosis) and are staged as distant metastatic (pM1b) disease (Figure 8.16).

## Distant Metastases

The M staging category is used to denote distant metastatic disease. Distant metastases include tumor deposits in nonregional lymph nodes that are usually designated by the surgeon, discontinuous peritoneal deposits distant from the primary tumor, and parenchymal metastases to other organs, such as the liver, lung, bone, and other sites. Distant metastases limited to a single organ are denoted pM1a, whereas multiple distant metastases and peritoneal tumor deposits are classified as pM1b. Previous staging systems advocated use of pM0 or pMx to denote the absence of distant metastases or a lack of knowledge regarding the presence, or absence, of metastatic disease, respectively. This practice is now discouraged since pM0 is a global designation that can only be determined with confidence when complete pathologic examination of all organs is performed (i.e., autopsy evaluation). Current guidelines suggest that pathologists comment on the M category only when the presence of distant metastases is pathologically confirmed (pM1).

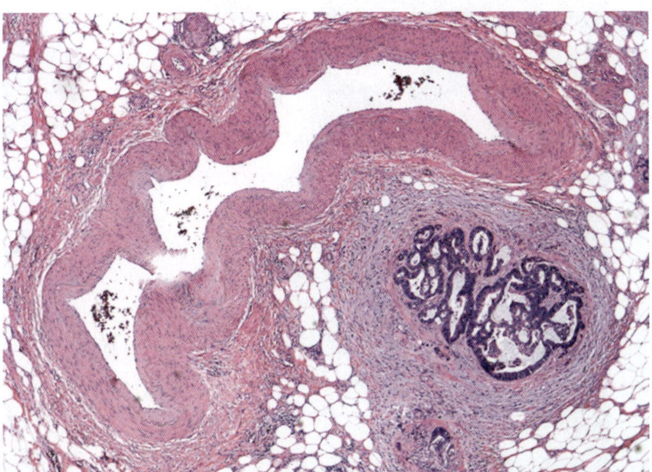

FIGURE 8.15: Tumor nodules located adjacent to arteries often represent large vein invasion by cancer, which can obliterate some, or all, of the vein wall and induce a fibroinflammatory response in surrounding soft tissue. These deposits should be denoted as satellite tumor nodules, and the presence of large vein invasion should also be reported.

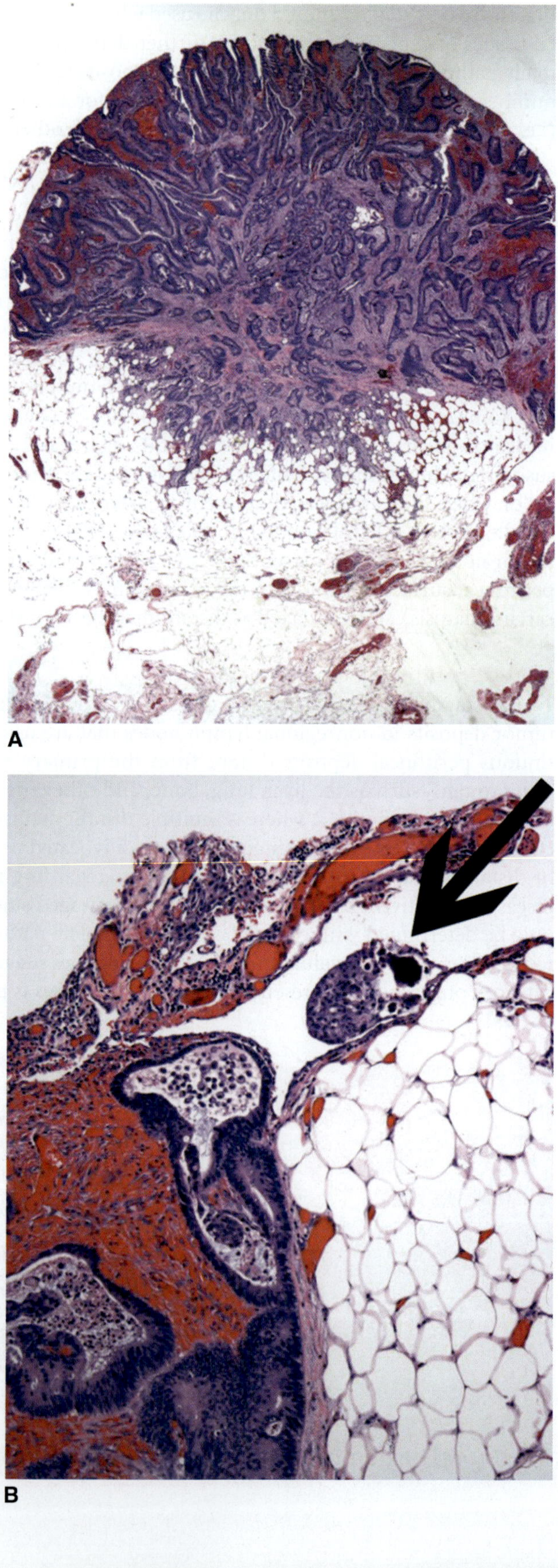

**FIGURE 8.16:** Tumor nodules in pericolic fat may reflect peritoneal carcinomatosis. In this case, innumerable tumor deposits were grossly apparent in the pericolic soft tissue, many of which had a mostly rounded appearance (**A**). Tumor deposits (**left**) on the peritoneal surface of pericolic fat distant from the tumor contained mesothelial hyperplasia with psammomatous calcifications (*arrow*) (**B**). These deposits are appropriately classified as peritoneal carcinomatosis and should be considered to represent distant metastatic disease (pM1b).

### Effects of Neoadjuvant Therapy on Pathologic Stage Assignment

Patients with locally advanced (pT3 or higher) rectal cancer routinely receive neoadjuvant chemotherapy, radiotherapy, or both, prior to definitive surgical resection. In this situation, pathologists should apply the "y" prefix (ypT, N, M) to pathologic stage assignment. Neoadjuvantly treated tumors typically show some degree of regression evidenced by replacement of invasive carcinoma by fibrosis, calcifications, and acellular mucin pools, but only extent of viable tumor is considered when assigning pathologic stage to the primary tumor. Similarly, regional lymph nodes that contain acellular mucin, or show features suggestive of a therapeutic effect, should not be considered when assessing for the presence of regional lymph node metastases. Issues related to handling of neoadjuvantly treated rectal cancers are discussed more fully in Chapters 6 and 9.

## SUMMARY AND CONCLUSIONS

Colorectal carcinoma is the most common carcinoma of the gastrointestinal tract, and more than 150,000 cases are diagnosed in the United States each year.[20] Surgical resection is the mainstay of therapy, but pathologic assessment is increasingly important to the subsequent management of patients. The primary role of pathologists is assignment of pathologic stage to resection specimens, as described in the AJCC/TNM seventh edition *Cancer Staging Manual* and enumerated in this chapter. However, pathologists also provide clinicians with prognostically important information regarding histologic features of colorectal cancers and may be called upon to provide quality assessment of surgical techniques. Key elements that pathologists should include in pathology reports are discussed in Chapter 9.

# References

1. Washington MK. Colorectal carcinoma: selected issues in pathologic examination and staging and determination of prognostic factors. *Arch Pathol Lab Med* 2008;132(10):1600–1607.
2. Washington MK, Berlin J, Branton PA, et al. Protocol for the examination of specimens from patients with primary carcinomas of the colon and rectum. *Arch Pathol Lab Med* 2008;132(7):1182–1193.
3. Colon and rectum. In: Edge S, Byrd D, Compton CC, et al., eds. *AJCC Cancer Staging Manual.* 7th ed. New York, NY: Springer; 2009:143–164.
4. Hamilton SR, Bosman FT, Boffetta P, et al. Tumors of the colon and rectum. In: Bosman FT, Carneiro F, Hruban RH, et al., eds. *WHO Classification of Tumours of the Digestive System.* 4th ed. Lyon, France: International Agency for Research on Cancer; 2010:134–146.
5. Haggitt RC, Glotzbach RE, Soffer EE, et al. Prognostic factors in colorectal carcinomas arising in adenomas: implications for lesions removed by endoscopic polypectomy. *Gastroenterology* 1985;89(2): 328–336.
6. Haggitt RC. Management of the patient with carcinoma in an adenoma. *Prog Clin Biol Res* 1988;279: 89–99.
7. Choi DH, Sohn DK, Chang HJ, et al. Indications for subsequent surgery after endoscopic resection of submucosally invasive colorectal carcinomas: a prospective cohort study. *Dis Colon Rectum* 2009;52(3):438–445.
8. Pollheimer MJ, Kornprat P, Pollheimer VS, et al. Clinical significance of pT sub-classification in surgical pathology of colorectal cancer. *Int J Colorectal Dis* 2010;25(2):187–196.
9. Merkel S, Mansmann U, Siassi M, et al. The prognostic inhomogeneity in pT3 rectal carcinomas. *Int J Colorectal Dis* 2001;16(5):298–304.
10. Colon and rectum. In: Green F, Page D, Fleming I, et al., eds. *AJCC Cancer Staging Manual.* 6th ed. Philadelphia, PA: Springer; 2002:113–124.
11. Shepherd NA, Baxter KJ, Love SB. The prognostic importance of peritoneal involvement in colonic cancer: a prospective evaluation. *Gastroenterology* 1997;112(4):1096–1102.

12. Kojima M, Nakajima K, Ishii G, et al. Peritoneal elastic laminal invasion of colorectal cancer: the diagnostic utility and clinicopathologic relationship. *Am J Surg Pathol* 2010;34(9):1351–1360.
13. Shinto E, Ueno H, Hashiguchi Y, et al. The subserosal elastic lamina: an anatomic landmark for stratifying pT3 colorectal cancer. *Dis Colon Rectum* 2004;47(4):467–473.
14. Swanson RS, Compton CC, Stewart AK, et al. The prognosis of T3N0 colon cancer is dependent on the number of lymph nodes examined. *Ann Surg Oncol* 2003;10(1):65–71.
15. Prandi M, Lionetto R, Bini A, et al. Prognostic evaluation of stage B colon cancer patients is improved by an adequate lymphadenectomy: results of a secondary analysis of a large scale adjuvant trial. *Ann Surg* 2002;235(4):458–463.
16. Scott KW, Grace RH. Detection of lymph node metastases in colorectal carcinoma before and after fat clearance. *Br J Surg* 1989;76(11):1165–1167.
17. Colon and rectum. In: Fleming ID, Cooper JS, Henson DE, et al., eds. *AJCC Cancer Staging Manual.* 5th ed. Philadelphia, PA: Lippincott-Raven; 1997:83–90.
18. Puppa G, Maisonneuve P, Sonzogni A, et al. Pathological assessment of pericolonic tumor deposits in advanced colonic carcinoma: relevance to prognosis and tumor staging. *Mod Pathol* 2007;20(8): 843–855.
19. Nagtegaal ID, Tot T, Jayne DG, et al. Lymph nodes, tumor deposits, and TNM: are we getting better? *J Clin Oncol* 2011;29(18):2487–2492.
20. Jemal A, Siegel R, Ward E, et al. Cancer statistics, 2008. *CA Cancer J Clin* 2008;58(2):71–96.

# Prognostically Important Features of Colorectal Carcinoma

# 9

Rhonda K. Yantiss

Although tumor stage is the single most important prognostic factor among patients with colorectal carcinoma, a number of other findings are clinically relevant. Some features, such as status of resection margins, adequacy of resection, number of detected lymph nodes, and tumor perforation, are evident at the time of gross examination. Histologic grade, small-vessel (lymphovascular and small vein) invasion, large-vessel invasion, perineural invasion, tumor configuration, tumor budding, and satellite tumor deposits are all associated with aggressive biologic behavior, and thus, comments regarding their presence or absence should be included in the surgical pathology report. Specific types of cancer are high-grade neoplasms at risk for biologically aggressive behavior, and others are associated with underlying molecular changes. Some features, such as a host inflammatory response to invasive carcinoma, are associated with a better prognosis or reflect underlying molecular alterations that impact patient management. The purpose of this chapter is to discuss characteristics of colorectal cancer that are associated with biologic behavior.

## INDEPENDENT PROGNOSTIC FACTORS DETECTED ON GROSS EXAMINATION

### Adequacy of Surgical Resection

The distance from the advancing edge of the primary tumor to the surgical resection margin is defined as tumor clearance, which should be documented for each resection margin on colorectal cancer specimens. Every colectomy specimen contains at least three surgical resection margins: the ends of the luminal bowel and a soft tissue resection margin. Proximal and distal resection margins that are greater than 5 cm from the tumor are rarely associated with anastomotic recurrences and, thus, represent adequate margins. However, low-lying rectal tumors are frequently removed with narrower clearance of the distal margin because wide surgical resection may compromise the anal sphincter. Most data suggest that at least 2-cm clearance is adequate for all rectal cancers, and clearance of 1 cm or greater is generally considered sufficient for carcinomas that invade no more deeply than the muscularis propria.[1,2]

Soft tissue resection margins are created by surgical dissection of the colon from surrounding connective tissues, and their nature varies depending on the type of specimen removed, as described in Chapter 6. The soft tissue resection margin of colonic segments that lie entirely within the peritoneal cavity is the mesenteric margin. Right and left colectomy specimens contain a mesenteric margin as well as posterior soft tissue margins reflecting dissection of the pericolic fat from the posterior abdominal wall at the hepatic and splenic flexures, respectively. The rectum lies below the peritoneal reflection and has a circumferential (radial) soft tissue resection margin. Adequate clearance of the circumferential margin is defined as a distance of at least 0.1 cm from the tumor and its value should be specifically stated. Clearance less than 0.1 cm is defined

**Table 9.1 Classification of Residual Disease in Resection Specimens for Colorectal Carcinoma (R)**

| Designation | Definition |
|---|---|
| RX | Presence of residual tumor cannot be assessed |
| R0 | No residual disease |
| R1 | Microscopically residual tumor |
| R2 | Macroscopically residual tumor |

as a positive margin. Status of the circumferential margin is the single most important factor in predicting local recurrence of rectal cancer. A positive circumferential margin is associated with nearly a fourfold increased risk of disease recurrence and twofold risk of death from disease compared to patients with negative circumferential margins.[3]

Some patients who undergo surgery with curative intent have residual disease after treatment. The AJCC/TNM seventh edition *Cancer Staging Manual* qualifies residual tumor after surgery with the R classification system (Table 9.1). Pathologists may use this system to denote margins of resection, thereby allowing treating physicians to make reasonable assumptions regarding residual tumor in the patient. Microscopically (R1) or macroscopically (R2) positive resection margins on colectomy specimens likely correspond to residual microscopic or macroscopic disease in the patient, respectively.[4] However, use of the R0 category to denote negative surgical margins represents a departure from prior staging systems. Previous classification schemes defined R0 as the absence of residual disease in the patient, but did not limit evaluation to the margins of a resection specimen. Pathologists were discouraged from using R0 to denote negative surgical margins because R0 status implied an absence of residual disease anywhere in the patient, including distant metastatic sites.[1]

## Complete Excision of the Mesorectal Envelope (Adequacy of Total Mesorectal Excision)

Advances in surgical techniques and introduction of the total mesorectal excision have improved local recurrence rates and overall survival among patients with rectal cancer.[5] Surgeons who perform a total mesorectal excision sharply dissect the perirectal soft tissues in the areolar plane outside the mesorectal (Waldeyer) fascia, such that the rectum, mesorectum, and all regional lymph nodes are removed entirely (Figure 9.1). Cancer operations performed in this fashion are associated with local recurrence and 5-year survival rates of 8% to 10% and 68%, respectively, compared to 20% to 30% and 48% among rectal cancers removed using older techniques.[5,6] Pathologic evaluation of rectal resection specimens effectively determines the adequacy of mesorectal excision and predicts both local recurrence and 5-year survival. Thus, pathologists are increasingly asked to grossly assess the mesorectum on resection specimens, as discussed in Chapter 6.

## Number of Harvested Regional Lymph Nodes

The number of lymph nodes detected in resection specimens positively correlates with overall survival among patients with stage II and stage III colorectal cancer. Five-year survival rates are approximately 76% when 18 or more lymph nodes are recovered from colorectal cancer patients with node-negative disease, compared to 62% when seven or fewer lymph nodes are detected.[7] Indeed, the relationship between number of recovered lymph nodes and prognosis

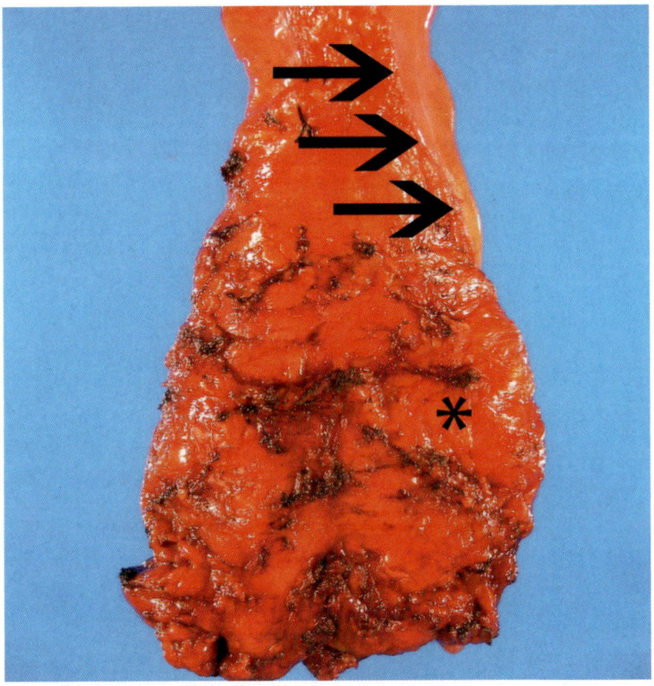


FIGURE 9.1: A total mesorectal excision specimen is surfaced by the mesorectal envelope (*asterisk*), which lies below the peritoneal reflection (*arrows*) and contains all the regional lymph nodes.

is so strong that the former may represent an important criterion used to stratify patients with T3N0 colorectal cancer who are under consideration for clinical trials.[8] The relationship between survival and number of harvested lymph nodes reflects a combination of two factors: stage migration and host immunity. Stage migration is a term used to describe the association between appropriate stage assessment and number of harvested lymph nodes. The likelihood of detecting metastatic lymph node deposits increases as more lymph nodes are identified, resulting in assignment to a higher pathologic stage grouping that more accurately predicts outcome. Alternatively, detection of numerous lymph nodes may reflect a host immune response to cancer, which is independently associated with improved survival.[9] A robust inflammatory response to colorectal cancer induces reactive enlargement of regional lymph nodes, which facilitates their detection.

## Tumor Perforation

Free tumor perforation is defined by the presence of transmural necrosis and perforation at the site of an invasive adenocarcinoma. Tumor perforation is always designated pT4a and is independently associated with poor outcome.[2] Although one frequently appreciates tumor perforation at the time of gross examination, tumor cells are not always readily demonstrable on the serosal surface in histologic sections.[10] Similar to nonneoplastic colonic perforation, free perforation through a tumor elicits an exuberant inflammatory reaction with abscesses, a fibroinflammatory tissue reaction, and fibrin at the site of penetration that mask contamination of the peritoneal surface (Figure 9.2). Findings such as these should prompt careful examination of the gross specimen, review of the clinical information, and additional tissue sections, as discussed in Chapter 8. Tumor perforation should be distinguished from perforation of the uninvolved colon proximal to an obstructing colon cancer. Although the latter is also associated with high mortality, poor outcome reflects the frequent occurrence of generalized peritonitis and sepsis in patients with colonic perforation, rather than tumor recurrence and death from disease.[2,11]

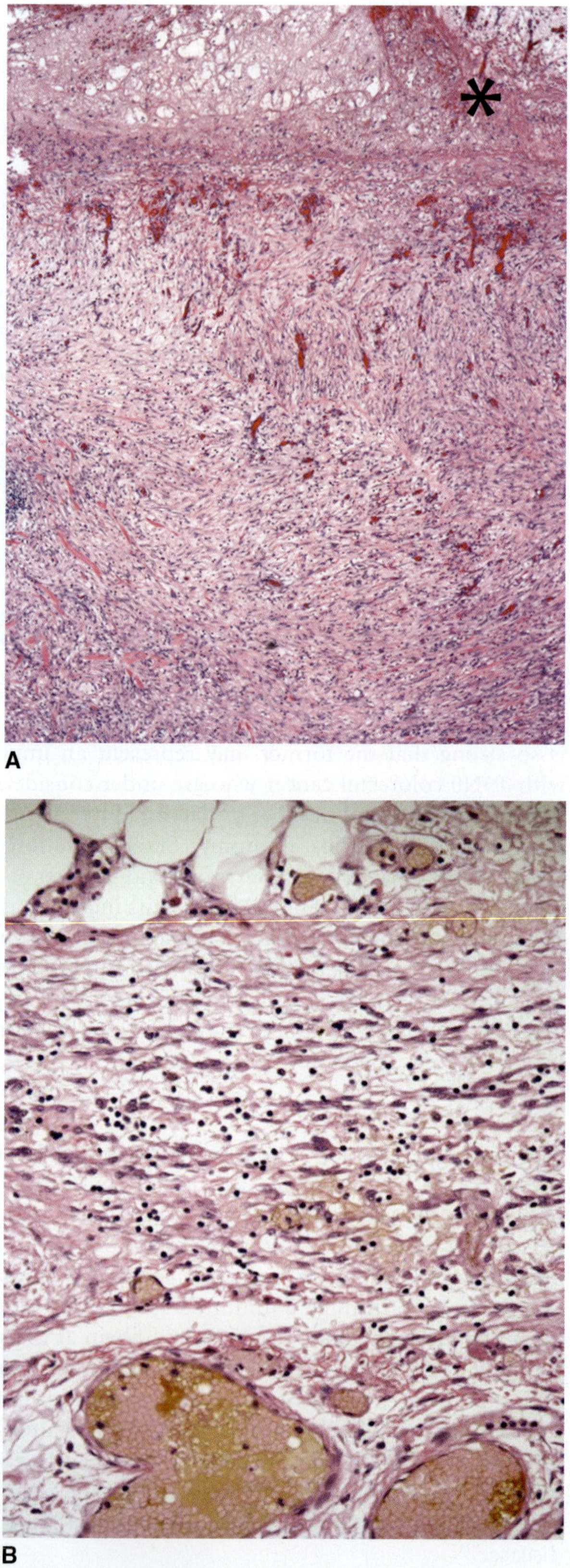

**FIGURE 9.2:** Perforated colonic carcinomas elicit an exuberant fibroinflammatory reaction that masks extent of disease. This patient presented with an acute abdomen and free peritoneal air. Sections demonstrate fibrin deposits (*asterisk*) and granulation tissue with perpendicularly oriented new vessels on the serosal surface (**A**). Entrapped mesothelial cells are visible within fibrin (**B**).

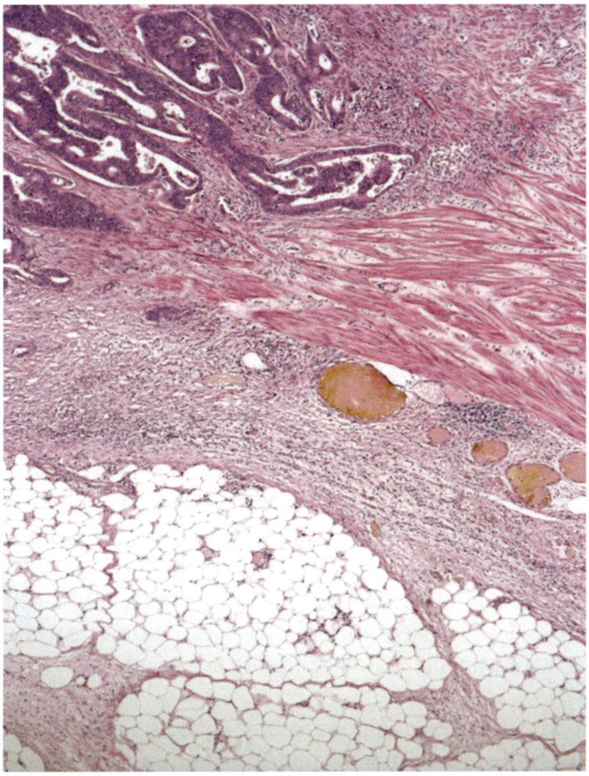

C

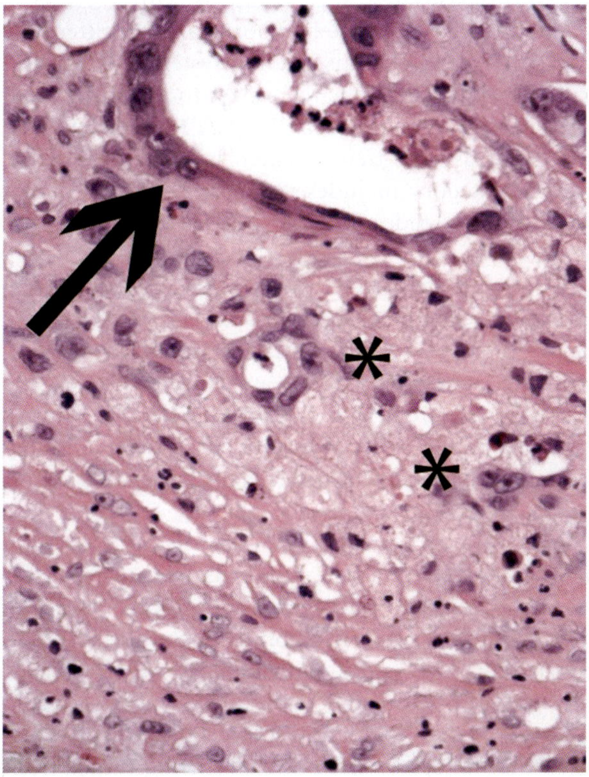

D

FIGURE 9.2: (*Continued*) Additional sections reveal tumor cells in close proximity to the serosal reaction (**C**), within which entrapped mesothelial cells (*asterisk*), tumor cells (*arrow*), and fibrin are detectable (**D**).

## HISTOLOGIC GRADING OF INVASIVE COLORECTAL CARCINOMA

Although many pathologists use "differentiation" and "grade" interchangeably, these designations are not synonymous. Differentiation describes the extent to which a cellular proliferation resembles the normal components of the organ of origin. For example, well-differentiated colonic adenocarcinomas contain mostly gland-forming elements that are similar in size and shape to nonneoplastic colonic glands, whereas poorly differentiated adenocarcinomas contain sheets of tumor cells that are not organized in well-formed glands and bear minimal, if any, resemblance to normal epithelial cells. Histologic grade, on the other hand, refers to severity of cytologic atypia as evidenced by a constellation of features including nuclear size and contour, chromatin pattern, nucleolar prominence, mitotic activity, and the presence, or absence, of necrosis. Low-grade cytologic atypia is characterized by slight nuclear enlargement with minimal nuclear membrane abnormalities, mostly dispersed chromatin, occasional prominent nucleoli, and scattered mitotic figures. Markedly enlarged, irregular, or folded nuclei with coarse chromatin and one or more large nucleoli represent high-grade cytologic features. High-grade tumors usually display easily detected mitotic figures and individual cell necrosis. Histologic grade and degree of differentiation are positively correlated in most colorectal carcinomas. Well-differentiated carcinomas tend to show low-grade cytologic features, whereas poorly differentiated carcinomas are generally high grade. However, most colorectal adenocarcinomas show a greater degree of cytologic atypia relative to gland formation compared to adenocarcinomas of other organs.

The most widely accepted colorectal cancer grading scheme is based solely on extent of glandular differentiation within the neoplasm because lack of gland formation has adverse prognostic significance independent of tumor stage.[12] The WHO considers carcinomas that contain >95% glandular elements to be well differentiated, whereas those with 50%–95%, 5%–49%, and <5% gland formation are classified as moderately, poorly, and undifferentiated carcinomas, respectively (Figure 9.3).[13] Unfortunately, this grading system suffers from a substantial degree of interobserver variability, particularly with respect to the distinction between well- and moderately differentiated carcinomas. Thus, the AJCC/TNM seventh edition *Cancer Staging Manual* recommends that this four-tiered system be collapsed into a two-tiered system (Table 9.2).[4] The low-grade category includes well-to-moderately differentiated carcinomas, whereas poorly and undifferentiated tumors are classified as high-grade malignancies.

The most recent WHO colorectal carcinoma grading system also incorporates defective mismatch repair mechanisms into its classification scheme.[13] Carcinomas that are microsatellite stable (MSS) are graded based solely on degree of glandular differentiation as described above, whereas those with high-frequency microsatellite instability (MSI-H) are considered to be low grade, regardless of the extent of gland formation (Figure 9.4). Inclusion of molecular features in histologic grading schemes represents a major departure from traditional criteria, although incorporating microsatellite status into grade assessment reflects the generally favorable prognosis associated with MSI-H tumors.[14,15]

Colorectal carcinomas are morphologically heterogeneous, and the methods used to assess grade vary widely among different practices. Colorectal carcinomas tend to be better differentiated superficially, whereas the invasive front typically shows less gland formation. Some pathologists base classification on the extent of gland formation throughout the tumor, whereas others limit their evaluation to areas that are less differentiated. The WHO considers the advancing edge of the tumor to be suboptimal for grade assessment, and as a result, pathologists have historically neglected this region when evaluating colorectal cancers for histologic grade.[13] However, recent data suggest that failure to assess the advancing tumor front likely underestimates biologic potential among colorectal carcinomas. Tumors composed of

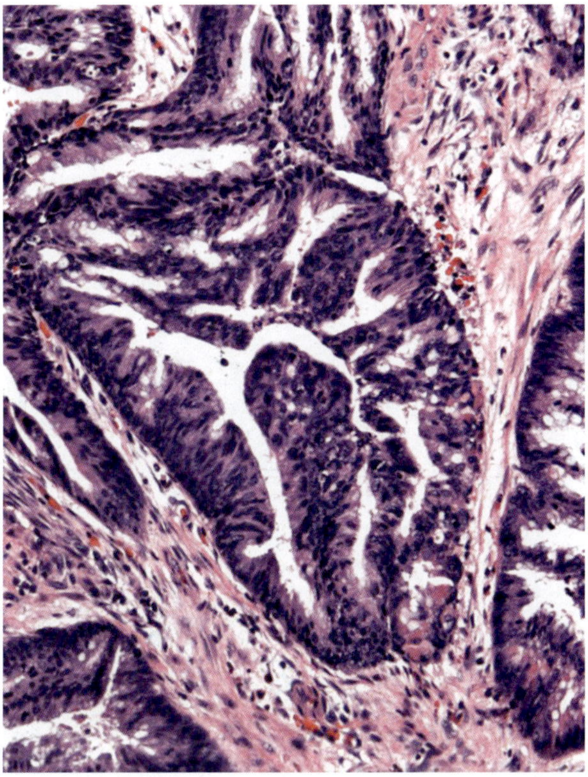

**A**

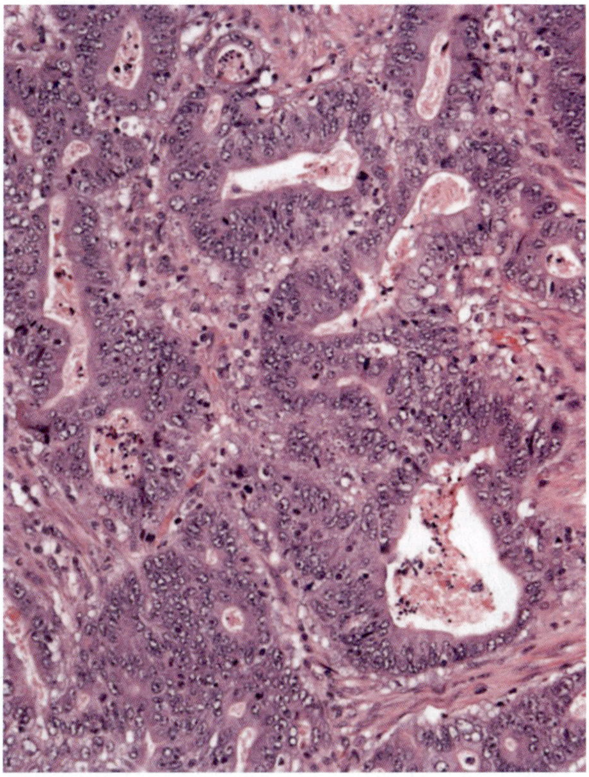

**B**

FIGURE 9.3: Low-grade adenocarcinomas include well- and moderately differentiated tumors that contain greater than 95% (**A**) and 50% to 95% (**B**) gland-forming elements, respectively.

**FIGURE 9.3:** (*Continued*) (**C**) High-grade carcinomas are poorly differentiated malignancies with less than 50% gland formation or undifferentiated cancers that show rare (<5%) glands (**D**).

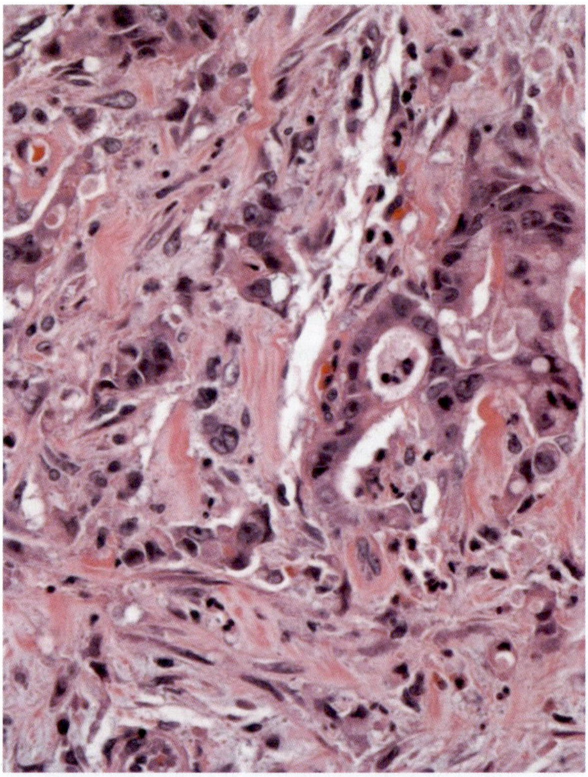

C

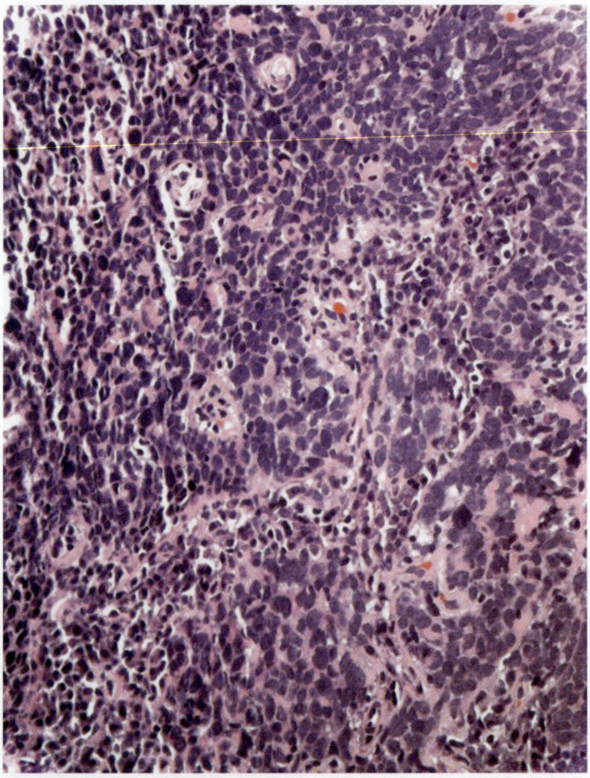

D

**Table 9.2 Grading Scheme for Classification of Colorectal Adenocarcinomas**

| Proposed Designation | Definition |
|---|---|
| Four-tiered system (WHO) | |
| Grade GX | Grade cannot be assessed |
| Grade G1 | Well differentiated (>95% gland forming) |
| Grade G2 | Moderately differentiated (50%–95% gland forming) |
| Grade G3 | Poorly differentiated (5%–49% gland forming) |
| Grade G4 | Undifferentiated (<5% gland forming) |
| Two-tiered system (AJCC) | |
| G1–G2 | Low grade (50%–100% gland forming) |
| G3–G4 | High grade (<50% gland forming) |

more than 50% gland-forming elements may behave aggressively, despite their classification as low-grade (moderately differentiated) cancers. Indeed, tumors that contain non–gland-forming elements occupying at least one high-power field (400× magnification) are associated with a 69% disease-related 5-year survival, compared to 99% 5-year survival among patients with cancers containing fewer than 10 solid tumor cell clusters per low-power field (40× magnification).[16] These observations have led to alternative grading schemes based on objective criteria that specifically assess extent of non–gland-forming elements, rather than glandular differentiation. One such model quantifies the number of solid cell clusters containing five or more tumor cells, regardless of where they are located in the mass (i.e., advancing edge or elsewhere). Tumors with <5, 5–9, and ≥10 cell clusters per intermediate power field (200× magnification) are classified as G1, G2, and G3, respectively. When applied to stage II and stage III colorectal carcinomas, these grade assignments are associated with 5-year disease-free survival rates of 96%, 85%, and 59%, respectively.[17]

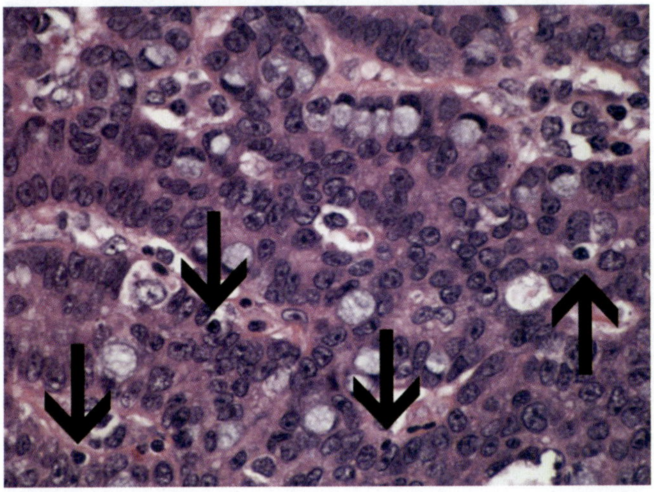

**FIGURE 9.4:** This cancer in the proximal colon contained cords and sheets of cells with large, irregular nuclei; open chromatin; and prominent nucleoli as well as scattered tumor cells with a signet ring cell appearance. Although such a tumor should be classified as a high-grade neoplasm due to a lack of gland formation, it is mismatch repair deficient and, thus, considered to be low-grade regardless of its morphologic features. Occasional tumor-infiltrating lymphocytes are present (*arrows*) and a clue to the presence of MSI-H.

# HISTOLOGIC GRADING OF SPECIFIC CANCER SUBTYPES

Some morphologic subtypes of colorectal carcinoma are, by definition, classified as low- or high-grade neoplasms based on their biologic behavior and molecular features. For example, medullary carcinomas are poorly differentiated inasmuch as they lack glandular differentiation, yet this phenotype is associated with improved survival compared to other colorectal carcinomas with minimal gland formation (Figure 9.5A). Medullary carcinomas are usually MSI-H and, thus, are classified by the WHO as low-grade carcinomas despite their lack of glandular differentiation.[13] On the other hand, signet ring cell, (neuro)endocrine (small cell), and undifferentiated colorectal carcinomas are considered to be high-grade malignancies because they are associated with poor survival (Figures 9.5B and 9.5C).[18,19] More than 75% of patients with signet ring cell carcinoma have regional lymph node metastases at the time of diagnosis, and 30% to 60% present with disseminated peritoneal disease.[20] Nearly 70% of patients with high-grade (neuro)endocrine carcinoma have metastatic disease at the time of diagnosis. One-, two-, and three-year survivals are approximately 46%, 26%, and 13%, respectively, and the mean survival is only 10.4 months.[18] Micropapillary carcinoma is an underrecognized colorectal cancer variant that is more aggressive than conventional adenocarcinoma.[21] Tumors with this growth pattern display lymphovascular invasion and lymph node metastases in more than 50% of cases.[22] Limited data suggest that the presence of a micropapillary component is an adverse prognostic factor among stage I and stage II colorectal carcinomas (Figure 9.5D).[23]

**FIGURE 9.5:** Medullary carcinomas of the colon do not show substantial glandular differentiation, but are usually mismatch repair deficient and, thus, classified as low-grade neoplasms according to the WHO (**A**).

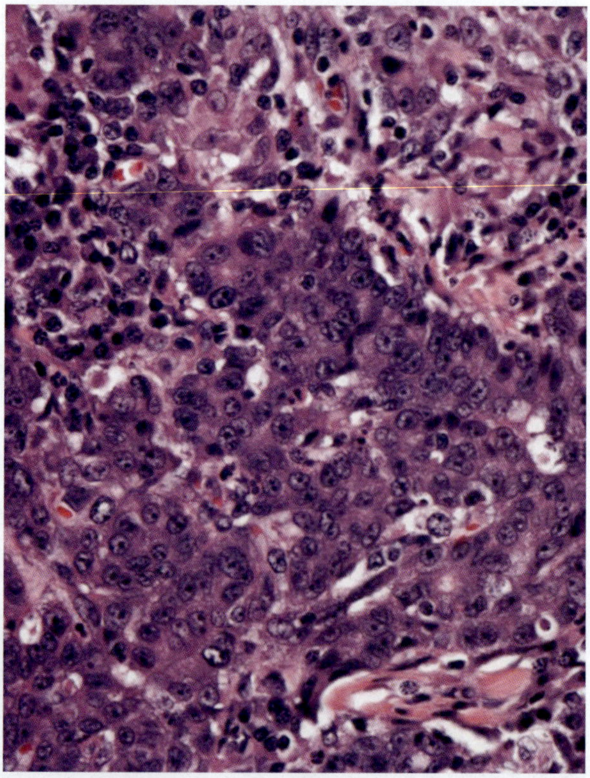

A

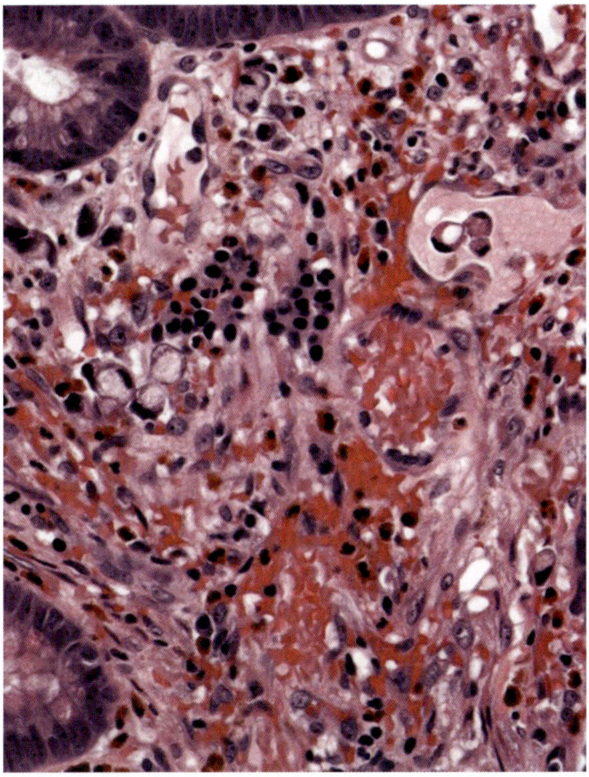

B

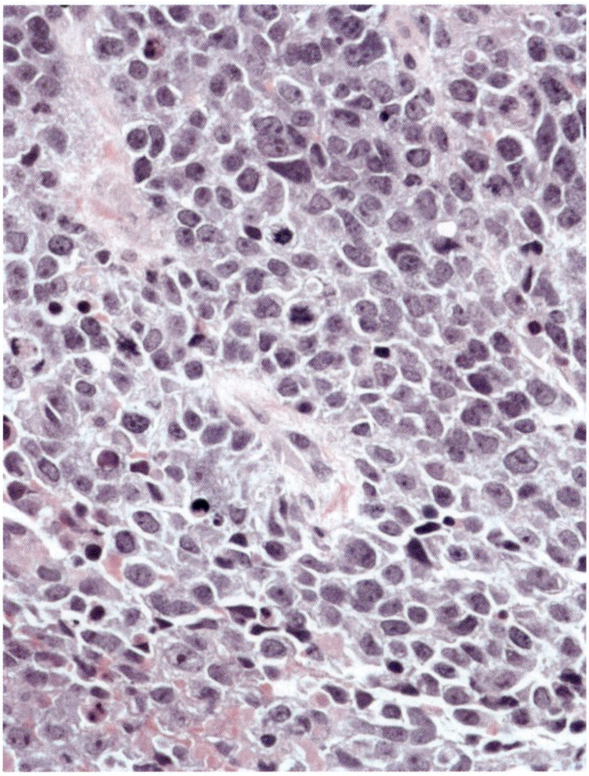

C

**FIGURE 9.5:** (*Continued*) Signet ring cell carcinomas of the colon (**B**) and high-grade (neuro) endocrine carcinoma (**C**) are always classified as high-grade malignant neoplasms.

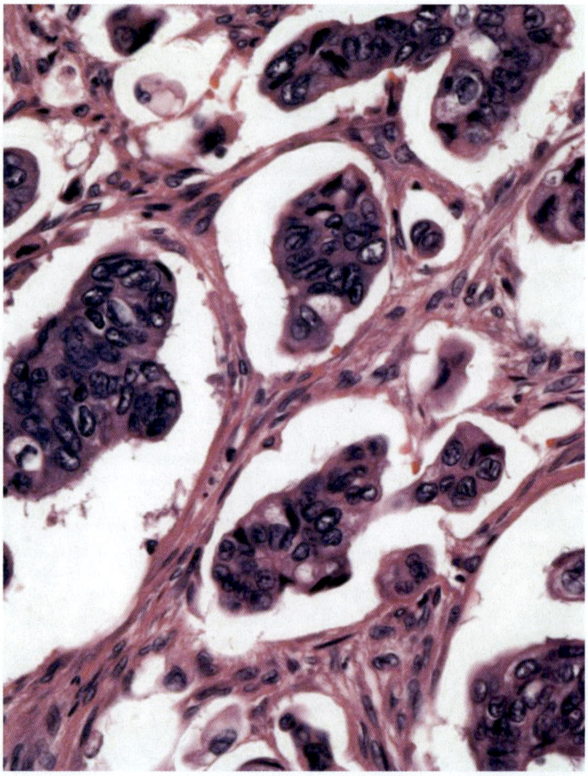

D

**FIGURE 9.5:** (*Continued*) Micropapillary carcinoma is an uncommon cancer variant with aggressive biologic behavior that is also considered to represent a high-grade malignancy (**D**).

# INDEPENDENT PROGNOSTIC FACTORS DETECTED ON HISTOLOGIC EXAMINATION

## Lymphovascular and Small-Vessel (Venous) Invasion

Lymphatic channels are normally present in all layers of the colonic wall, but are limited to the deep crypt region of the normal mucosa. Colorectal carcinomas induce lymphangiogenesis within the tumor as well as vascular growth in all areas of the adjacent mucosa. Lymphangiogenesis results from the complex interplay between lymphatic endothelial receptor tyrosine kinase (VEGFR-3) and its ligands, VEGF-C and VEGF-D.[24] Increased microvessel density, as determined by the presence of D240 immunopositive vascular channels in and around a cancer, is associated with a variety of parameters linked to overall prognosis. Features that are positively correlated with microvessel density include depth of tumor invasion (pT), lymphatic vessel invasion by carcinoma, regional lymph node metastases, and liver metastases.[25]

Both lymphovascular and venous invasion are of prognostic importance in colorectal carcinoma by univariate and multivariate analysis.[1,26] Some studies have shown lymphatic vessel invasion to be more strongly associated with clinical outcome than venous invasion, whereas the converse is true in other studies. The diagnosis of lymphovascular/small-vessel invasion requires identification of single or clustered tumor cell emboli within endothelium-lined spaces, although its recognition and distinction from potential mimics can be difficult in some cases. Retraction artifacts around tumor cell clusters within connective tissue can simulate the appearance of lymphovascular invasion, particularly in cancers with a micropapillary appearance (Figure 9.5D). The destructive nature of colorectal cancers also obscures lymphovascular invasion in the center of the tumor, and thus, permeation of lymphatic channels may be better appreciated at the advancing edge of the tumor or in the adjacent mucosa (Figure 9.6). Ancillary stains for endothelial

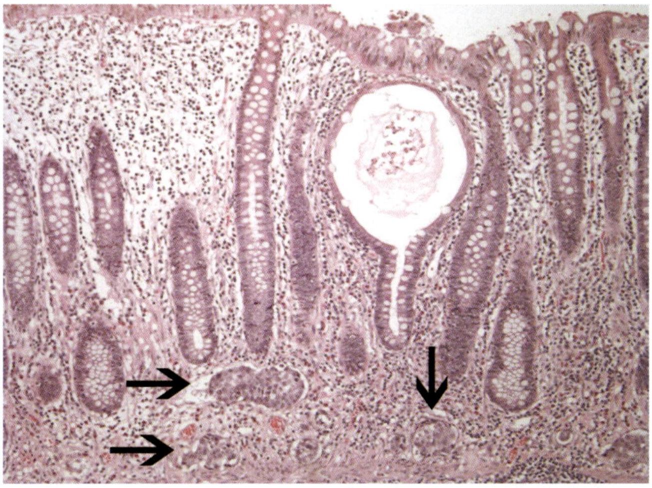

FIGURE 9.6: Tumor emboli are present in lymphatic vessels (*arrows*) in the mucosa adjacent to an invasive colonic adenocarcinoma.

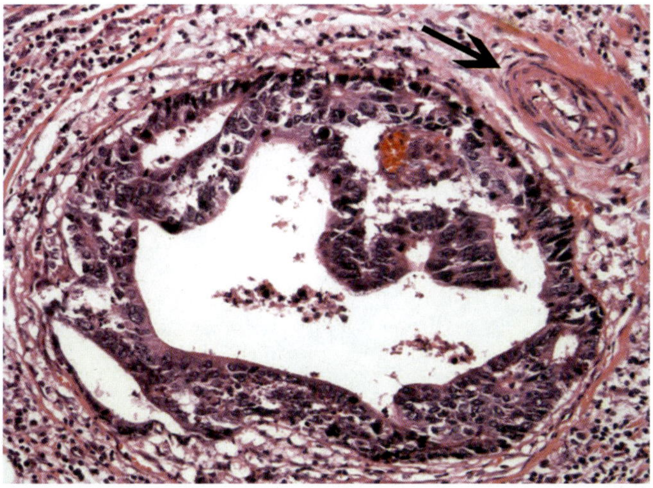

FIGURE 9.7: A large vein distended by tumor cells has a smooth, round contour that simulates the appearance of a satellite tumor deposit or lymph node metastasis. A clue to the nature of this nodule is its close proximity to a paired artery (*arrow*).

markers, such as D240, facilitate detection of lymphatic vessel invasion in some cases, whereas elastin stains aid identification of venous invasion in others.[27] The AJCC/TNM seventh edition *Cancer Staging Manual* considers both lymphatic vessel and small vein invasion together in the "lymphovascular invasion" (L) category.

## Large-Vessel (Venous) Invasion

Large vein invasion is separately denoted (V) in the AJCC/TNM seventh edition *Cancer Staging Manual* and is independently associated with poor prognosis.[4,28] Venous invasion may be limited to areas within the tumor in up to one-third of colorectal cancers, in which case its detection can be enhanced by addition of elastin stains.[27] Immunohistochemical stains are of limited value in detecting large vein invasion, since the endothelium is often destroyed by invasive carcinoma. Vascular invasion produces round or serpiginous nodules associated with remnants of the vein wall, an inflammatory response, or an accompanying artery (Figure 9.7).

## Perineural Invasion

Perineural invasion is detected in approximately 10% of colorectal carcinomas (Figure 9.8). It is more commonly observed in combination with other features associated with poor outcome

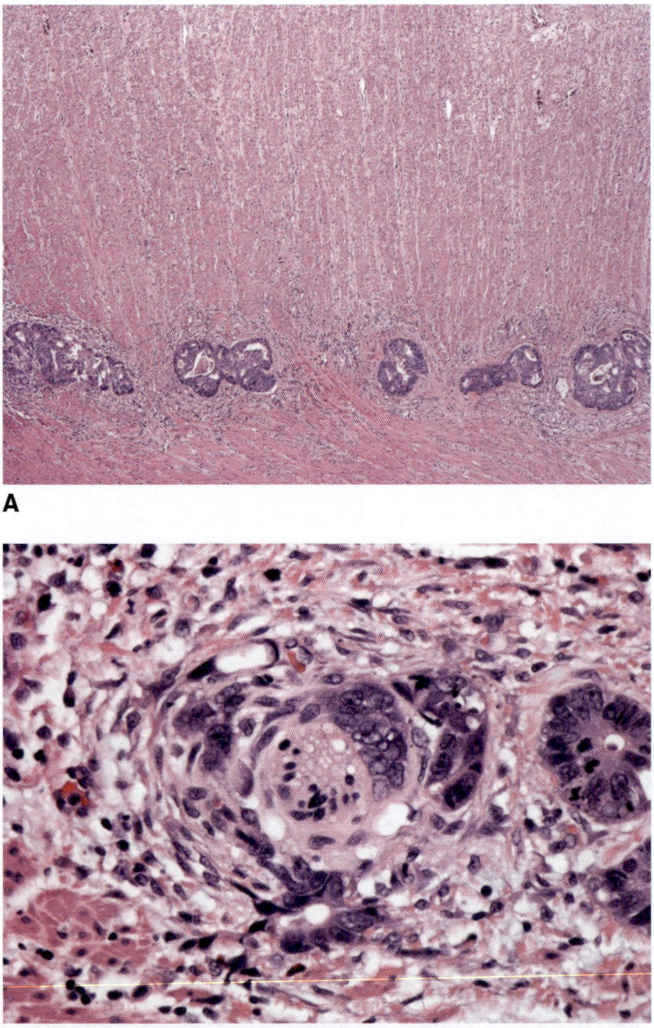

A

B

FIGURE 9.8: Perineural invasion involving the myenteric plexus appears as tumor nodules between layers of the muscularis propria (**A**). Nests of tumor cells surround bundles of nerves (**B**).

such as high-grade histology, lymphovascular involvement, or venous invasion, and occurs more frequently among tumors that extend into the muscularis propria or beyond. The biologic implications of perineural invasion are not entirely clear, although an emerging body of evidence suggests that it is a poor prognostic indicator that is independently associated with regional lymph node metastases and decreased survival.[29] Patients with stage II rectal cancer and perineural invasion have a more than 2.5-fold increased risk of local disease recurrence than patients without perineural invasion, indicating that this feature is a marker of more aggressive disease in a subset of patients who may require more intensive therapy.[30]

## Tumor Border Configuration

Colorectal carcinomas are classified as having an expansile or infiltrative border based on their low-power appearance.[31] Tumors with an expansile appearance have a smooth, pushing border with a lobulated configuration, whereas those with an infiltrative pattern have an irregular advancing front (Figure 9.9). The latter typically lack a sharp demarcation between the advancing edge of the tumor and adjacent nonneoplastic tissue and may contain tumor cells that dissect through the muscularis propria or pericolic fat without a substantial stromal response. An infiltrative growth pattern is associated with decreased survival among colorectal cancer patients.[32]

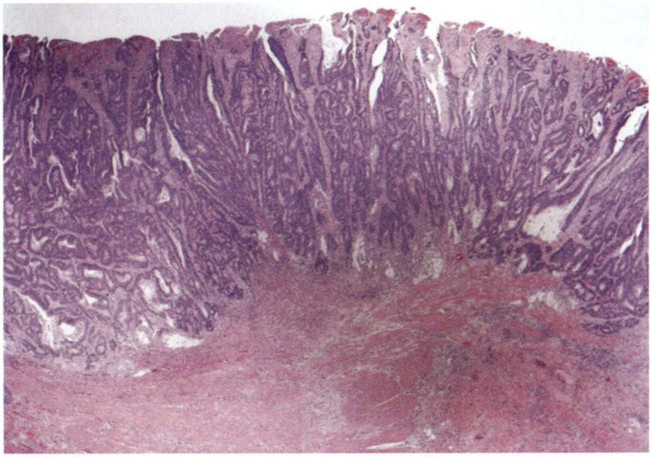

A

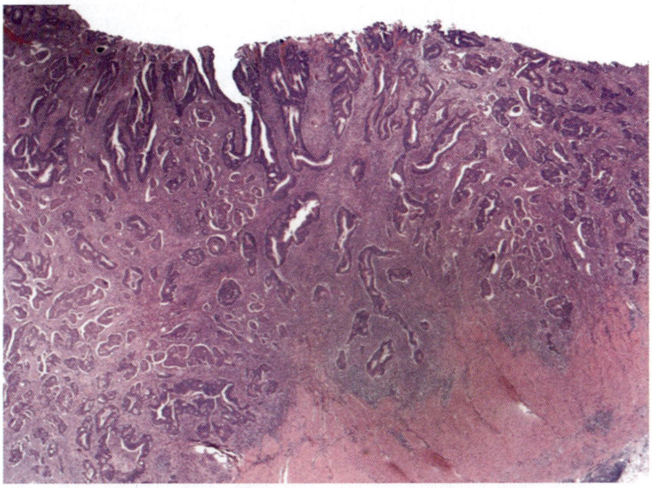

B

FIGURE 9.9: Invasive adenocarcinomas with a well-circumscribed, smooth advancing front are associated with improved overall survival (**A**). Carcinomas with ill-defined, infiltrative borders are more aggressive (**B**).

## Tumor Budding

Tumor budding is defined by the presence of single infiltrating cells or cell clusters (up to five tumor cells per group) enmeshed in desmoplastic stroma at the advancing edge of the tumor (Figure 9.10).[33] Tumor cells within areas of budding may appear elongated, or spindled, and merge imperceptibly with the surrounding desmoplastic stroma, a finding that has been termed "epithelial–mesenchymal transformation." Tumor budding results from loss of intercellular junctions and interactions between tumor cells and stroma. It is often accompanied by expression of stem cell markers such as CD133 and LGR5.[34,35] Tumor budding is more common among MSS than MSI-H colorectal cancers, and among MSI-H tumors, it is more frequently observed in Lynch-related cancers than sporadic tumors.[31]

Tumor budding is independently associated with poor prognosis among patients with colorectal carcinoma, including patients with stage I and stage II disease. Marked tumor budding (present along more than two-thirds of the advancing tumor front) correlates with high histologic grade, regional lymph node metastases, and advanced TNM stage, as well as decreased 5-year cancer-related survival compared to mild (less than one-third of advancing tumor front) or moderate (one-third to two-thirds of advancing tumor front) tumor budding.[36] Patients with stage II colorectal carcinomas that show tumor budding have a poorer prognosis than stage II tumors without budding, and in fact, the survival curves of the former closely approximate

FIGURE 9.10: Tumor budding is evaluated at the advancing edge of the carcinoma (**A**). Single cells and clusters of tumor cells surround infiltrating malignant glands (**B**).

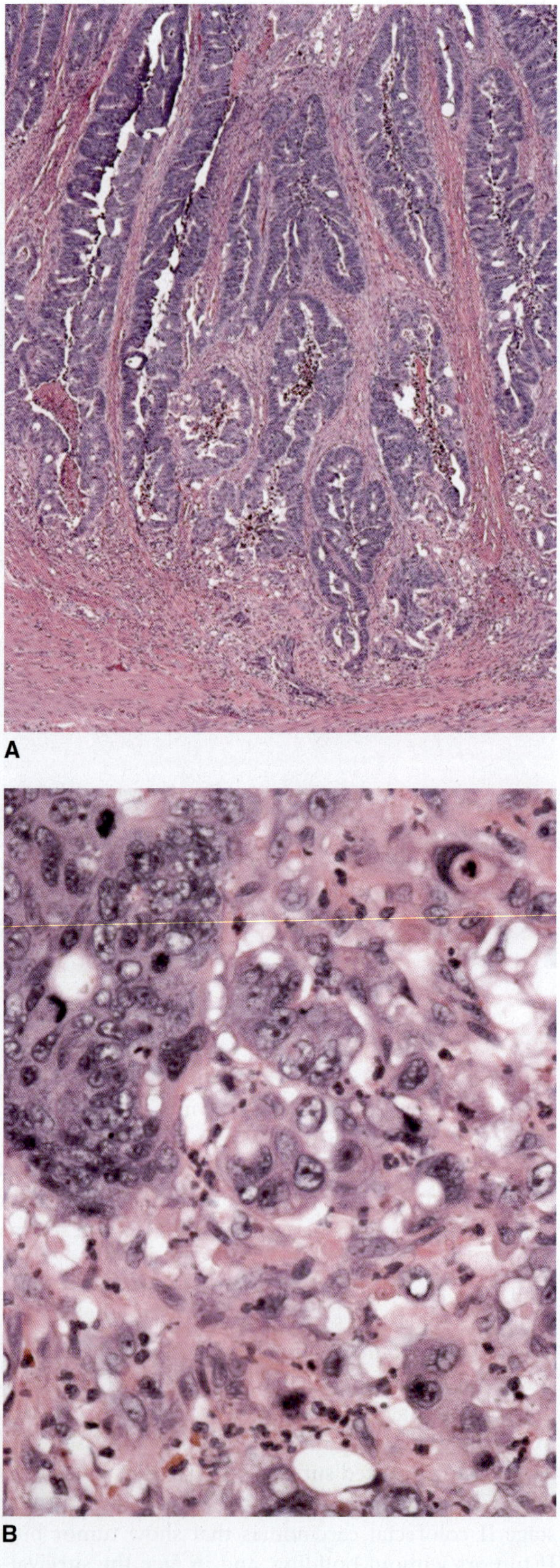

those of stage III tumors.[37] These data suggest that tumor budding represents a useful marker of high-risk stage II colorectal carcinomas.

## Satellite Tumor Deposits

Irregular tumor nodules in soft tissue surrounding the colorectum usually result from discontinuous extramural growth, extension of vascular or perineural invasion into soft tissue, or complete effacement of lymph nodes by metastatic disease.[38] Satellite tumor deposits are independently associated with poor prognosis among colorectal cancer patients, and thus, the AJCC/TNM seventh edition *Cancer Staging Manual* and CAP now require pathologists to comment upon their presence, or absence, in surgical pathology reports.[4] Tumor nodules that are interpreted to represent completely effaced lymph nodes are classified in the pN category, whereas those that are not believed to represent lymph nodes are counted and their number documented in the body of the pathology report. Tumor nodules that occur in cancers that are otherwise unassociated with regional nodal metastases are qualified using the pN1c category, as described in Chapter 8.

## Host Immune Response

The AJCC/TNM seventh edition *Cancer Staging Manual* and CAP recognize two types of host immune (lymphoid) response: Crohn-like lymphoid response and tumor-infiltrating lymphocytes. Both are associated with improved prognosis and MSI-H, although the relationship between host immune response and clinical outcome is independent of microsatellite status and DNA methylation.[39] Indeed, MSI-H colonic carcinomas lacking a host immune response are associated with survival rates similar to those of stage-matched MSS cancers (Joel K. Greenson, *personal communication*).

The Crohn-like lymphoid response is characterized by rounded lymphoid aggregates, some of which contain germinal centers, enmeshed in stellate fibrosis. Lymphoid aggregates are usually located one or more millimeters from the advancing edge of the tumor and are more common among cancers that penetrate the muscularis propria or extend beyond the colonic wall (Figure 9.11). However, one should be cautious when evaluating this finding in neoadjuvantly treated rectal cancers, since therapy induces a similar inflammatory response to invasive carcinoma that does not correlate with the presence of MSI-H or outcome. Tumor-infiltrating lymphocytes represent another type of host immune response commonly seen in MSI-H tumors, in which case they reflect a response to neoantigens generated by MSI-H. Tumor-infiltrating lymphocytes interdigitate between tumor cells and are usually present in high numbers, although as few as two tumor-infiltrating lymphocytes/high-power field (400× magnification) may be seen in MSI-H cancers (Figure 9.12).[40,41]

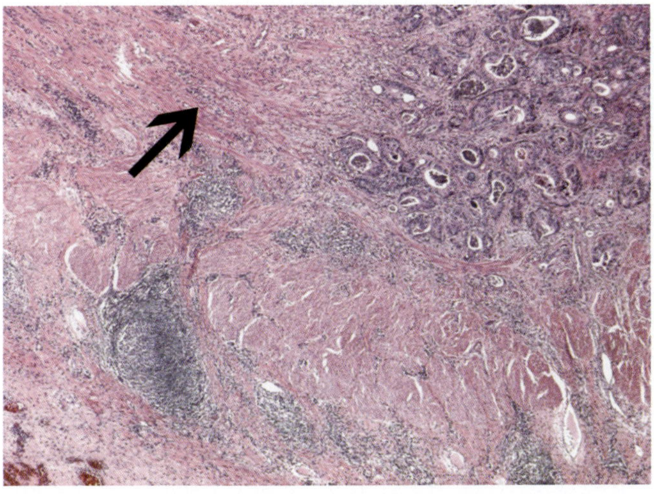

**FIGURE 9.11:** A Crohn-like host immune response consists of round lymphoid aggregates peripheral to the advancing edge of the carcinoma. Single infiltrating lymphocytes within the tumor and peritumoral fibrosis (*arrow*) also comprise the inflammatory reaction.

Extent of host immune response to colorectal cancer can be evaluated in order to better predict survival and underlying MSI-H. A Crohn-like lymphoid response is defined by the presence of at least four lymphoid aggregates in one low-power field (40× magnification), although some investigators recommend that the extent of response be specifically evaluated.[41] A three-tiered system is usually employed for evaluating a Crohn-like lymphoid response. Cases with no lymphoid aggregates at the tumor periphery (absent response) are separated from those with occasional aggregates and scattered lymphocytes at the advancing tumor edge (mild response) and those with numerous lymphoid aggregates with, or without, germinal centers and a prominent band of peritumoral lymphocytes (marked response). A pronounced inflammatory response is associated with better prognosis: a marked Crohn-like lymphoid response is associated with a decreased incidence of regional lymph node metastases and significantly improved 10-year survival.[42] Minimal criteria for quantifying tumor-infiltrating lymphocytes are not well defined. Statistical modeling studies aimed at developing criteria for MSI-H detection have suggested that a minimum of five tumor-infiltrating lymphocytes be identified per high-power field (400× magnification) and that at least 10 high-power fields be examined.[41] However, MSI-H cancers may contain fewer than five tumor-infiltrating lymphocytes per high-power field, and thus, current guidelines suggest that extent of tumor-infiltrating lymphocytes be graded as absent, mild (one or two tumor-infiltrating lymphocytes/high-power field [400× magnification]), or marked (three or more tumor-infiltrating lymphocytes/high-power field [400× magnification]).[2,40]

## Features of Microsatellite Instability

Pathologists are encouraged to identify colorectal carcinomas that display MSI-H for several reasons. First, these tumors may be associated with Lynch syndrome (hereditary nonpolyposis colorectal cancer), which predisposes patients to extracolonic malignancies and has important implications for patient family members. Second, approximately 15% to 25% of sporadic colorectal carcinomas also show MSI-H, and in this situation, MSI-H status is associated with improved survival. Third, sporadic MSI-H colorectal cancers show a suboptimal response to conventional 5-fluorouracil–based chemotherapy, and thus, detection of MSI-H can potentially impact patient management.[15] Most institutions do not routinely perform mismatch repair protein immunohistochemistry or PCR for microsatellite status on all colorectal carcinomas. Thus, pathologists must rely on key morphologic features that suggest underlying MSI-H in colorectal cancer resection and biopsy specimens.

Microsatellite unstable tumors typically elicit a host immune response, either in the form of a Crohn-like lymphoid response (Figure 9.11) or tumor-infiltrating lymphocytes (Figure 9.12). These neoplasms also show characteristic histologic features, including signet ring cell, mucinous, medullary, and poor differentiation (Figure 9.13). Carcinomas with MSI-H are often

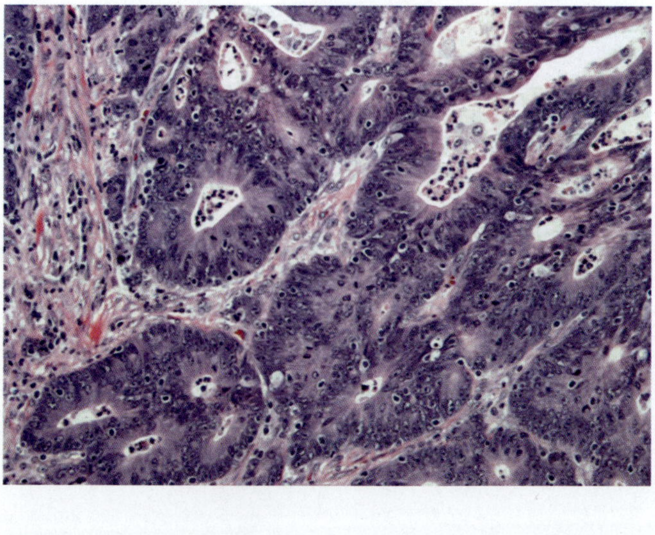

**FIGURE 9.12:** Tumor-infiltrating lymphocytes are a sensitive marker of MSI-H. Mature lymphocytes intercalate between epithelial cells within tumor glands.

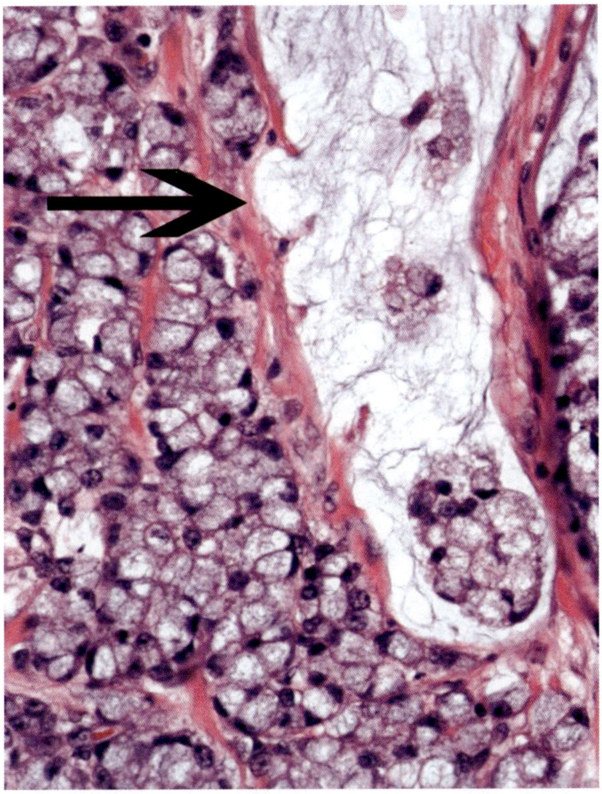

A

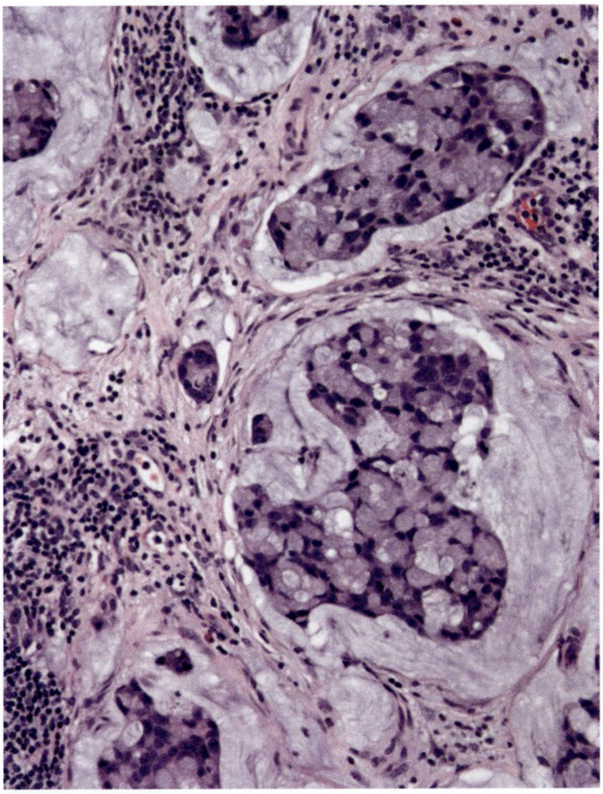

B

FIGURE 9.13: Microsatellite unstable tumors show a variety of characteristic morphologic features that may be present in combination within a tumor. Signet ring cell carcinomas are often associated with mucinous components (*arrow*) and typically grow as clusters, cords, and nests of cells with large mucin vacuoles (**A**). Mucinous carcinomas consist of mucin pools containing clusters and nests of tumor cells, many of which are distended by abundant mucin that imparts a signet ring cell appearance (**B**).

**FIGURE 9.13:** (*Continued*) Medullary carcinomas do not form glands. They contain cords and trabeculae of tumor cells with abundant cytoplasm and large round nuclei with open chromatin and prominent nucleoli (**C**). Although tumor-infiltrating lymphocytes are typically found in medullary carcinomas, they are also present in gland-forming adenocarcinomas with underlying MSI-H (**D**).

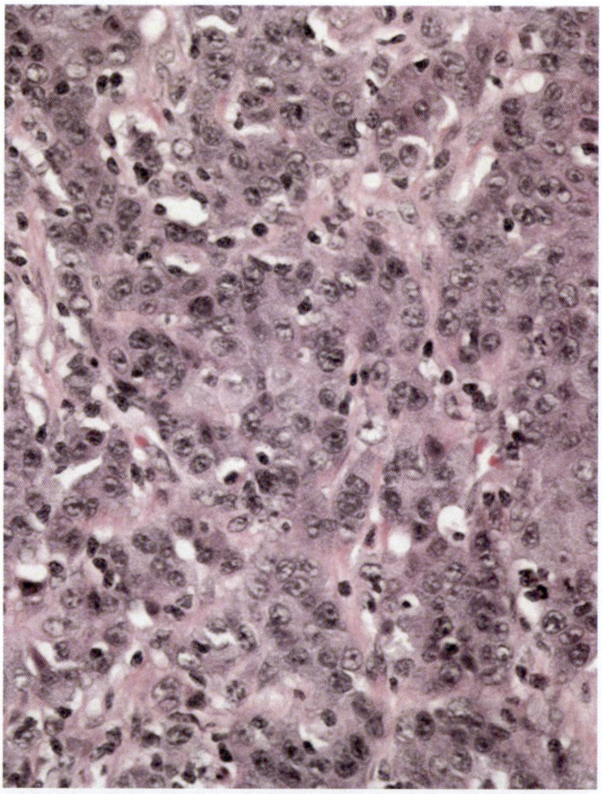

C

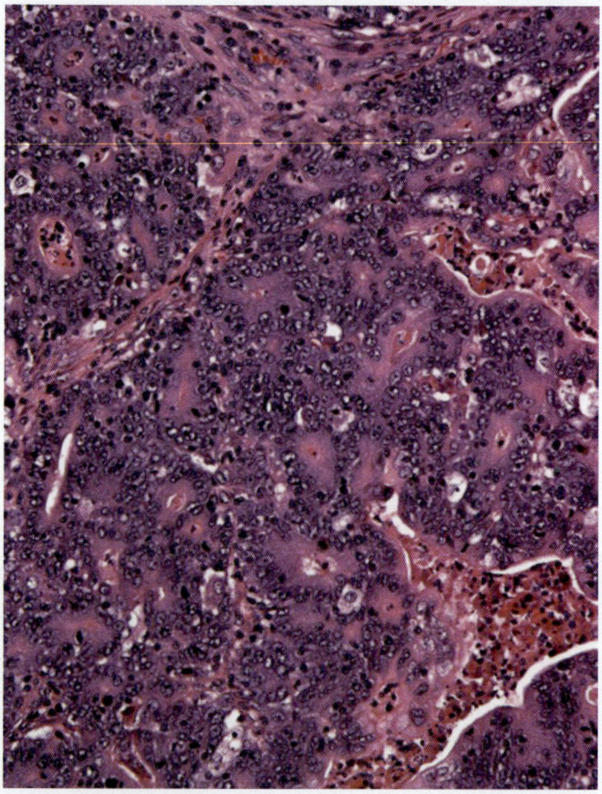

D

heterogeneous and display a combination of growth patterns. Less commonly described features of these lesions include a lack of "dirty necrosis" typical of most colorectal carcinomas, areas of well-differentiated carcinoma, and any amount of mucinous differentiation.[40] Overall, medullary carcinoma, tumor-infiltrating lymphocytes, and poor differentiation are the best discriminators between MSI-H and MSS colorectal carcinomas, and a medullary appearance is particularly associated with MSI-H (specificity, 99%).[40,43]

# POLYPECTOMY SPECIMENS

## Intramucosal High-Grade Carcinoma

Most colorectal carcinomas are derived from neoplastic precursor lesions (adenomas) that develop progressively severe dysplasia and infiltration of the mucosa. Tumors that are limited to the muscularis mucosae (intramucosal carcinoma) have no potential for malignant behavior and are essentially cured by complete excision. Most are well-differentiated adenocarcinomas with extensive glandular differentiation that expand the lamina propria, but do not elicit a desmoplastic stromal response (Figure 9.14). However, rare cases show high-grade cytologic features, including a sheet-like growth of tumor cells or signet ring cells that permeate the mucosa (Figure 9.15). Although the biologic behavior of intramucosal high-grade carcinoma has not been extensively studied, data from one small, retrospective study suggest that it is adequately treated by complete excision.[44] Despite these preliminary reports, the diagnosis of high-grade intramucosal carcinoma should only be made when one is confident that the entire lesion has

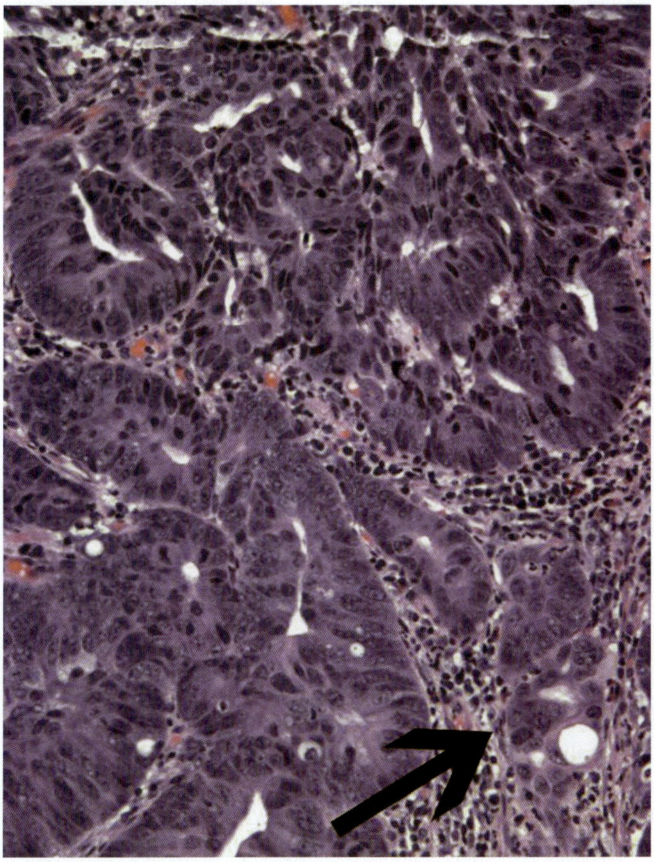

**FIGURE 9.14:** Intramucosal adenocarcinoma is usually identified in polypectomy specimens and contains well-formed glands arranged in confluent groups our single infiltrating glands (*arrow*). Tumor cells that infiltrate the lamina propria do not elicit a desmoplastic stromal response in most cases. The tumor cells contain large, irregular, and hyperchromatic nuclei with prominent nucleoli and easily identifiable mitotic figures.

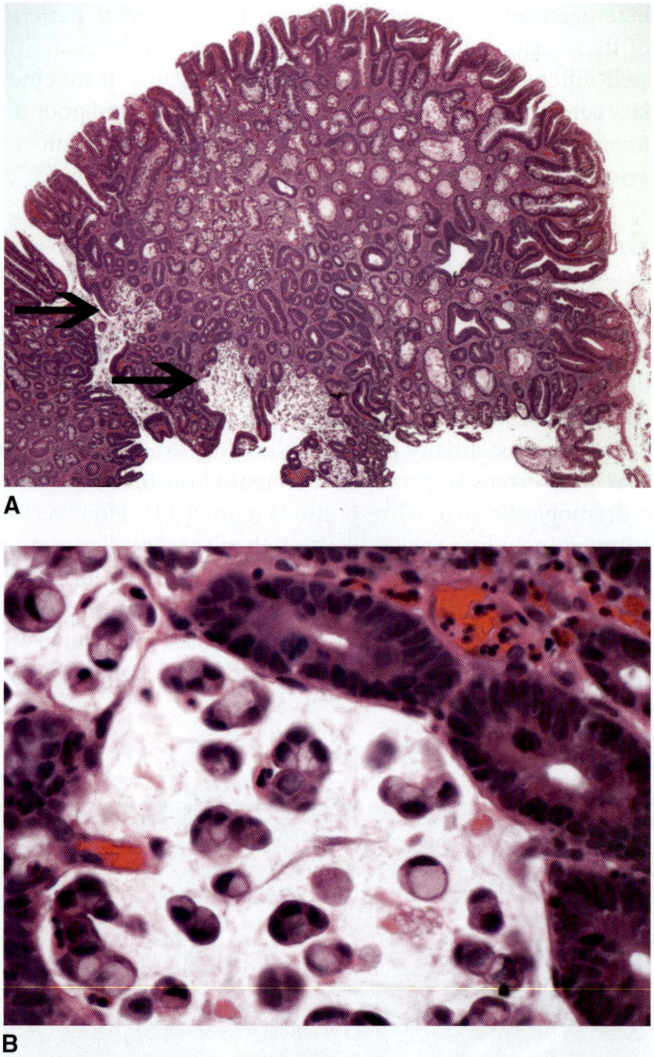

**FIGURE 9.15:** Rare colonic adenomas contain foci of a high-grade carcinoma (*arrows*) in the mucosa (**A**). Signet ring cells and clusters of malignant cells are dispersed in mucin pools confined to the lamina propria (**B**).

been histologically evaluated. Metastatic cancers, deeply situated colorectal carcinomas, and perianal Paget disease can all colonize the mucosa, in which case they do not elicit a desmoplastic stromal response and often simulate either high-grade dysplasia or intramucosal carcinoma.[45] High-grade intramucosal carcinoma that develops in the setting of inflammatory bowel disease has not been prospectively investigated, although patients with ulcerative colitis and dysplasia have increased numbers of mucosal lymphatic vessels compared to uninflamed colonic mucosae.[46] Thus, it is possible that inflammatory bowel disease–related intramucosal carcinoma is biologically different than that associated with sporadic adenomas. Patients with inflammatory bowel disease and intramucosal carcinoma should be carefully evaluated and strongly consider surgical intervention.

## Invasive Adenocarcinoma

Colorectal adenomas that contain adenocarcinomas invasive of the submucosa (malignant polyps) are amenable to complete excision followed by surveillance in some situations. Histologic features that predict adverse outcome following polypectomy include histologic tumor grade, lymphovascular or venous invasion, status of the resection margin, and extent of submucosal invasion. Prior studies have described classification schemes to assess depth of cancer invasion

**Table 9.3 Classification Scheme for Invasive Adenocarcinomas Present in Pedunculated and Sessile Adenomas**

| Proposed Designation | Depth of Invasion |
|---|---|
| Pedunculated adenomas | |
| Level 0 | Intramucosal carcinoma (pTis) |
| Level 1 | Tumor invades submucosa and limited to polyp head |
| Level 2 | Tumor invades submucosa and neck of polyp |
| Level 3 | Tumor invades submucosa in stalk of polyp |
| Level 4 | Tumor invades below polyp stalk into bowel wall |
| Sessile adenomas | |
| $Sm_1$ | Invasion limited to upper third of mucosa |
| $Sm_2$ | Invasion limited to middle third of mucosa |
| $Sm_3$ | Invasion limited to lower third of mucosa |

in pedunculated and sessile adenomas with invasive carcinoma in order to predict likelihood of residual disease following polypectomy (Table 9.3).[47] Carcinomas arising in pedunculated adenomas are adequately treated with polypectomy alone, provided the invasive carcinoma is entirely low-grade, lacks vascular invasion, and is limited to the polyp stalk at least 1 mm from the cauterized base of the polyp.[47–49] Fewer than 1% of malignant polyps that meet these criteria are associated with regional lymph node metastases. Pedunculated polyps with cancer below the level of the stalk (level 4) and sessile malignant polyps with cancer limited to the inner two-thirds of the submucosa ($Sm_1$ or $Sm_2$) may be conservatively managed, provided the margin is greater than 2 mm from the advancing edge of the tumor and both high-grade features and lymphovascular invasion are lacking.[50] Alternatively, approximately 15% of malignant polyps that show high-grade histology, lymphovascular invasion, or close (<1 mm) resection margins are associated with regional lymph node metastases or residual tumor in subsequent colectomy specimens and, thus, generally require further surgical intervention.[49,51] Recent studies have also identified tumor budding at the advancing front of the carcinoma as an important predictor of regional lymph node metastases.[49,52] Thus, surgical pathology reports for malignant polyps should specifically include comments regarding each of these parameters: histologic grade, presence or absence of lymphatic and/or venous invasion, distance from the tumor to the resection margin, and tumor budding. Other features, such as an expansile, irregular tumor growth, the pedunculated or sessile appearance of the polyp, and the nature of the noninvasive precursor lesion (e.g., tubular adenoma, villous adenoma, serrated adenoma, sessile serrated polyp), may be reported, but their clinical importance has yet to be determined.[2]

## PROGNOSTIC IMPORTANCE OF RESPONSE TO NEOADJUVANT THERAPY

Patients with locally advanced rectal cancer routinely receive neoadjuvant therapy prior to definitive surgical resection in order to downstage the tumor, improve surgical outcome, and enhance postsurgical quality of life.[6] Neoadjuvantly treated tumors usually show evidence of regression with mural fibrosis, dystrophic calcifications, and pools of mucin. These changes may be present in the primary tumor as well as lymph node deposits, and the extent of regression is predictive of prognosis.[53] Tumors that show a striking response to therapy are associated with improved disease-free survival compared to cases in which grossly evident viable tumor remains after neoadjuvant treatment.[54] A variety of regression scoring systems have been proposed. The grading system endorsed by the AJCC/TNM seventh edition *Cancer Staging Manual* applies the lowest

**Table 9.4 Classification of Residual Disease in Rectal Resection Specimens Following Neoadjuvant Therapy**

| Tumor Regression Grade | Definition |
|---|---|
| 0 (Complete response) | No viable cancer cells |
| 1 (Moderate response) | Single cells or small groups of cancer cells |
| 2 (Minimal response) | Residual cancer outgrown by fibrosis |
| 3 (Poor response) | Extensive residual cancer with minimal, or no, tumor response |

grade to the best treatment response and highest grade to the poorest response. Tumors are considered to show a grade 0 response when complete tumor regression is noted, whereas grades 1, 2, and 3 reflect a marked, moderate, and poor reduction in viable tumor volume, respectively (Table 9.4).[55] Assessment of tumor regression is only performed on the primary tumor. Lymph node deposits that show a therapeutic response are not considered when grading tumor regression or are they counted toward the assignment of pN stage if no viable tumor is identified within the lymph node.[2]

## SUMMARY AND CONCLUSIONS

A number of pathologic features may be prognostically important and should be commented upon in colorectal carcinoma surgical pathology reports. Some of these features are readily apparent upon gross examination of the resection specimen. Adequacy of surgical resection is a major predictor of local recurrence and death due to disease, particularly among locally advanced rectal cancers. Free perforation through the tumor is associated with poor outcome, as is detection of inadequate numbers of regional lymph nodes. Specific types of cancer, such as signet ring cell, high-grade (neuro)endocrine, micropapillary, and undifferentiated carcinomas, are high-grade neoplasms at risk for biologically aggressive behavior, whereas tumors with MSI-H are, by definition, low-grade. Lymphovascular and venous invasion are associated with regional and distant metastases, and both perineural invasion and satellite tumor deposits predict poorer overall survival. Colorectal carcinomas that invade with an infiltrative border or show tumor budding are more aggressive than those that lack these findings, whereas a host immune response and histologic features suggestive of MSI-H are associated with improved patient survival.

# References

1. Compton CC, Greene FL. The staging of colorectal cancer: 2004 and beyond. *CA Cancer J Clin* 2004; 54(6):295–308.
2. Washington MK, Berlin J, Branton PA, et al. Protocol for the examination of specimens from patients with primary carcinomas of the colon and rectum. *Arch Pathol Lab Med* 2008;132(7):1182–1193.
3. Birbeck KF, Macklin CP, Tiffin NJ, et al. Rates of circumferential resection margin involvement vary between surgeons and predict outcomes in rectal cancer surgery. *Ann Surg* 2002;235(4):449–457.
4. Colon and rectum. In: Edge S, Byrd D, Compton CC, et al., eds. *AJCC Cancer Staging Manual.* 7th ed. New York, NY: Springer; 2009:143–164.
5. Arbman G, Nilsson E, Hallbook O, et al. Local recurrence following total mesorectal excision for rectal cancer. *Br J Surg* 1996;83(3):375–379.
6. Kapiteijn E, Marijnen CA, Nagtegaal ID, et al. Preoperative radiotherapy combined with total mesorectal excision for resectable rectal cancer. *N Engl J Med* 2001;345(9):638–646.

7. Goldstein NS. Lymph node recoveries from 2427 pT3 colorectal resection specimens spanning 45 years: recommendations for a minimum number of recovered lymph nodes based on predictive probabilities. *Am J Surg Pathol* 2002;26(2):179–189.
8. Swanson RS, Compton CC, Stewart AK, et al. The prognosis of T3N0 colon cancer is dependent on the number of lymph nodes examined. *Ann Surg Oncol* 2003;10(1):65–71.
9. George S, Primrose J, Talbot R, et al. Will Rogers revisited: prospective observational study of survival of 3592 patients with colorectal cancer according to number of nodes examined by pathologists. *Br J Cancer* 2006;95(7):841–847.
10. Shepherd NA, Baxter KJ, Love SB. The prognostic importance of peritoneal involvement in colonic cancer: a prospective evaluation. *Gastroenterology* 1997;112(4):1096–1102.
11. Anwar MA, D'Souza F, Coulter R, et al. Outcome of acutely perforated colorectal cancers: experience of a single district general hospital. *Surg Oncol* 2006;15(2):91–96.
12. Ogawa M, Watanabe M, Eto K, et al. Poorly differentiated adenocarcinoma of the colon and rectum: clinical characteristics. *Hepatogastroenterology* 2008;55(84):907–911.
13. Hamilton SR, Bosman FT, Boffetta P, et al. Tumors of the colon and rectum. In: Bosman FT, Carneiro F, Hruban RH, et al., eds. *WHO Classification of Tumours of the Digestive System.* 4th ed. Lyon, France: International Agency for Research on Cancer; 2010:134–146.
14. Parc Y, Gueroult S, Mourra N, et al. Prognostic significance of microsatellite instability determined by immunohistochemical staining of MSH2 and MLH1 in sporadic T3N0M0 colon cancer. *Gut* 2004;53(3):371–375.
15. Ribic CM, Sargent DJ, Moore MJ, et al. Tumor microsatellite-instability status as a predictor of benefit from fluorouracil-based adjuvant chemotherapy for colon cancer. *N Engl J Med* 2003;349(3):247–257.
16. Ueno H, Mochizuki H, Hashiguchi Y, et al. Histological grading of colorectal cancer: a simple and objective method. *Ann Surg* 2008;247(5):811–818.
17. Ueno H, Kajiwara Y, Shimazaki H, et al. New criteria for histologic grading of colorectal cancer. *Am J Surg Pathol* 2012;36(2):193–201.
18. Bernick PE, Klimstra DS, Shia J, et al. Neuroendocrine carcinomas of the colon and rectum. *Dis Colon Rectum* 2004;47(2):163–169.
19. Wachtel MS, Haynes AL III, Griswold JA. Signet ring, high grade, and undifferentiated colorectal adenocarcinomas differ. *J Surg Res* 2010;163(2):250–256.
20. Makino T, Tsujinaka T, Mishima H, et al. Primary signet-ring cell carcinoma of the colon and rectum: report of eight cases and review of 154 Japanese cases. *Hepatogastroenterology* 2006;53(72):845–849.
21. Lino-Silva LS, Hernandez RA, Caro-Sanchez CH. Colonic micropapillary carcinoma, a recently recognized subtype associated with histologic adverse factors. Clinicopathologic analysis of 15 cases. *Colorectal Dis* 2012;14(9):e567–e572.
22. Verdu M, Roman R, Calvo M, et al. Clinicopathological and molecular characterization of colorectal micropapillary carcinoma. *Mod Pathol* 2011;24(5):729–738.
23. Xu F, Xu J, Lou Z, et al. Micropapillary component in colorectal carcinoma is associated with lymph node metastasis in T1 and T2 Stages and decreased survival time in TNM stages I and II. *Am J Surg Pathol* 2009;33(9):1287–1292.
24. Schoppmann SF. Lymphangiogenesis, inflammation and metastasis. *Anticancer Res* 2005;25(6C): 4503–4511.
25. Saad RS, Kordunsky L, Liu YL, et al. Lymphatic microvessel density as prognostic marker in colorectal cancer. *Mod Pathol* 2006;19(10):1317–1323.
26. Yamamoto S, Watanabe M, Hasegawa H, et al. The risk of lymph node metastasis in T1 colorectal carcinoma. *Hepatogastroenterology* 2004;51(58):998–1000.
27. Sternberg A, Amar M, Alfici R, et al. Conclusions from a study of venous invasion in stage IV colorectal adenocarcinoma. *J Clin Pathol* 2002;55(1):17–21.
28. Puppa G, Caneva A, Colombari R. Venous invasion detection in colorectal cancer: which approach, which technique? *J Clin Pathol* 2009;62(2):102–103.
29. Huh JW, Kim HR, Kim YJ. Lymphovascular or perineural invasion may predict lymph node metastasis in patients with T1 and T2 colorectal cancer. *J Gastrointest Surg* 2010;14(7):1074–1080.
30. Peng J, Sheng W, Huang D, et al. Perineural invasion in pT3N0 rectal cancer: the incidence and its prognostic effect. *Cancer* 2011;117(7):1415–1421.
31. Prall F, Weirich V, Ostwald C. Phenotypes of invasion in sporadic colorectal carcinomas related to aberrations of the adenomatous polyposis coli (APC) gene. *Histopathology* 2007;50(3):318–330.

32. Halvorsen TB, Seim E. Association between invasiveness, inflammatory reaction, desmoplasia and survival in colorectal cancer. *J Clin Pathol* 1989;42(2):162–166.
33. Ueno H, Murphy J, Jass JR, et al. Tumour 'budding' as an index to estimate the potential of aggressiveness in rectal cancer. *Histopathology* 2002;40(2):127–132.
34. Ricci-Vitiani L, Lombardi DG, Pilozzi E, et al. Identification and expansion of human colon-cancer-initiating cells. *Nature* 2007;445(7123):111–115.
35. Vermeulen L, Todaro M, de Sousa Mello F, et al. Single-cell cloning of colon cancer stem cells reveals a multi-lineage differentiation capacity. *Proc Natl Acad Sci U S A* 2008;105(36):13427–13432.
36. Kanazawa H, Mitomi H, Nishiyama Y, et al. Tumour budding at invasive margins and outcome in colorectal cancer. *Colorectal Dis* 2008;10(1):41–47.
37. Okuyama T, Nakamura T, Yamaguchi M. Budding is useful to select high-risk patients in stage II well-differentiated or moderately differentiated colon adenocarcinoma. *Dis Colon Rectum* 2003;46(10):1400–1406.
38. Puppa G, Maisonneuve P, Sonzogni A, et al. Pathological assessment of pericolonic tumor deposits in advanced colonic carcinoma: relevance to prognosis and tumor staging. *Mod Pathol* 2007;20(8):843–855.
39. Ogino S, Nosho K, Irahara N, et al. Lymphocytic reaction to colorectal cancer is associated with longer survival, independent of lymph node count, microsatellite instability, and CpG island methylator phenotype. *Clin Cancer Res* 2009;15(20):6412–6420.
40. Greenson JK, Bonner JD, Ben-Yzhak O, et al. Phenotype of microsatellite unstable colorectal carcinomas: Well-differentiated and focally mucinous tumors and the absence of dirty necrosis correlate with microsatellite instability. *Am J Surg Pathol* 2003;27(5):563–570.
41. Sinicrope F, Foster NR, Sargent DJ, et al. Model-based prediction of defective DNA mismatch repair using clinicopathological variables in sporadic colon cancer patients. *Cancer* 2010;116(7):1691–1698.
42. Graham DM, Appelman HD. Crohn's-like lymphoid reaction and colorectal carcinoma: a potential histologic prognosticator. *Mod Pathol* 1990;3(3):332–335.
43. Alexander J, Watanabe T, Wu TT, et al. Histopathological identification of colon cancer with microsatellite instability. *Am J Pathol* 2001;158(2):527–535.
44. Lewin MR, Fenton H, Burkart AL, et al. Poorly differentiated colorectal carcinoma with invasion restricted to lamina propria (intramucosal carcinoma): a follow-up study of 15 cases. *Am J Surg Pathol* 2007;31(12):1882–1886.
45. Estrella JS, Wu TT, Rashid A, et al. Mucosal colonization by metastatic carcinoma in the gastrointestinal tract: a potential mimic of primary neoplasia. *Am J Surg Pathol* 2011;35(4):563–572.
46. Kaiserling E, Krober S, Geleff S. Lymphatic vessels in the colonic mucosa in ulcerative colitis. *Lymphology* 2003;36(2):52–61.
47. Haggitt RC, Glotzbach RE, Soffer EE, et al. Prognostic factors in colorectal carcinomas arising in adenomas: implications for lesions removed by endoscopic polypectomy. *Gastroenterology* 1985;89(2):328–336.
48. Haggitt RC. Management of the patient with carcinoma in an adenoma. *Prog Clin Biol Res* 1988;279:89–99.
49. Choi DH, Sohn DK, Chang HJ, et al. Indications for subsequent surgery after endoscopic resection of submucosally invasive colorectal carcinomas: a prospective cohort study. *Dis Colon Rectum* 2009;52(3):438–445.
50. Kudo S. Endoscopic mucosal resection of flat and depressed types of early colorectal cancer. *Endoscopy* 1993;25(7):455–461.
51. Butte JM, Tang P, Gonen M, et al. Rate of residual disease after complete endoscopic resection of malignant colonic polyp. *Dis Colon Rectum* 2012;55(2):122–127.
52. Tateishi Y, Nakanishi Y, Taniguchi H, et al. Pathological prognostic factors predicting lymph node metastasis in submucosal invasive (T1) colorectal carcinoma. *Mod Pathol* 2010;23(8):1068–1072.
53. Kuo LJ, Liu MC, Jian JJ, et al. Is final TNM staging a predictor for survival in locally advanced rectal cancer after preoperative chemoradiation therapy? *Ann Surg Oncol* 2007;14(10):2766–2772.
54. Ruo L, Tickoo S, Klimstra DS, et al. Long-term prognostic significance of extent of rectal cancer response to preoperative radiation and chemotherapy. *Ann Surg* 2002;236(1):75–81.
55. Ryan R, Gibbons D, Hyland JM, et al. Pathological response following long-course neoadjuvant chemoradiotherapy for locally advanced rectal cancer. *Histopathology* 2005;47(2):141–146.

# Differential Diagnosis of Colorectal Carcinoma

# 10

Rhonda K. Yantiss

The recognition of colorectal carcinoma and its distinction from potential mimics poses several challenges, particularly in endoscopically obtained samples. For example, early invasive adenocarcinoma in colorectal adenomas may be difficult to distinguish from inflammatory changes in traumatized polyps. The colon is also a common site for primary and metastatic carcinomas that must be appropriately classified because therapeutic regimens for colorectal cancer differ from those for cancers originating in other organs. Management of primary colorectal carcinoma consists of complete surgical removal, if possible, with the addition of radiation and/or chemotherapy for local and systemic control, respectively. In contrast, metastases to the colorectum are managed with chemotherapy, and surgery and radiation are reserved for patients who require symptomatic relief of obstruction or bleeding. In this chapter we discuss the differential diagnosis of colorectal carcinoma as well as the ancillary immunohistochemical stains that aid in its identification.

## DISTINCTION BETWEEN IN SITU AND INVASIVE LESIONS

Colorectal adenomas that show high-grade dysplasia (intraepithelial carcinoma) and carcinomas limited by the muscularis mucosae (intramucosal carcinoma) are staged as carcinomas in situ (pTis) and adequately treated by polypectomy. The World Health Organization (WHO) classifies such lesions as intraepithelial and intramucosal neoplasia, respectively, in order to avoid terminology that may trigger overly aggressive management.[1] However, invasive adenocarcinoma can mimic "in situ" neoplasia when it grows in the mucosa (Figure 10.1). It frequently colonizes the basement membrane, which induces maturation of malignant epithelium and simulates the appearance of an adenoma with high-grade dysplasia. Invasive adenocarcinoma also lacks a desmoplastic stromal response when it extends into the lamina propria, mimicking the appearance of intramucosal carcinoma (Figure 10.2). Several helpful features distinguish between primary neoplasia and colonization of the mucosa by invasive carcinoma. Most colorectal adenomas with high-grade dysplasia also show low-grade dysplasia, so a complete absence of the latter raises the possibility of mucosal colonization by a more deeply invasive tumor. Microvesicular or foamy cytoplasm is unusual in intestinal adenomas, but is characteristic of some secondary tumors that show a predilection to colonize the basement membrane, such as pancreatic carcinoma (Figure 10.3). Since most invasive carcinomas associated with adenomas are well-to-moderately differentiated, the presence of a high-grade tumor that infiltrates the lamina propria raises the possibility of metastasis.[2] Given the propensity for invasive carcinomas to mimic in situ lesions in mucosal biopsies, diagnoses of high-grade dysplasia and intramucosal carcinoma should only be made when one is confident that the entire lesion has been removed (i.e., polypectomy specimens).

## MIMICS OF INVASIVE ADENOCARCINOMA

Most superficially invasive adenocarcinomas are identified in polypectomy specimens. Recognition of submucosal invasion is generally straightforward, although potential mimics do occur. Large pedunculated polyps, particularly those in the distal colon that are subjected

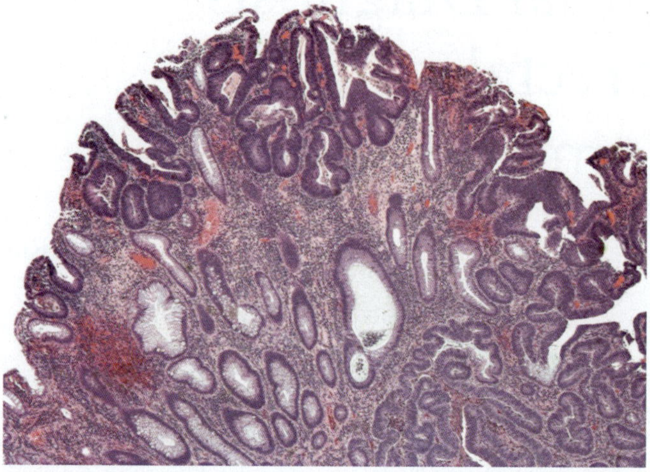

**FIGURE 10.1:** Invasive colonic carcinomas can colonize the mucosa and grow along the basement membrane. This tumor in the distal colon simulated the appearance of an adenoma in mucosal biopsies because it appeared to be confined to the basement membrane in biopsy samples. However, the carcinoma deeply invaded the colonic wall and was associated with regional lymph node metastases in the resection specimen.

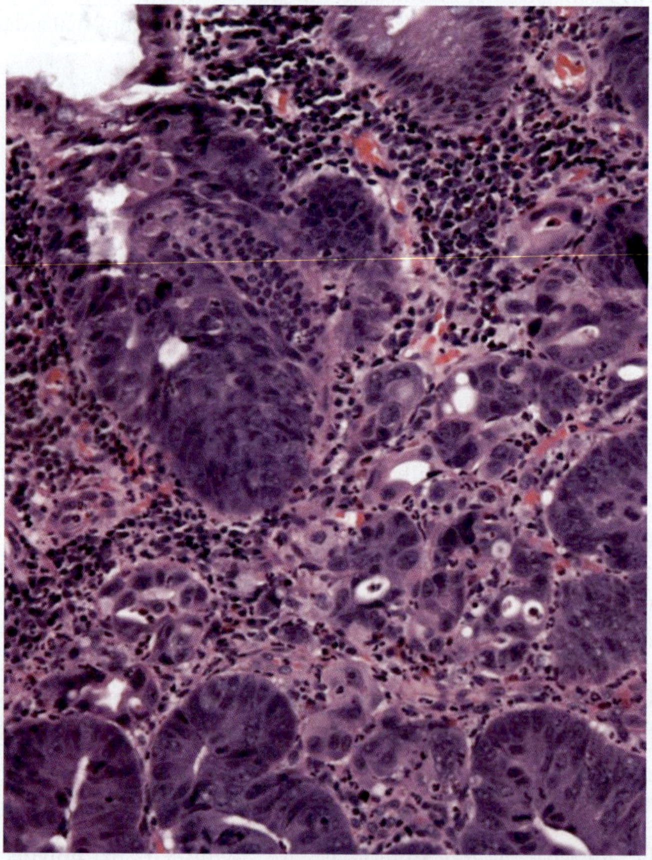

**FIGURE 10.2:** Invasive adenocarcinoma does not elicit a desmoplastic response when it extends into the lamina propria. This rectal polyp occurred in a patient with invasive colonic adenocarcinoma and multiple mucosal metastases. It contains glands that simulate an adenoma surrounded by a diffuse proliferation of high-grade tumor cells.

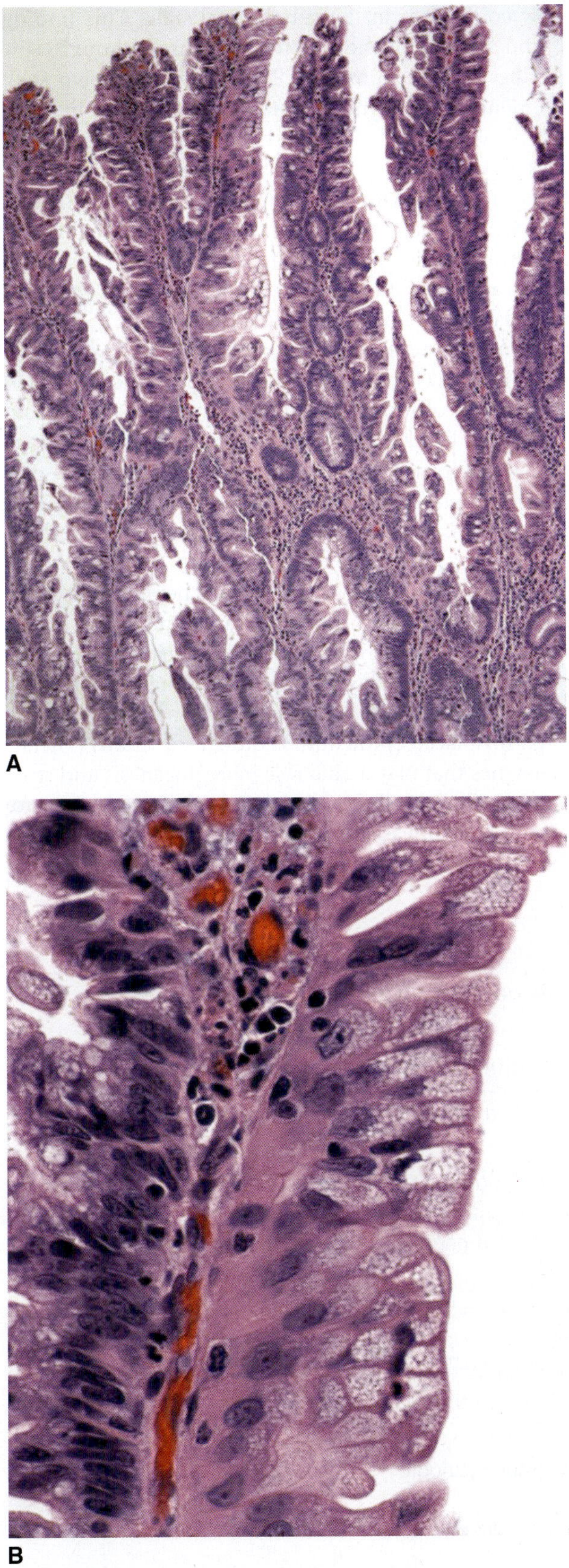

FIGURE 10.3: Metastatic pancreatic adenocarcinoma assumes a villiform growth pattern in the mucosa with micropapillae and high-grade cytologic features (**A**). Some of the tumor cells simulate the appearance of an intestinal primary and contain elongated, hyperchromatic nuclei (left), whereas others contain microvesicular, foamy cytoplasm (right) typical of pancreaticobiliary tumors (**B**).

to luminal or endoscopic trauma, can show epithelium in the submucosal stalk. This finding has been termed "epithelial misplacement" and "pseudoinvasion" in the literature, although "epithelial displacement" more accurately describes this phenomenon. Twisting of the polyp stalk presumably causes herniation of mucosal elements through the muscularis mucosae into the submucosa. The histologic distinction between displaced epithelium and invasive adenocarcinoma has significant clinical implications because some superficial adenocarcinomas require colectomy and staging of regional lymph nodes, whereas adenomas with epithelial misplacement are treated adequately by simple polypectomy, as discussed in Chapter 9. Several features help distinguish adenomas with displaced epithelium from invasive adenocarcinoma (Table 10.1).[3,4] Displaced submucosal epithelium has a lobular configuration with a distinct rim of lamina propria and resembles the epithelium at the polyp surface (Figure 10.4A). Benign, displaced crypts in the submucosa dilate and rupture, inciting an inflammatory response to extruded mucin, and stromal hemorrhage and hemosiderin deposits are common (Figure 10.4B). Endoscopic manipulation of large adenomas also causes traumatic herniation of mucosa into the submucosa with mucin extrusion, scarring, and hemorrhage (Figure 10.5). Unlike displaced benign epithelium, invasive adenocarcinoma typically grows in an expansile, infiltrative fashion (Figure 10.6A). It is unassociated with lamina propria tissue and incites a desmoplastic stromal response. Malignant epithelial cells are cytologically atypical with high-grade nuclei, nuclear pleomorphism, and clumped chromatin (Figure 10.6B).

Morphologic assessment alone may be inadequate to distinguish displaced benign epithelium from invasive adenocarcinoma in some cases, such as those in which displaced epithelium shows high-grade dysplasia.[3] Immunohistochemical expression of several biomarkers can facilitate detection of invasive adenocarcinoma. Invasive adenocarcinoma in adenomas shows increased nuclear staining for TP53 when compared with the surface adenomatous epithelium in nearly two-thirds of cases, whereas increased staining of benign misplaced epithelium is quite rare.[5] Matrix metalloproteinases, which comprise a family of enzymes that play a vital role in angiogenesis and stromal breakdown and aid invasion of malignant epithelial cells into highly vascularized stroma, are overexpressed in the stroma and epithelium of most invasive adenocarcinomas.[6] These include matrix metalloproteinase-1 and stromelysin-3, which are strongly expressed in most carcinomas

**Table 10.1** Features That Aid Distinction Between Misplaced Epithelium and Invasive Adenocarcinoma in Colorectal Polyps

| Features of Submucosal Epithelium | Misplaced Epithelium | Invasive Adenocarcinoma |
|---|---|---|
| Gland arrangement | Well-circumscribed lobules | Irregular, expansile aggregates<br>Infiltrating glands and cells |
| Extracellular mucin | Acellular mucin pools with inflammatory reaction<br>Any epithelium is at periphery of mucin pool | Mucin pools contain strips or clusters of floating epithelium |
| Stromal features | Fresh hemorrhage and/or hemosiderin<br>Inflammation and fibrosis<br>Lamina propria surrounds epithelium | No lamina propria<br>Desmoplasia |
| Epithelium | Usually low-grade cytologic features<br>Similar to that of overlying mucosa | Cytologically malignant |

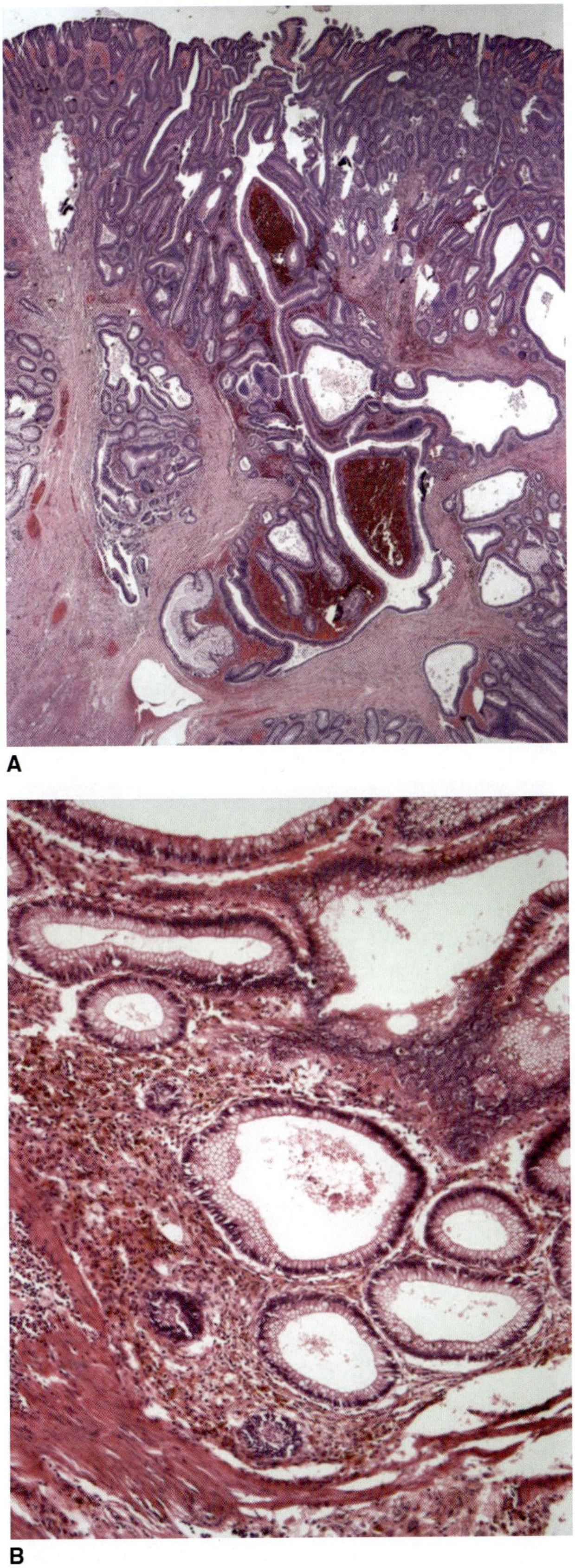

A

B

FIGURE 10.4: Epithelial misplacement results from trauma to pedunculated colonic adenomas and appears as lobules of mucosa within the submucosa (**A**). Herniated mucosal elements contain cystically dilated glands, hemorrhage, and hemosiderin with associated lamina propria (**B**).

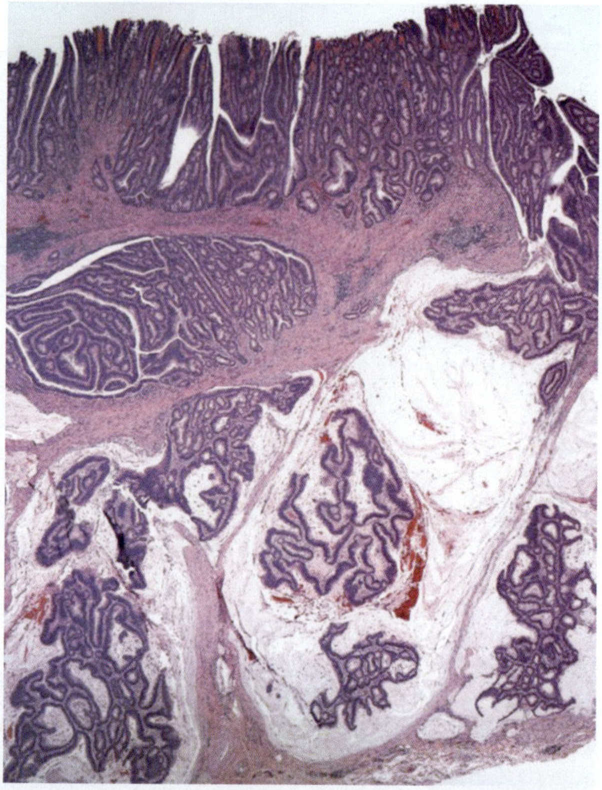

A

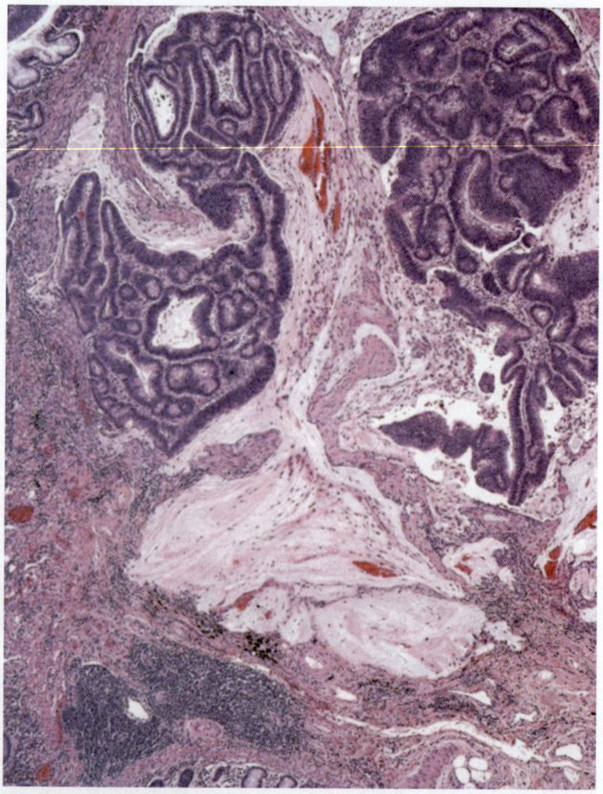

B

FIGURE 10.5: Endoscopic biopsy of large polyps may induce herniation of mucosal elements into the submucosa (A). Round aggregates of neoplastic epithelium are associated with lamina propria and extruded mucin (B). The submucosa is inflamed and fibrotic.

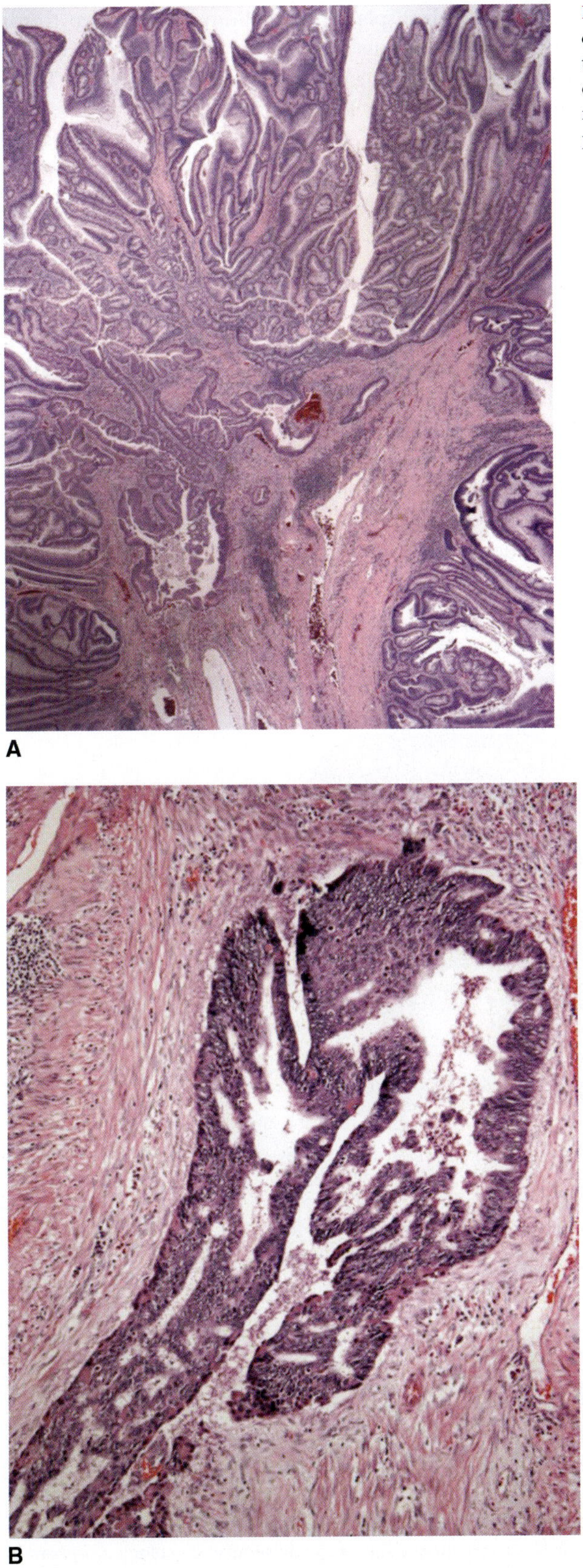

A

B

FIGURE 10.6: Invasive adenocarcinomas are expansile tumors composed of irregularly distributed glands with an ill-defined advancing edge (**A**). Invasive glands contain cytologically malignant cells and are surrounded by desmoplastic stroma (**B**).

in comparison with less than 50% of adenomas with displaced epithelium.[7] Nearly two-thirds of invasive adenocarcinomas show diminished membranous staining for E-cadherin, and more than 90% show discontinuous, or absent, collagen IV staining of the basement membrane. These markers remain unaltered in adenomatous epithelium in any location.[4,8–10]

# DISTINGUISHING PRIMARY COLORECTAL CARCINOMA FROM OTHER ENTITIES

## General Features

When metastases from another site involve the colonic mucosa, they may be difficult to distinguish from primary colonic cancers. Features suggestive of a primary malignancy include a concurrent adenomatous precursor lesion, regional lymph node involvement, and location of the tumor epicenter in the luminal aspect of the bowel wall. Multicentricity is more typical of a metastasis than primary colorectal cancer. However, none of these features is exclusively seen in either primary or secondary tumors. Metastatic tumors may colonize the mucosa and grow along the basement membrane, mimicking the appearance of an adenomatous component, as previously described (Figure 10.3). Mucosal colonization is a common feature of metastases of gastrointestinal origin and of endometrioid adenocarcinomas of müllerian origin (Figure 10.7). More than a third of metastases to the colon also involve regional pericolic lymph nodes, thereby simulating the disease distribution of a primary cancer.[11]

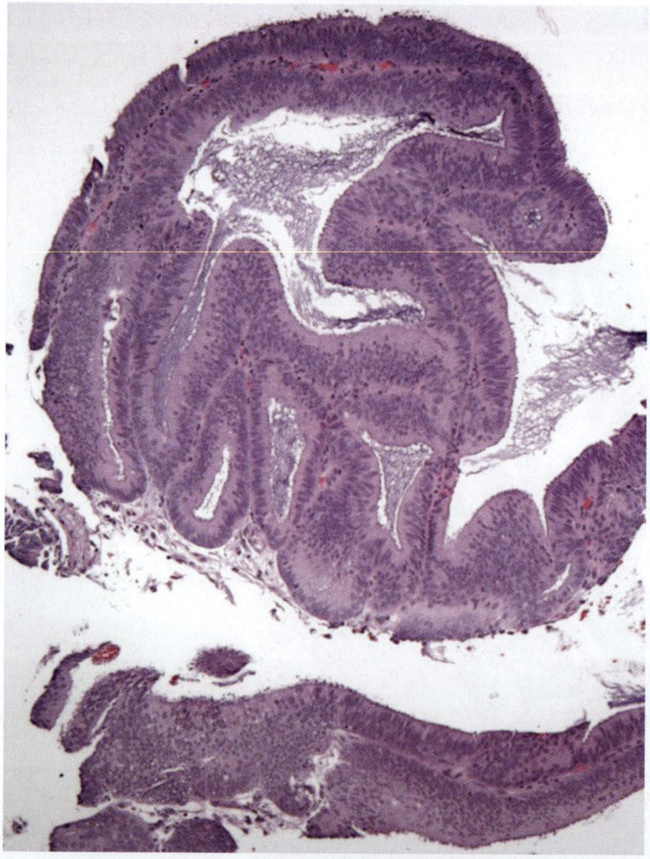

A

FIGURE 10.7: Endometrioid adenocarcinoma from a primary uterine tumor closely simulates a colonic neoplasm in mucosal biopsies (A).

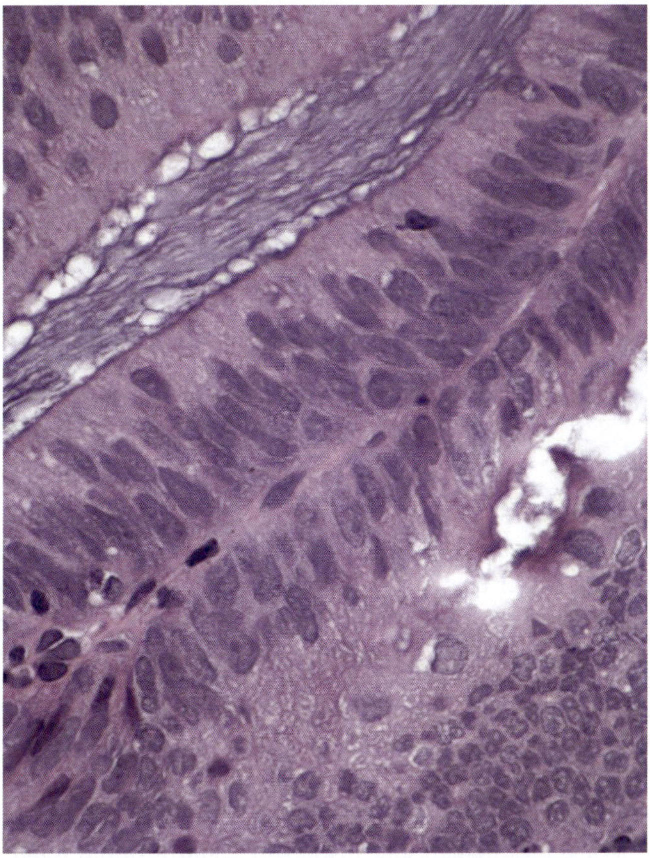


FIGURE 10.7: (*Continued*) Colonization of the colonic surface induces maturation in this gynecologic cancer such that the features closely simulate those of a colorectal neoplasm (**B**).

Immunohistochemical stains are effective in distinguishing primary from metastatic carcinomas, particularly when the differential diagnosis includes tumors of nonintestinal origin. Cytokeratin 20 and CDX-2 positivity combined with negativity for cytokeratin 7 are specific for tumors of colorectal origin, whereas other combinations suggest a different primary site. Cadherin-17 (CDH17) is also a helpful marker of intestinal differentiation.[12] This molecule is under the transcriptional control of CDX-2 and manifests a membranous staining pattern in intestinal epithelium.

## Multifocal Colorectal Carcinoma

Two or more tumors at the time of diagnosis are present in fewer than 5% of patients with colorectal carcinoma. Possible etiologies include synchronous primary tumors and mucosal metastases from a primary colonic malignancy. Synchronous primary tumors are more likely to occur in patients with long-standing inflammatory bowel disease and heritable cancer syndromes, but may also develop in patients without underlying cancer risk factors. Although detection of a precursor lesion is considered evidence of its primary location, metastatic tumor deposits may colonize the mucosa and simulate an adenoma, as previously described (Figure 10.8). Metastasis also induces hyperplasia of the adjacent nonneoplastic mucosa, which simulates a serrated precursor lesion. Features that suggest a metastasis include extensive lymphovascular invasion and dissimilar morphology among synchronous tumor nodules. Unfortunately, the latter is rarely helpful since most colorectal carcinomas display an intestinal phenotype. Differences among tumors with respect to mismatch repair protein immunohistochemistry also indicate the presence of synchronous primary neoplasms.

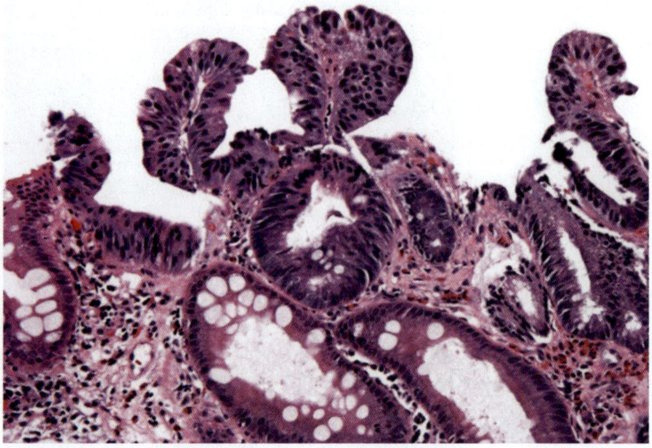

FIGURE 10.8: Carcinomas that metastasize to the colon colonize the mucosa and grow along the basement membrane. This metastasis from the proximal colon simulates the appearance of an adenoma, although extensive high-grade cytologic atypia without a low-grade component should raise suspicion for secondary mucosal involvement by malignancy.

## Recurrent Carcinoma versus Metachronous Neoplasia

Patients with a history of colorectal carcinoma are at risk for development of subsequent cancers. Distinguishing recurrent cancer from a new primary tumor may be challenging in some cases. Extensive lymphovascular invasion and location at the surgical anastomosis both suggest recurrent carcinoma. The absence of an adenomatous precursor may also signal a tumor recurrence, but recurrent cancer may colonize the mucosa and simulate a precursor lesion.

## Differential Diagnosis of Intestinal-Type Adenocarcinoma

### *Endometriosis*

The vast majority of colorectal carcinomas are intestinal-type adenocarcinomas, and thus, the differential diagnosis includes benign and malignant gland-forming lesions that involve the colorectum. Endometriosis affects up to 15% of menstruating women and also affects postmenopausal women. Approximately 15% to 37% of patients with pelvic endometriosis also have involvement of the gastrointestinal tract, most commonly in the rectosigmoid colon.[13] Subserosal deposits of endometriosis are usually detected as incidental findings in colectomy specimens. Mural endometriosis produces hypertrophy and scarring of the muscularis propria with obstructive symptoms, whereas mucosal disease induces pseudopolyps and ulcers that may simulate carcinoma (Figure 10.9A). The histologic appearance of endometriosis comprises rounded aggregates of endometrioid glands associated with cellular stroma and hemorrhage, distinct from the desmoplastic stroma of invasive adenocarcinoma (Figure 10.9B). Endometriotic foci involving the mucosa simulate an adenoma or dysplasia, although the former lack cytoplasmic mucin and often display cilia (Figure 10.9C and D).[14] Immunohistochemical stains for cytokeratins 7 and 20 distinguish endometriosis from colonic neoplasia: Endometriotic epithelium shows cytokeratin 7 positivity and negativity for cytokeratin 20, which is the opposite pattern of intestinal epithelium.

### *Involvement of the Colorectum by Müllerian Neoplasms*

Müllerian carcinomas involve the colorectum *via* direct extension from the gynecologic tract, peritoneal seeding from carcinomatosis, or as primary neoplasia arising from preexisting endometriosis. The diagnosis is straightforward when patients have an established history of gynecologic malignancy, but may not be obvious in patients who have not been extensively evaluated. Müllerian carcinomas can show squamous, serous, endometrioid, or mucinous differentiation. Tumors that directly extend into the rectosigmoid colon from the gynecologic tract are usually squamous cell carcinomas and mucinous adenocarcinomas originating in the uterine cervix, while most endometrial malignancies that secondarily affect the colorectum are endometrioid. Distinction between müllerian squamous cell carcinoma and rectal carcinoma is

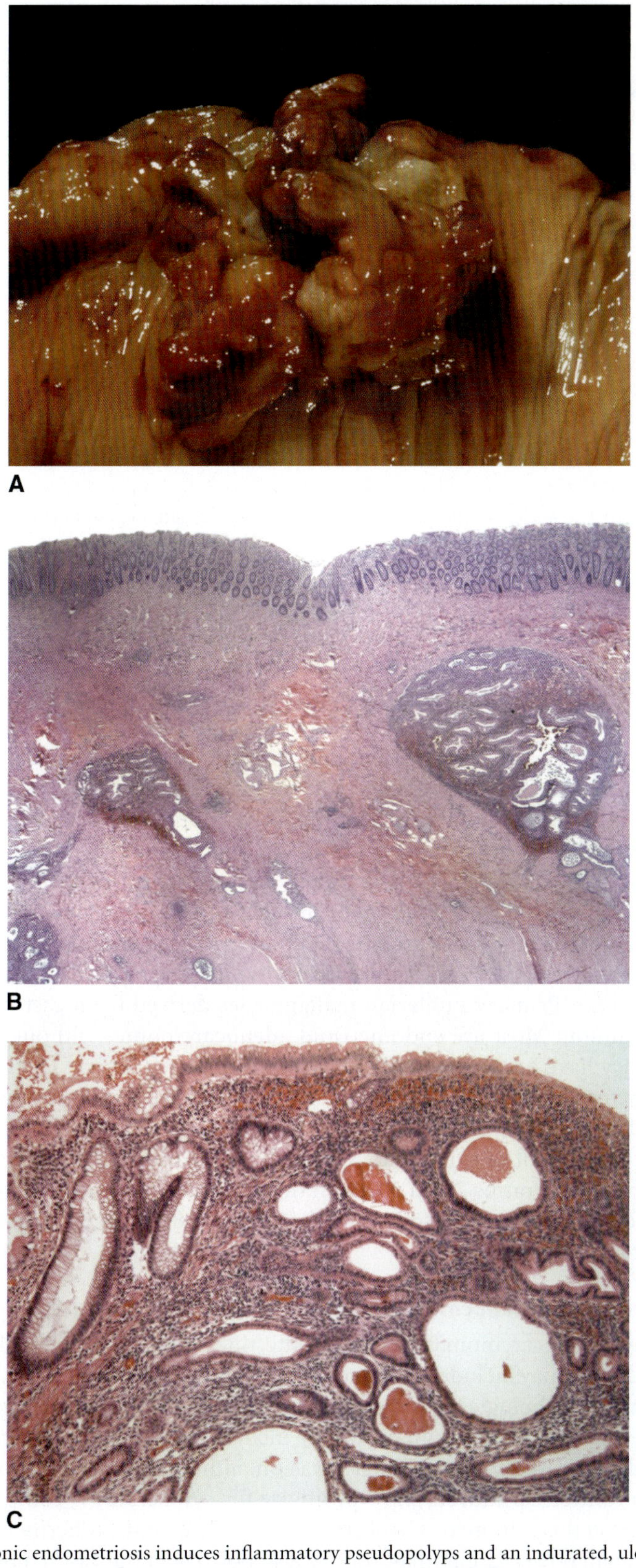

A

B

C

FIGURE 10.9: Colonic endometriosis induces inflammatory pseudopolyps and an indurated, ulcerated mass that simulate malignancy (**A**). Round aggregates of endometriotic glands surrounded by cellular stroma and hemorrhage are present in the submucosa and muscularis propria (**B**). Polypoid endometriosis in the mucosa contains numerous irregularly spaced crypts composed of nonmucinous epithelial cells with large nuclei that simulate a neoplasm (**C**).

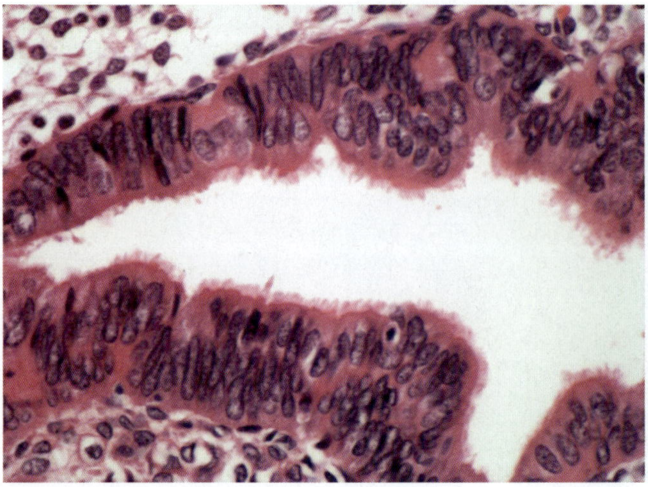

D

FIGURE 10.9: (*Continued*) The nuclei are elongated with coarse chromatin, although mitotic figures are rare and cilia are present (**D**).

straightforward since squamous differentiation among colorectal adenocarcinomas is extremely uncommon. Indeed, the presence of squamous differentiation in a colorectal carcinoma should lead one to investigate the possibility of secondary involvement from another site, particularly if the squamous elements also show p16 nuclear immunopositivity. Müllerian endometrioid and mucinous adenocarcinomas may be difficult to distinguish from intestinal-type adenocarcinomas in mucosal biopsies. Features that suggest a secondary müllerian neoplasm include architectural growth patterns that are unusual in conventional and serrated adenomas, such as micropapillary projections, solid nests of tumor cells, and small glandular proliferation, as well as high-grade cytologic changes with abundant intraepithelial neutrophils (Figure 10.10). Müllerian tumors that involve the colon *via* peritoneal spread are usually serous carcinomas with solid, papillary, or micropapillary growth and high-grade cytologic features (Figure 10.11). They often contain small nests of tumor cells with eosinophilic cytoplasm and occasional psammomatous calcifications. Primary müllerian malignancies derived from gastrointestinal endometriosis are uncommon. Most are endometrioid adenocarcinomas, although many types of müllerian malignancy have been described in colorectal endometriosis.[15] Distinction from primary colorectal carcinomas is clinically important, since endometriosis-associated carcinomas tend to be low grade and respond to resection alone, whereas colorectal carcinomas that extensively involve the colonic wall may be treated with a combination of chemotherapy, radiation therapy, and surgery. Cytokeratins 7 and 20 aid in the recognition of most müllerian malignancies, although a broader panel may also include WT-1, PAX-8, estrogen receptor, CDX-2, and cadherin-17 (Figure 10.11).[12,16–18]

### *Primary Small-Intestinal Adenocarcinoma Involving the Colorectum*

Patients with invasive adenocarcinoma of the small intestine typically present with advanced stage disease. Recurrent disease may include secondary involvement of the colorectum. Small-intestinal adenocarcinomas are morphologically indistinguishable from colorectal intestinal-type cancers. Features that suggest a noncolonic primary tumor include the absence of a precursor (adenomatous) lesion and extensive lymphovascular invasion, although these may not be detected in all cases. Most small-intestinal cancers show positivity for cytokeratin 7, compared to approximately 10% of colorectal carcinomas. Cytokeratin 20, CDX-2, and cadherin-17 are positive in more than 50% of small bowel carcinomas, but are also positive in the vast majority of colorectal carcinomas.[19]

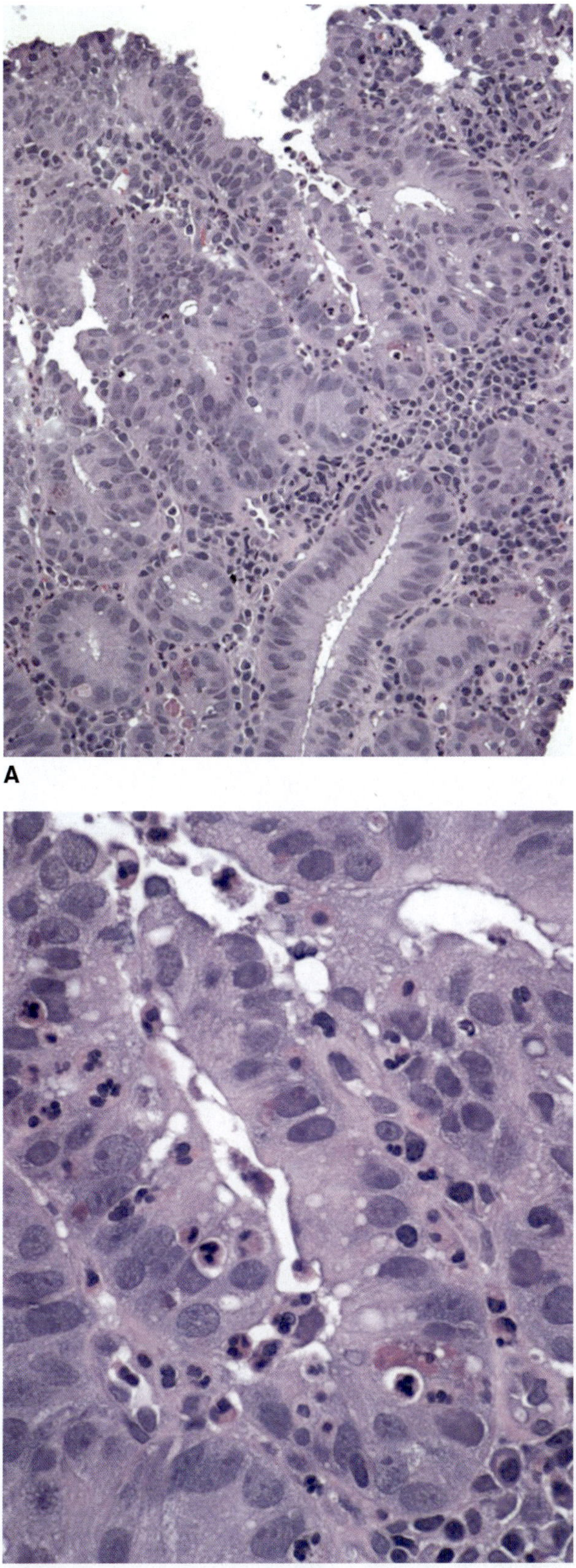

A

B

FIGURE 10.10: Endometrioid adenocarcinoma directly invades the rectum and extends to the mucosal surface, simulating an adenoma in biopsy samples. The tumor is composed of architecturally complex glands with vague micropapillae (**A**). The tumor cells show malignant cytologic features with enlarged round nuclei and prominent nucleoli (**B**). Neutrophils are evident throughout the lesion, though uncommon in most colorectal adenomas.

**FIGURE 10.11:** Serous carcinoma that invades the colonic wall colonizes the mucosa, thereby mimicking a primary neoplasm. This tumor contains solid nests of cells below the muscularis mucosae (**A**) with overtly malignant cytologic features, large nuclei with prominent nucleoli (**B**), and rare psammomatous calcifications (*arrow*).

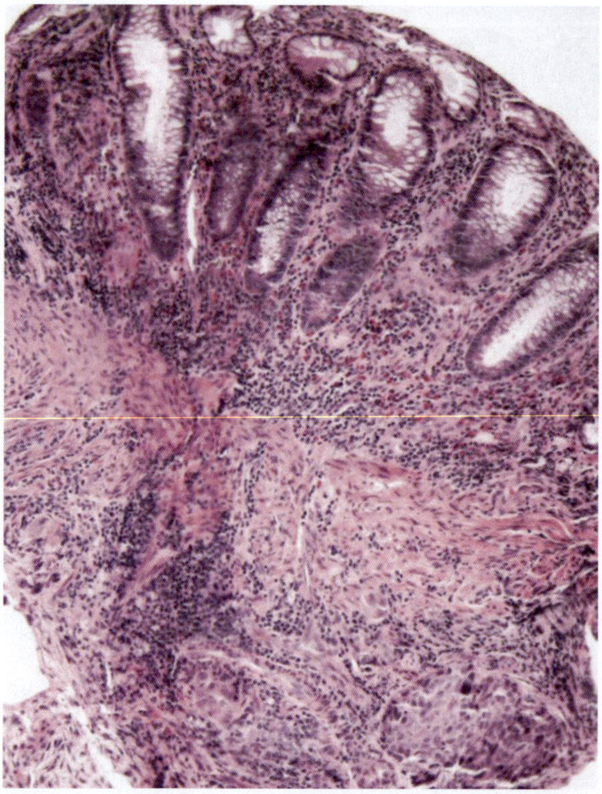

A

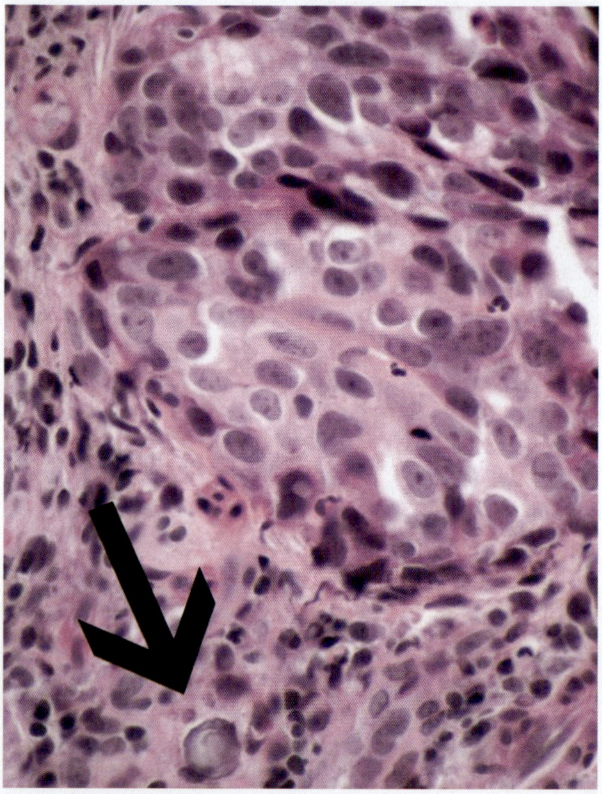

B

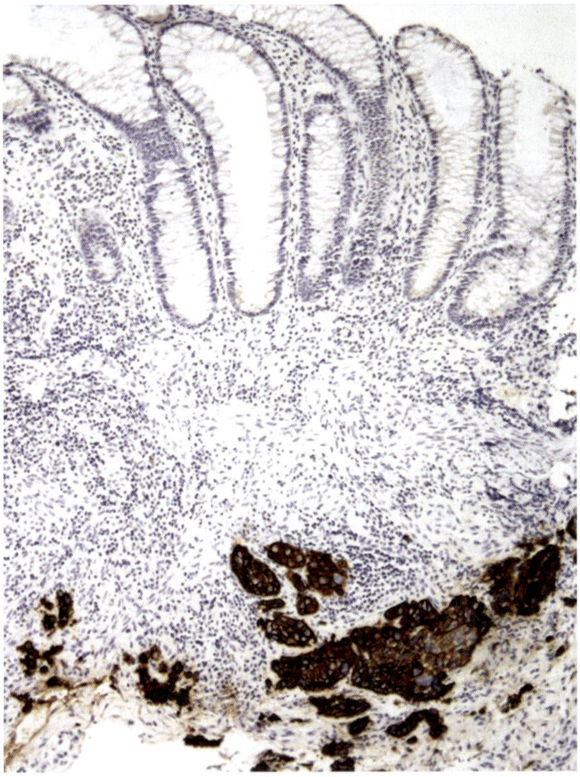

C

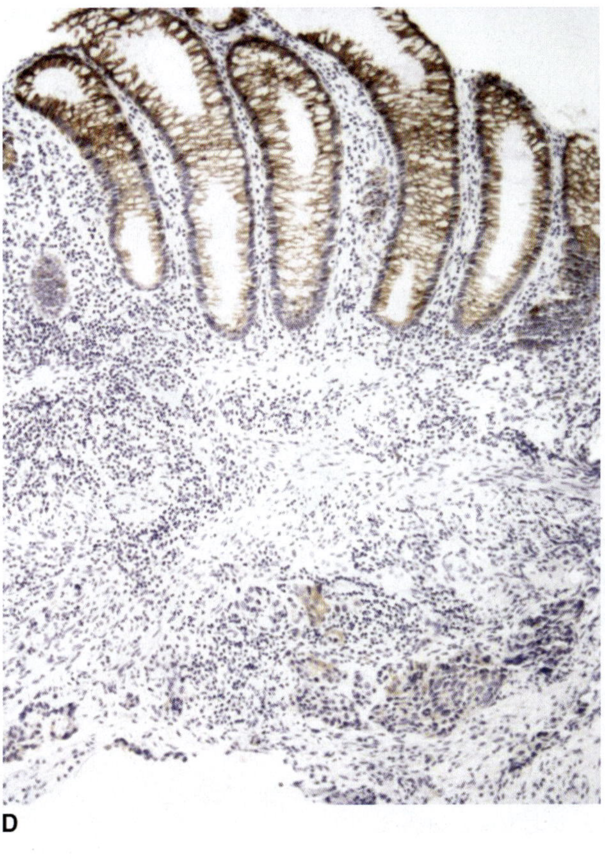

D

FIGURE 10.11: (*Continued*) The tumor cells are strongly positive for cytokeratin 7 (**C**), but negative for cytokeratin 20 (**D**).

## Diagnosis of Mucinous Carcinoma

Mucinous adenocarcinomas of the colon are rarely confused with metastases, but a lack of consensus regarding diagnostic criteria causes difficulty in distinguishing it from other colorectal cancer variants. The WHO defines mucinous adenocarcinoma as a tumor with more than 50% mucinous differentiation, comprising mucin pools that contain strips and clusters of globoid, mucin-filled cells (Figure 10.12A).[1] This designation is not applied to intestinal-type adenocarcinomas that contain glands distended by copious extracellular mucin (Figure 10.12B). High-grade mucinous carcinomas contain mucin pools with single and clustered signet ring cells (Figure 10.12C). Such tumors are distinguished from signet ring cell carcinomas that consist of single infiltrating tumor cells in desmoplastic stroma, as discussed in Chapter 7 (Figure 10.12D).

## Signet Ring Cell and Undifferentiated Carcinoma

Signet ring cell carcinomas that are associated with high-grade mucinous carcinomas are readily recognized as primary colorectal neoplasms. Primary signet ring cell carcinomas unaccompanied by mucinous neoplasia are uncommon in the colon, as are colorectal tumors composed entirely of poorly differentiated and undifferentiated carcinoma (<5% gland forming elements). Any high-grade carcinoma comprising a diffuse growth pattern, without gland formation, or unusual features should prompt consideration of the possibility of metastasis and potential immunohistochemical evaluation (Table 10.2).[12,20–25] Malignancies that commonly metastasize to the colorectum include carcinomas of lung, stomach, small intestine, breast, and melanoma.

Pulmonary and gastric metastases to the colon are typically high-grade lesions that occur in the terminal stages of disease, whereas metastasis to the colon may be the first manifestation of breast cancer or develop following a prolonged disease-free interval. Metastatic breast cancer

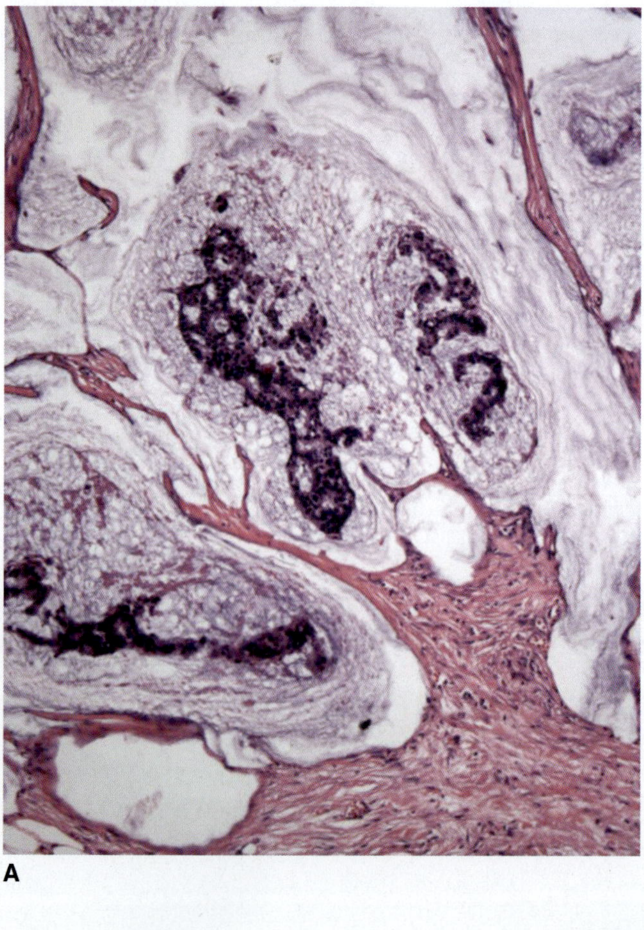

A

FIGURE 10.12: Mucinous carcinomas of the colorectum consist of clusters and glands composed of mucinous epithelium floating in pools of extracellular mucin (**A**).

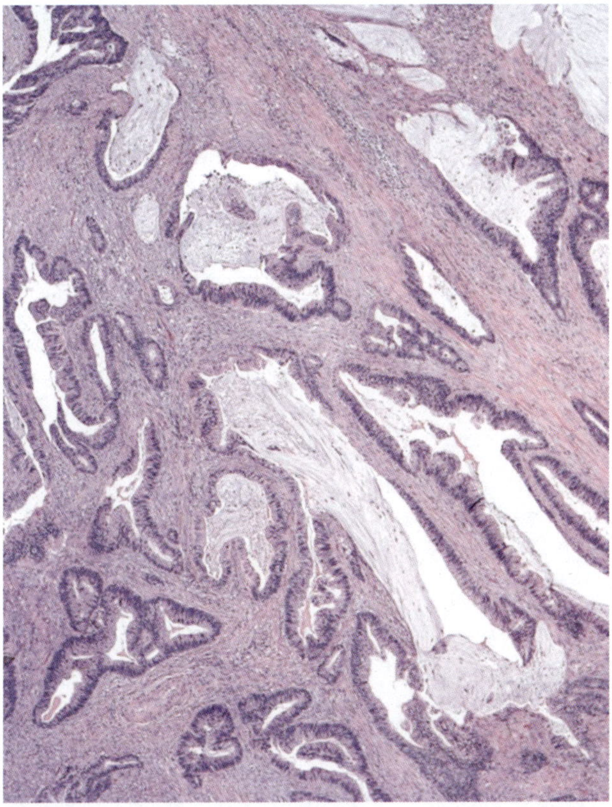

B

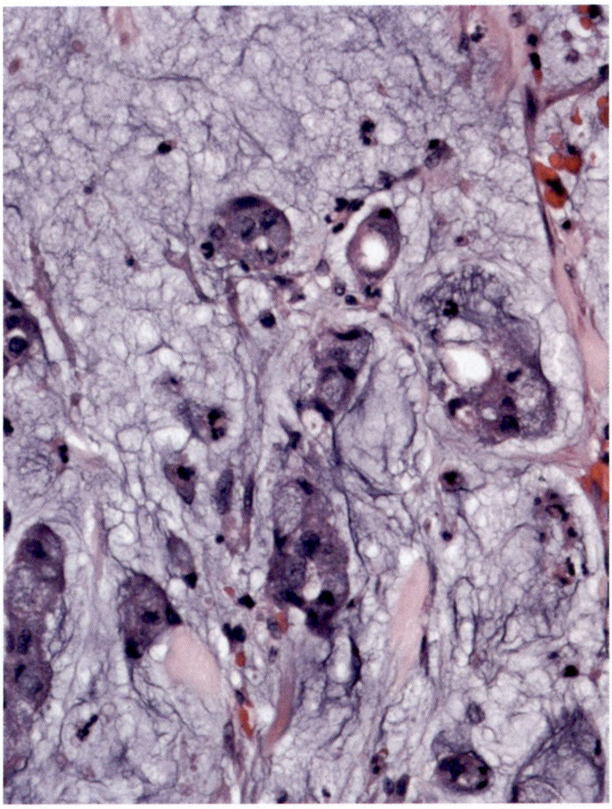

C

FIGURE 10.12: (*Continued*) Intestinal-type cancers that contain distended glands are not classified as mucinous carcinomas (**B**). Some high-grade mucinous carcinomas contain small clusters and signet ring cells (**C**).

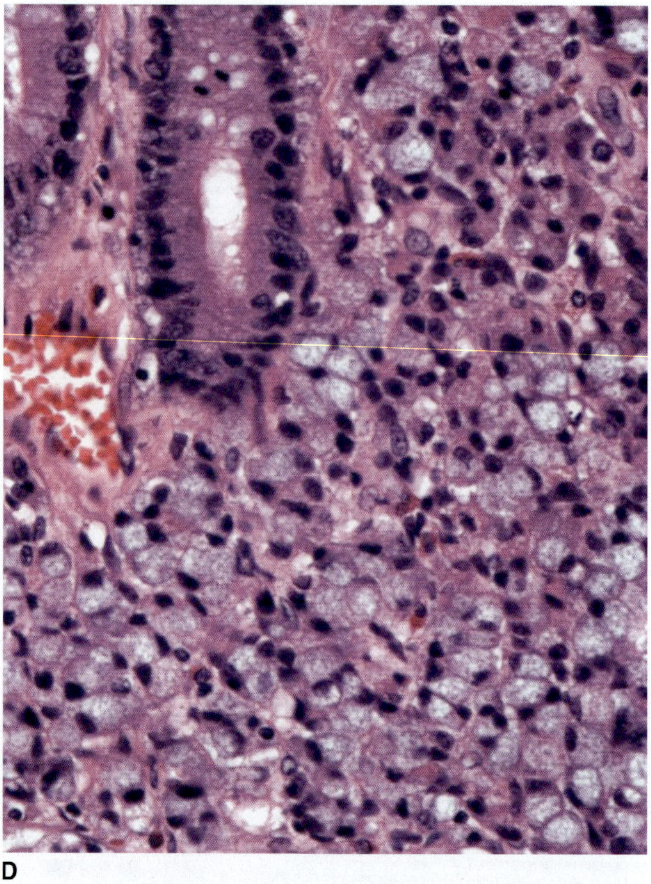

FIGURE 10.12: (*Continued*) The signet ring cell designation is reserved for tumors containing infiltrating signet ring cells unassociated with abundant extracellular mucin (**D**).

usually involves the outer aspects of the colon and produces obstructive symptoms, although it may appear as one or more mucosal polyps. Metastasis is usually of the lobular phenotype, even when the primary tumor contains ductal elements. Metastatic breast cancer cells typically insinuate between colonic crypts without crypt destruction (Figure 10.13). The tumor cells often stain for estrogen receptor and cytokeratin 7, but are negative for cytokeratin 20 and CDX-2.[26]

Most nonepithelial colonic metastases are melanomas, which show as predilection for the entire gastrointestinal tract. Approximately 30% of patients with gastrointestinal metastases do not have a history of cutaneous melanoma: most of these are presumed to have undetected, or regressed, skin lesions. Nearly 50% of metastases are entirely, or mostly, amelanotic. Because the metastatic foci contain a mixed population of spindled and epithelioid cells, the differential diagnosis includes gastrointestinal stromal tumor and other sarcomas, rather than carcinoma. Melanomas with a predominant epithelioid cell population have a nested or sheet-like growth pattern. The tumor cells are large, with abundant eosinophilic or clear cytoplasm, round-to-elongated nuclei, and prominent nucleoli. Plasmacytoid and multinucleated cells are a clue to the diagnosis (Figure 10.14). Immunohistochemical studies usually show the tumor cells to be S-100 positive with variable staining for other melanoma markers, but keratin stains are negative.

Hematopoietic malignancies may simulate a primary colorectal neoplasm as well as metastatic melanoma. Low-grade lesions are readily distinguished from carcinomas, but anaplastic lymphomas and myeloid tumors simulate the clinical and histologic features of primary colonic malignancies. Hematopoietic neoplasms should always be considered in immunosuppressed patients with new-onset colorectal masses. A limited panel of immunostains against keratins, S-100, CD45, CD20, CD3, and myeloid markers is appropriate as an initial evaluation, and additional stains may be considered as necessary. In situ hybridization for Epstein-Barr virus–encoded RNAs is useful when applied to lymphomas in immunocompromised patients.

**Table 10.2 Immunohistochemical Markers Used to Distinguish Between Colorectal Carcinomas and Secondary Neoplasms**

| Immunostain | Positivity in Colorectal Carcinoma | Staining in Extracolonic Tumors |
|---|---|---|
| **Markers of Intestinal Differentiation** | | |
| Cytokeratin 20 | >95% | >50% upper gastrointestinal carcinomas<br>20%–30% pancreaticobiliary carcinomas |
| CDX-2 | >95% | ~33% upper gastrointestinal carcinomas<br>25% pancreaticobiliary carcinomas<br>20%–30% endometrial and ovarian carcinomas<br><10% carcinomas of lung and thyroid |
| Cadherin-17 | >95% | >80% upper gastrointestinal adenocarcinomas<br>50% pancreaticobiliary carcinomas<br><10% lung and endometrial carcinomas<br><1% other carcinomas outside gastrointestinal tract |
| **Markers of Extracolonic Malignancy** | | |
| Cytokeratin 7 | <10% | Lung, breast, pancreaticobiliary, upper gastrointestinal tract |
| TTF-1 | <5% | Lung adenocarcinomas |
| Napsin-A | <5% | Lung adenocarcinomas |
| Estrogen receptor | <1% | Breast and müllerian carcinomas |
| WT-1 | Negative | Mullerian serous carcinomas |
| PAX-8 | Negative | Mullerian, thyroid, renal, thymic carcinomas |
| S-100 | Negative | Malignant melanoma |

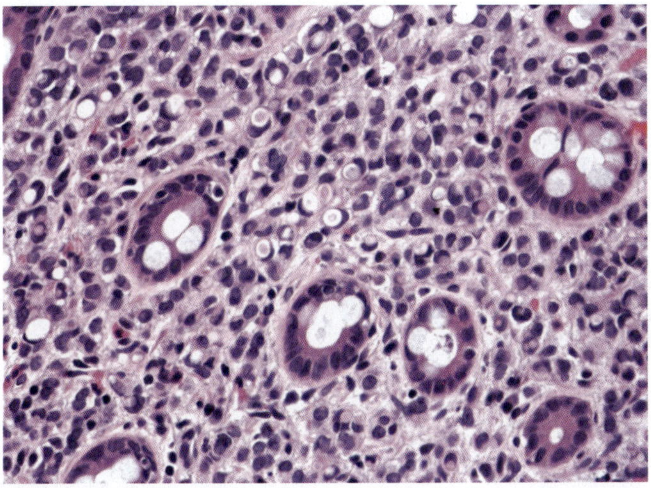

FIGURE 10.13: Metastatic breast cancer in the colon usually has a lobular phenotype. Tumor cells infiltrate between colonic crypts, rather than destroying them. Some tumor cells have a signet ring cell appearance with targetoid inclusions. These cytoplasmic vacuoles do not contain mucin, but, rather, represent abortive lumina.

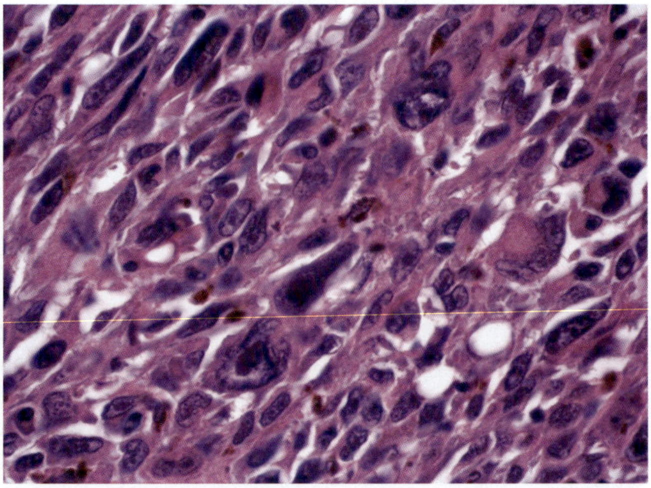

FIGURE 10.14: Metastatic melanoma displays a pleomorphic population of cells with scant melanin pigment. The tumor cells contain abundant eosinophilic cytoplasm and large nuclei with macronucleoli. Multinucleated cells are also present (**right**).

## Rare Variants of Colonic Adenocarcinoma and Their Mimics

Some colorectal cancer variants display unique morphologic features that may resemble malignancies from other sites. Clear cell carcinomas of the intestine comprise large cells with faintly eosinophilic or clear cytoplasm and large subnuclear vacuoles. Unlike ovarian clear cell carcinomas, the tumor cells are columnar and display elongated nuclei with prominent nucleoli. Most colonic clear cell carcinomas also show extensive glandular differentiation and luminal necrosis, similar to intestinal-type carcinomas without clear cells (Figure 10.15). Such tumors are distinct from clear cell carcinomas of renal origin, which generally do not contain glands, show lower grade nuclear features without cellular necrosis, and display a characteristic vascular pattern with hemorrhage. Medullary carcinomas of the colon show a syncytial growth pattern with intraepithelial lymphocytes that aid in their recognition, as described in Chapter 7. The tumor cells have round nuclei with relatively open chromatin and conspicuous nucleoli that can resemble high-grade (neuro)endocrine carcinomas. The latter may also contain necrotic tumor cells that simulate infiltrating lymphocytes (Figure 10.16). Distinguishing features of the former include a pronounced host lymphoid response around the periphery of the tumor and occasional gland forming elements or cytoplasmic mucin. Immunostains for endocrine markers, such as chromogranin A and synaptophysin, are helpful in challenging cases.

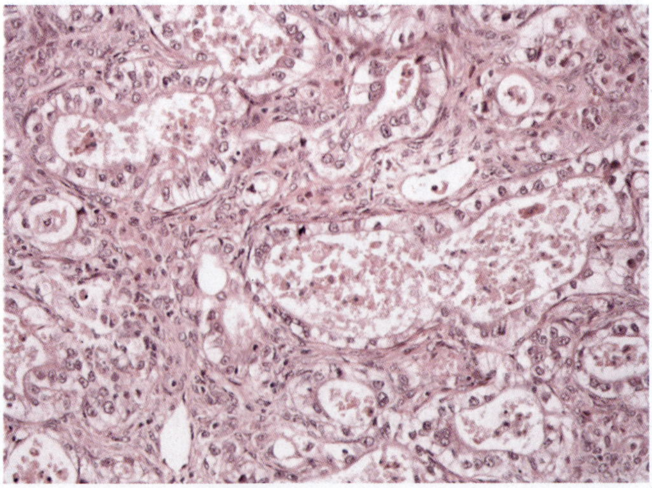

FIGURE 10.15: Clear cell carcinoma of the colon is a gland-forming tumor composed of intestinal-type cells with abundant faintly eosinophilic, or clear, cytoplasm. The tumor cells contain subnuclear vacuoles and large, round nuclei with prominent nucleoli. Luminal necrotic debris is readily apparent.

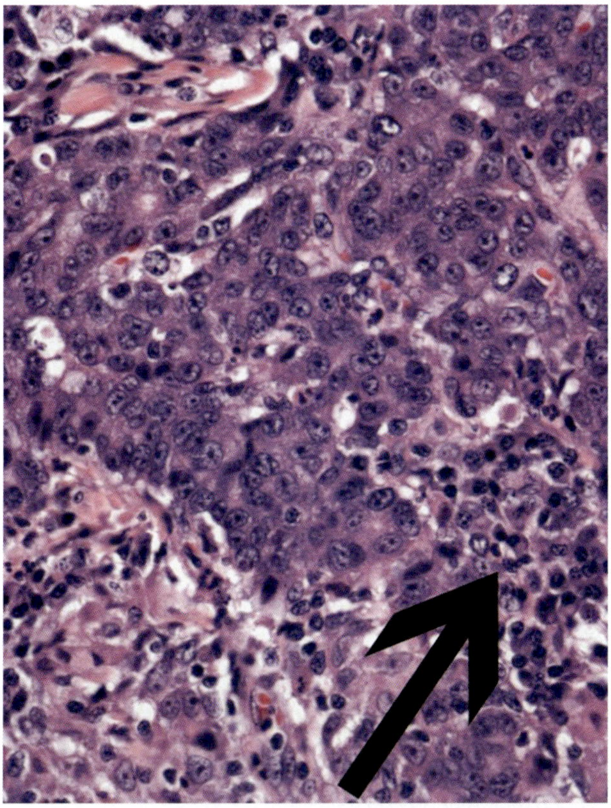

A

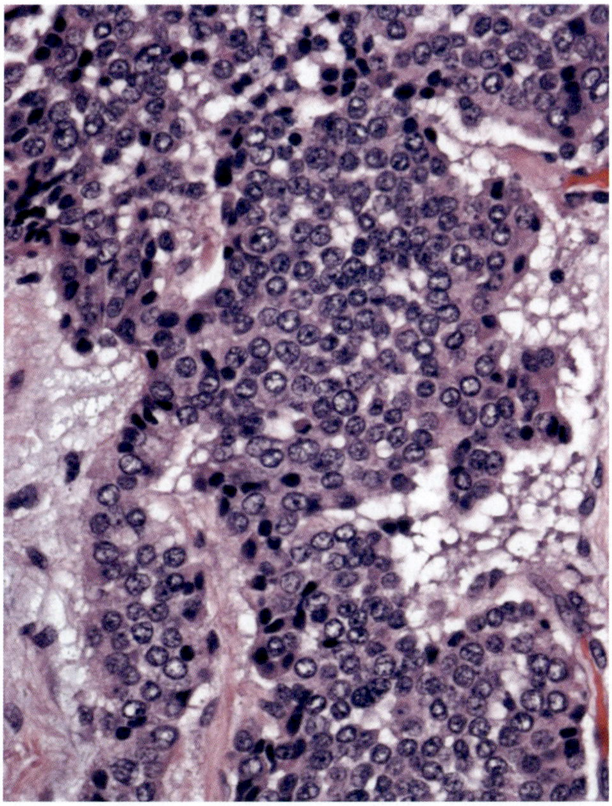

B

FIGURE 10.16: The cytologic features of medullary carcinoma (**A**) can overlap considerably with those of high-grade (neuro)endocrine carcinoma (**B**), particularly if the latter contains necrotic epithelial cells that simulate lymphocytes. Infiltrating lymphocytes are present in the epithelium and stroma of medullary carcinomas (*arrow*).

## SUMMARY AND CONCLUSIONS

The morphologic diagnosis of colorectal carcinoma is generally straightforward, without the need for immunohistochemical studies. Routine use of immunohistochemistry for TP53, CDX-2, cytokeratin 7, cytokeratin 20, Ki-67, and other markers may lead to erroneous conclusions when aberrant staining is detected. Immunohistochemical stains are most useful when applied to specific cancer subtypes, for which appropriate treatment depends on accurate classification, such as (neuro)endocrine carcinomas and metastatic malignancies. Confirmatory immunohistochemical stains for intestinal markers (i.e., CDX-2, cytokeratin 20, cadherin-17) as well as a limited panel of other antibodies to exclude morphologically similar tumors from other sites are appropriate in these instances. However, ancillary stains are no substitute for review of radiographic findings and clinical information, the latter of which should always be obtained in diagnostically challenging cases.

# References

1. Hamilton SR, Bosman FT, Boffetta P, et al. Tumors of the colon and rectum. In: Bosman FT, Carneiro F, Hruban RH, et al., eds. *WHO Classification of Tumours of the Digestive System*. 4th ed. Lyon, France: International Agency for Research on Cancer; 2010:134–146.
2. Lewin MR, Fenton H, Burkart AL, et al. Poorly differentiated colorectal carcinoma with invasion restricted to lamina propria (intramucosal carcinoma): a follow-up study of 15 cases. *Am J Surg Pathol* 2007;31(12):1882–1886.
3. Pascal RR, Hertzler G, Hunter S, et al. Pseudoinvasion with high-grade dysplasia in a colonic adenoma. Distinction from adenocarcinoma. *Am J Surg Pathol* 1990;14(7):694–697.
4. Yantiss RK, Bosenberg MW, Antonioli DA, et al. Utility of MMP-1, p53, E-cadherin, and collagen IV immunohistochemical stains in the differential diagnosis of adenomas with misplaced epithelium versus adenomas with invasive adenocarcinoma. *Am J Surg Pathol* 2002;26(2):206–215.
5. Wolber R, Owen D. Differential expression of p53 protein in colonic adenomas containing invasive carcinoma, in situ carcinoma and pseudoinvasion. *Mod Pathol* 1994;7:68A.
6. Shiozawa J, Ito M, Nakayama T, et al. Expression of matrix metalloproteinase-1 in human colorectal carcinoma. *Mod Pathol* [Comparative Study] 2000;13(9):925–933.
7. Mueller J, Mueller E, Arras E, et al. Stromelysin-3 expression in early (pT1) carcinomas and pseudoinvasive lesions of the colorectum. *Virchows Arch* 1997;430(3):213–219.
8. Valizadeh A, Karayiannakis AJ, el-Hariry I, et al. Expression of E-cadherin-associated molecules (alpha-, beta-, and gamma-catenins and p120) in colorectal polyps. *Am J Pathol* [Research Support, Non-U.S. Gov't] 1997;150(6):1977–1984.
9. Visser R, Arends JW, Leigh IM, et al. Patterns and composition of basement membranes in colon adenomas and adenocarcinomas. *J Pathol* 1993;170(3):285–290.
10. Jiang WG. E-cadherin and its associated protein catenins, cancer invasion and metastasis. *Br J Surg* [Research Support, Non-U.S. Gov't Review] 1996;83(4):437–446.
11. Estrella JS, Wu TT, Rashid A, et al. Mucosal colonization by metastatic carcinoma in the gastrointestinal tract: a potential mimic of primary neoplasia. *Am J Surg Pathol* 2011;35(4):563–572.
12. Su MC, Yuan RH, Lin CY, et al. Cadherin-17 is a useful diagnostic marker for adenocarcinomas of the digestive system. *Mod Pathol* 2008;21(11):1379–1386.
13. Prystowsky JB, Stryker SJ, Ujiki GT, et al. Gastrointestinal endometriosis. Incidence and indications for resection. *Arch Surg* 1988;123(7):855–858.
14. Yantiss RK, Clement PB, Young RH. Endometriosis of the intestinal tract: a study of 44 cases of a disease that may cause diverse challenges in clinical and pathologic evaluation. *Am J Surg Pathol* 2001;25(4):445–454.
15. Yantiss RK, Clement PB, Young RH. Neoplastic and pre-neoplastic changes in gastrointestinal endometriosis: a study of 17 cases. *Am J Surg Pathol* 2000;24(4):513–524.
16. Chu P, Wu E, Weiss LM. Cytokeratin 7 and cytokeratin 20 expression in epithelial neoplasms: a survey of 435 cases. *Mod Pathol* 2000;13(9):962–972.

17. Lewis MR, Deavers MT, Silva EG, et al. Ovarian involvement by metastatic colorectal adenocarcinoma: still a diagnostic challenge. *Am J Surg Pathol* 2006;30(2):177–184.
18. Lee BH, Hecht JL, Pinkus JL, et al. WT1, estrogen receptor, and progesterone receptor as markers for breast or ovarian primary sites in metastatic adenocarcinoma to body fluids. *Am J Clin Pathol* 2002;117(5):745–750.
19. Chen ZM, Wang HL. Alteration of cytokeratin 7 and cytokeratin 20 expression profile is uniquely associated with tumorigenesis of primary adenocarcinoma of the small intestine. *Am J Surg Pathol* 2004;28(10):1352–1359.
20. Werling RW, Yaziji H, Bacchi CE, et al. CDX2, a highly sensitive and specific marker of adenocarcinomas of intestinal origin: an immunohistochemical survey of 476 primary and metastatic carcinomas. *Am J Surg Pathol* [Comparative Study Evaluation Studies] 2003;27(3):303–310.
21. Dettmer M, Kim TE, Jung CK, et al. Thyroid transcription factor-1 expression in colorectal adenocarcinomas. *Pathol Res Pract* [Research Support, Non-U.S. Gov't] 2011;207(11):686–690.
22. Turner BM, Cagle PT, Sainz IM, et al. Napsin A, a new marker for lung adenocarcinoma, is complementary and more sensitive and specific than thyroid transcription factor 1 in the differential diagnosis of primary pulmonary carcinoma: evaluation of 1674 cases by tissue microarray. *Arch Pathol Lab Med* 2012;136(2):163–171.
23. Hwang H, Quenneville L, Yaziji H, et al. Wilms tumor gene product: sensitive and contextually specific marker of serous carcinomas of ovarian surface epithelial origin. *Appl Immunohistochem Mol Morphol* 2004;12(2):122–126.
24. Laury AR, Perets R, Piao H, et al. A comprehensive analysis of PAX8 expression in human epithelial tumors. *Am J Surg Pathol* [Research Support, Non-U.S. Gov't] 2011;35(6):816–826.
25. Bayrak R, Haltas H, Yenidunya S. The value of CDX2 and cytokeratins 7 and 20 expression in differentiating colorectal adenocarcinomas from extraintestinal gastrointestinal adenocarcinomas: cytokeratin 7-/20+ phenotype is more specific than CDX2 antibody. *Diagn Pathol* 2012;7:9.
26. O'Connell FP, Wang HH, Odze RD. Utility of immunohistochemistry in distinguishing primary adenocarcinomas from metastatic breast carcinomas in the gastrointestinal tract. *Arch Pathol Lab Med* 2005;129(3):338–347.

SECTION

# IV

# Molecular Pathology of Colorectal Carcinoma

# Molecular Mechanisms of Colorectal Carcinogenesis

# 11

Jinru Shia
Rhonda K. Yantiss

Colorectal carcinomas evolve *via* heterogeneous mechanisms and most arise from preexisting neoplasms, namely, adenomas. We now believe that colorectal cancer is essentially a genetic disease driven by an array of complex genetic and epigenetic perturbations.[1] Cancer cells obtain early mutations that deleteriously affect genome stability and propagate additional changes, thereby generating a pool of alterations that enable cancer cells to proliferate and spread. Two major types of genomic instability have been widely studied in colorectal carcinoma: chromosomal instability and microsatellite instability (MSI). Elucidation of these mechanisms has been facilitated by study of two familial syndromes, familial adenomatous polyposis and Lynch syndrome (hereditary nonpolyposis colorectal cancer), respectively, resulting in recognition of several clinically important molecular aberrations. Some changes, such as mutations affecting tumor suppressor or DNA repair genes, aid identification of patients and family members with heritable cancer risk, whereas others have therapeutic implications, as discussed in Chapter 16.

## KEY PLAYERS IN COLORECTAL CARCINOGENESIS

### Oncogenes

Protooncogenes encode proteins that regulate embryogenesis and development, proliferation, differentiation, and apoptosis; and include growth factors, growth factor receptors, members of signal transduction pathways, and transcription factors. These proteins are normally produced in small quantities and rapidly degraded. Dysregulated protooncogenes are classified as oncogenes and develop *via* point mutations, chromosomal translocations, or other alterations. All of these changes increase gene expression, enhance protein activity, or confer resistance to degradation, resulting in an overall "gain of function" with respect to oncogenic activity. Thus, alteration of only one allele is sufficient to cause oncoprotein dysregulation.

### Tumor Suppressor Genes

In contrast to oncogenes that drive cell proliferation and prolonged cell survival, tumor suppressor genes encode proteins that suppress transcription of protooncogenes and diminish the potency of their products. Tumor suppressor genes are highly conserved across species because their absence, or disrupted function, prevents inhibition of protooncogenic activity and leads to uncontrolled expansion of cell populations. Changes that affect tumor suppressor gene potency include mutations, translocations, loss of heterozygosity, and transcriptional silencing *via* promoter hypermethylation. In contrast to oncogenes that drive cell growth with only one altered allele, both tumor suppressor gene alleles must be defective in order to impact cell proliferation; the presence of one intact allele is generally sufficient to regulate protooncogenes. Most heritable cancer syndromes result from tumor suppressor gene germline mutations, in which case each cell harbors one dysfunctional allele. Loss or mutation of the second allele promotes neoplasia.

## MicroRNAs

MicroRNAs comprise a recently recognized class of molecules that plays a major role in the post-transcriptional regulation of protein expression. These short, noncoding sequences participate in complexes that bind to, and prevent translation of, mRNA strands. Decreased expression of microRNAs that normally suppress translation of oncogenic mRNA transcripts will lead to an overall increase in oncoprotein activity. Alternatively, increased expression of microRNAs that regulate transcripts from tumor suppressor genes will further diminish regulation of cell growth. MicroRNAs are further discussed in Chapter 13.

# APC/WNT SIGNALING AND THE CHROMOSOMAL INSTABILITY PATHWAY

## Overview

Chromosomal instability underlies the stepwise genetic model developed to explain the progression from adenoma to invasive carcinoma.[2] Biallelic inactivation of *adenomatous polyposis coli* (*APC*) on chromosome 5q facilitates adenoma formation, whereas subsequently mutations in *KRAS*, losses of large amounts of genetic material from chromosome 18q, and *TP53* inactivation accompany the transition from adenoma to carcinoma (Figure 11.1). Tumors that develop *via* this mechanism are characterized by gains and losses of whole, or large portions of, chromosomes or loss of heterozygosity that results in karyotypic variability among tumor cells (i.e., chromosomal instability). The role of *APC* is of particular significance to this cancer model. Mutations in *APC* occur early in colorectal cancers and presumably exert their pathogenetic effects through a variety of mechanisms, including the Wnt signaling pathway as discussed below.

## Familial Adenomatous Polyposis Due to *APC* Mutations

Familial adenomatous polyposis is a dominantly inherited condition. Patients with typical familial adenomatous polyposis have hundreds to thousands of adenomatous polyps in the colorectum, and virtually 100% of affected individuals develop colorectal cancer by the age of 30 years. Patients with

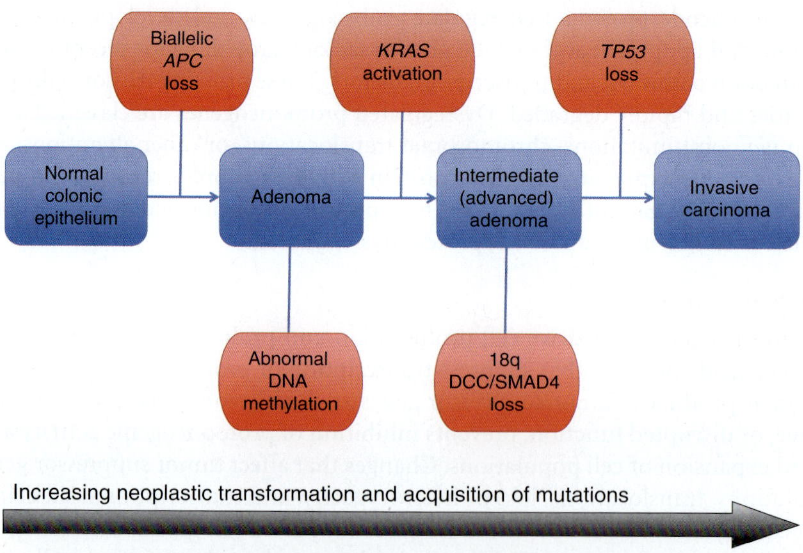


**FIGURE 11.1:** The chromosomal instability pathway of colorectal carcinogenesis proposes that adenomas develop as a result of biallelic inactivation of *APC*. Loss of APC function promotes additional genetic changes, including *KRAS* mutations, losses from chromosome 18q, and alterations affecting *TP53*. These subsequent changes typically occur *via* losses of large amounts of genetic material (loss of heterozygosity) and represent the molecular counterpart to the adenoma–carcinoma sequence.

familial adenomatous polyposis are at risk for upper gastrointestinal polyps as well as a variety of extraintestinal manifestations. Two named syndromes represent subtypes of familial adenomatous polyposis with different extraintestinal manifestations: Gardner syndrome and Crail syndrome. Features of Gardner syndrome include osteomas, intraabdominal desmoid tumors (mesenteric fibromatosis), cutaneous cysts, lipomas, and dental abnormalities. The combination of polyposis and medulloblastomas is referred to as Crail syndrome, although this constellation of findings is sometimes mislabeled Turcot syndrome. Turcot syndrome is more appropriately used to describe a subtype of Lynch syndrome, in which patients develop microsatellite unstable intestinal cancers and glioblastoma multiforme, not medulloblastoma. Familial adenomatous polyposis patients are also at risk for hepatoblastoma, gastric adenocarcinoma, adrenal cortical adenoma, nasopharyngeal angiofibroma, and papillary thyroid carcinoma, particularly the cribriform–morular variant.[3]

Most *APC* mutations are either nonsense or frameshift mutations.[4] Nonsense mutations introduce a premature stop codon and produce a truncated protein, whereas frameshift mutations result from insertions or deletions. Large deletions affect bigger portions of the gene and result in loss of some, or all, of chromosome 5 (loss of heterozygosity). Different types of *APC* mutations are associated with variably severe gastrointestinal polyposis and extracolorectal manifestations. Approximately 70% to 90% of patients have truncating *APC* mutations that show a predilection for the mutation cluster region. The most severe phenotypes are associated with mutations in the c1290-1400 regions.

## Deviation from the Classic Tumor Suppressor Model

The traditional "Vogelgram" model of colorectal carcinogenesis illustrates many principles that have proven true regarding colorectal neoplasia, but several developments since its description provide proof of variations to this paradigm. Attenuated forms of familial adenomatous polyposis are characterized by relatively few polyps (<100) and later onset of colorectal cancer. They result from mutations at the extreme 3′ (c78-167) and 5′ (c1581-2843) ends, producing a protein with partial function from the germline-mutated allele.[5,6] A third hit mechanism is required for removal of residual *APC* function in these cases. The first hit is the germline mutation, the second hit inactivates the wild-type allele, and the third hit is a second, more traditional mutation in the germline-mutated allele that removes any residual function from the *APC* gene and promotes further tumor growth.[6] A third hit also occurs in development of some sporadic colorectal carcinomas that contain one inactive and one partially functional allele for similar reasons.[7]

The concept that biallelic inactivation of *APC* occurs *via* independent events is also incorrect. Recent evidences suggest that the type of acquired *APC* mutation depends upon the location of the preceding germline alteration due to selection for at least one mutation between codons 1250 and 1450.[8] Germline mutations in this region are followed by mutations in the second allele that result in complete loss of the gene (loss of heterozygosity), whereas germline mutations outside this region are associated with somatic mutations between codons 1250 and 1450, suggesting some level of interdependence between these events. Selection for at least one mutation between codons 1250 and 1450 ensures that mutant APC protein retains some of the 20 amino acid repeats required to bind β-catenin and provides adequate Wnt/β-catenin signaling to promote tumor formation.[9] *DCC* apparently plays a less significant role in colorectal carcinogenesis than previously believed, as described below.

## Familial Adenomatous Polyposis Due to MYH Mutations

Some patients with a colonic phenotype that suggests familial adenomatous polyposis do not have detectable *APC* mutations. Biallelic inactivating mutations in the base excision repair gene, *MYH*, have been identified as the cause of some previously unexplained polyposis cases. This gene is located at 1p32-34 and contains mutational hotspots, such that most germline mutations are Y165C and G382D missense mutations. Patients with inactive *MYH* acquire somatic *APC* mutations as a consequence of impaired base excision repair function. The *MLH1* gene is also a reported target of *MUTYH*-associated transversions, in which case resultant tumors have the MSI phenotype.[10]

## APC and Wnt Signaling in Colorectal Carcinogenesis

Activation of Wnt signaling occurs early in the progression of sporadic adenomas to adenocarcinomas of the colorectum.[11] The *APC* protein product consists of 2,843 amino acids and performs several complex functions. It is normally expressed in nonproliferating colorectal epithelium and is essential for maintaining normal growth control and differentiation. Loss of *APC* function exerts a tumorigenic effect mainly through its impact on the Wnt signaling pathway, which is an evolutionarily conserved mechanism that interacts with several other signaling pathways important to colorectal neoplasia. In the absence of Wnt signaling, the APC–axin–GSK3ß cytoplasmic complex induces phosphorylation of serine and tyrosine residues on β-catenin, thereby targeting it for ubiquitination and ultimate destruction and preventing its stimulating effects on cell proliferation. However, active Wnt signaling promotes the effects of β-catenin. Wnt proteins are likely secreted by adjacent subepithelial cells and bind to an epithelial cell surface receptor complex that includes the Frizzled receptor and the LDL receptor–related protein coreceptor.[12] Coupling these molecules induces an interaction between axin and LDL receptor–related protein that drives phosphorylation of the cytoplasmic protein, Dishevelled. This protein subsequently interferes with the APC–axin–GSK3ß cytoplasmic complex and prevents phosphorylation and ubiquitination of β-catenin, resulting in its cytoplasmic accumulation. Excess β-catenin is then translocated to the nucleus where it associates with T cell factor (TCF) and lymphoid enhancer factor, forming a complex that promotes expression of several important cell cycle regulating genes (Figure 11.2). Thus, APC negatively regulates Wnt signaling *via*

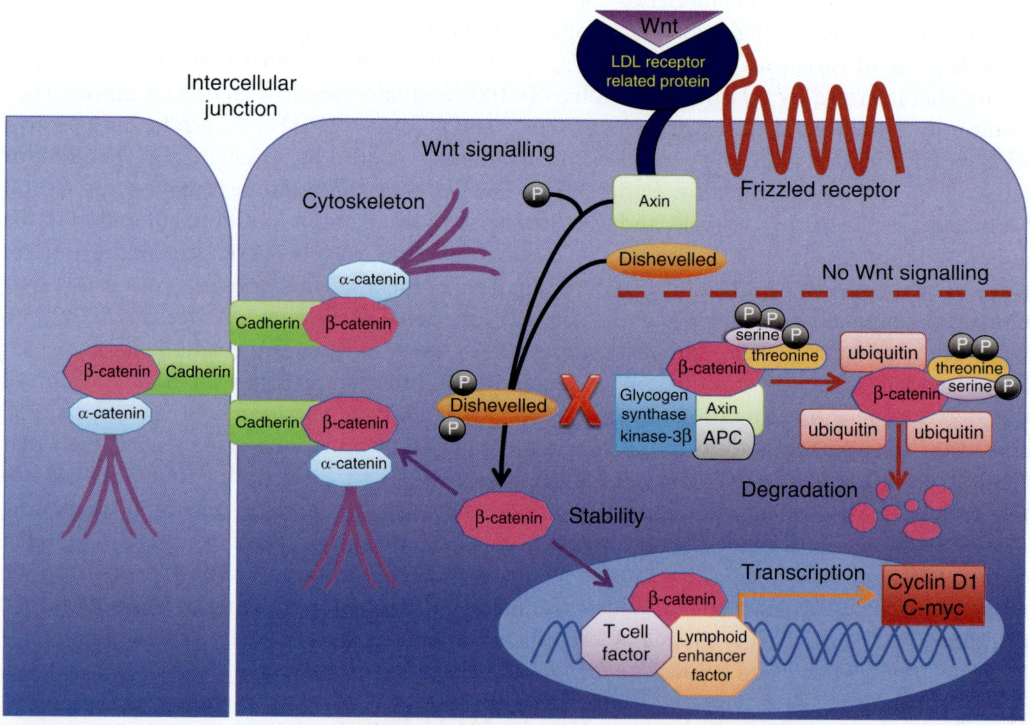


**FIGURE 11.2:** Cytoplasmic APC forms a complex with axin and glycogen synthase kinase-3β (GSK-3β) that promotes β-catenin degradation in the absence of Wnt signaling. Phosphorylation of serine and threonine residues on β-catenin by this complex leads to coupling of β-catenin with ubiquitin, thereby targeting it for destruction. However, activation of Wnt signaling leads to coupling of LDL receptor–related protein with axin and phosphorylation of Dishevelled. Phosphorylated Dishevelled interacts with the APC/axin/GSK-3 complex, thereby inhibiting β-catenin degradation and promoting its accumulation in the cytoplasm. Cytoplasmic β-catenin is then transported to the nucleus where it forms a complex with TCF and lymphoid enhancer factor to promote transcription of several genes involved in cell proliferation and prolonged survival. Loss of APC function prevents destruction of β-catenin, so it accumulates in the cytoplasm and nucleus to drive transcription of genes that represent endpoints of activated Wnt signaling.

participation in the APC–axin–GSK3ß destruction complex that promotes β-catenin degradation.[13] Immunohistochemical stains for β-catenin can serve as surrogate markers of Wnt signaling. Staining for β-catenin is limited to epithelial cell membranes with weak cytoplasmic staining in the absence of Wnt signaling, but strong staining of the nucleus and cytoplasm suggests that the pathway is activated.

The antitumorigenic effects of APC are not limited to degradation of β-catenin. It also suppresses Wnt signaling by acting on promoters of Wnt responsive genes and shuttling β-catenin out of the nucleus for destruction.[14] APC exerts effects through cytoskeletal interactions and chromosomal dynamics. It negatively regulates cell cycling by blocking entry from G0/G1 into the S phase and/or progression through S phase and participates in directed cell migration *via* binding to microtubules and F-actin.[15,16] Finally, APC regulates mitosis by interfering with microtubule dynamics.[17] Cells with mutated *APC* are predisposed to mitotic errors due to defects in mitotic spindles and, thus, have an increased likelihood of aneuploidy.[18]

### Other Molecules Involved in Chromosomal Instability Pathway of Colorectal Carcinoma

Inactivation of *APC* promotes additional major genetic and chromosomal alterations involving *KRAS2* (12p12), genes in chromosome 18q, and *TP53* (17q13). Activating *KRAS* mutations are important to cancer development. This gene encodes a GTP-binding protein that loses GTPase activity when mutated, thereby impairing hydrolysis of active GTP into inactive GDP and resulting in constitutive signaling through the downstream pathway. The original "Vogelgram" depicted *KRAS* mutations occurring in an intermediate adenoma after *APC* inactivation (Figure 11.1). Indeed, *KRAS* mutations can be detected in up to 40% of advanced adenomas (i.e., those with high-grade dysplasia, villous architecture, or size >1 cm), comparable to their frequency in carcinomas. Allelic loss at 18q is found in up to 60% of colorectal carcinomas, affecting the region that contains *SMAD2*, *SMAD4*, and *DCC*.[19] Both *SMAD2* and *SMAD4* are involved in the TGF-β signaling pathway, which is important for growth regulation and programmed cell death. *DCC* encodes a transmembrane receptor that promotes apoptosis and has been implicated as a key driver of carcinogenesis. However, mutations in *DCC* and *SMAD2* are rare in colorectal carcinoma, whereas *SMAD4* may be more influential.[20] Indeed, germline *SMAD4* mutations are found in a substantial number of patients with juvenile polyposis syndrome, as discussed in Chapter 4. Loss of *TP53* is a late event in the adenoma–carcinoma sequence and usually occurs through allelic loss of 17p.[21] Functional TP53 protein, which is stabilized by DNA damage, is an important transcription factor. It increases expression of cell cycle retarding genes and slows the cell cycle, thereby providing sufficient time for DNA repair following occasional genetic insults. This protein is also capable of inducing proapoptotic genes in the event that genetic damage is too great for the cell to successfully repair itself.[22]

## MISMATCH REPAIR DEFICIENCY AND MICROSATELLITE INSTABILITY

### Overview

Up to 20% of colorectal carcinomas lack chromosomal instability and are diploid, rather than aneuploid. These tumors display morphologic and molecular heterogeneity distinct from features typical of tumors with Wnt signaling abnormalities and chromosomal instability. In 1993, several groups independently identified MSI as a central mechanism of carcinogenesis.[23] Similar to carcinomas with Wnt signaling abnormalities, early studies of tumors with MSI focused on those with a heritable component (i.e., Lynch syndrome), which account for approximately 2% to 4% of all colorectal carcinomas. Approximately 10% to 15% of sporadic colorectal carcinomas show high-frequency MSI.

## Lynch Syndrome (Hereditary Nonpolyposis Colon Cancer, HNPCC)

Lynch syndrome is an autosomal dominantly inherited disease characterized by early-onset colonic carcinoma that usually develops in the proximal colon. Patients with Lynch syndrome have an increased risk for a number of extracolonic cancers, including carcinomas of the endometrium, ovary, renal pelvis and ureter, small intestine, stomach, and hepatobiliary tract. Colorectal carcinomas associated with Lynch syndrome often show unusual histologic features, such as medullary growth, mucinous differentiation, and signet ring cells, as discussed in Chapter 8. It is not uncommon to encounter multiple growth patterns in the same tumor, and, in fact, heterogeneity within a carcinoma is one feature that should prompt suspicion for underlying MSI. These cancers also elicit a host immune response in the form of tumor-infiltrating lymphocytes and a Crohn-like lymphoid response. There are two named Lynch syndrome variants: Muir-Torre syndrome and Turcot syndrome. The former is characterized by internal malignancies associated with sebaceous neoplasms, whereas patients with the latter have colorectal carcinomas in association with glioblastoma multiforme.[3]

Lynch syndrome–associated carcinomas develop from preexisting adenomas that show inactivation of *APC* or β-*catenin* mutations, mainly in exon 3.[24,25] Patients with germline mutations affecting one mismatch repair allele develop adenomas at rates comparable to those in the general population, but inactivation of the second allele results in rapid progression of adenomas to invasive carcinoma. Thus, Lynch syndrome–associated tumors show activation of both the Wnt signaling pathway and MSI. They may harbor *KRAS* mutations, but *BRAF* mutations are extremely rare, being described only in *PMS2*-mutated tumors.[26]

Lynch syndrome results from inactivating germline mutations in mismatch repair genes, usually in the form of knockout or missense mutations.[27] There are at least four mismatch repair genes that, when mutated, are responsible for Lynch syndrome: *MutL homolog 1* (*MLH1*), *MutS homolog 2* (*MSH2*), *MutS homolog 6* (*MSH6*), and *postmeiotic segregation increased 2* (*PMS2*). These genes encode proteins that form complexes with specific binding partners and patrol the genome to correct replicative errors. First, MSH2 and MSH6 form a heterodimer that recognizes and binds to mismatched base pairs and then recruits the MLH1/PMS2 heterodimer to repair the mismatch.[13] Most Lynch syndrome–related colon cancers result from *MLH1* or *MSH2* mutations. Mismatch errors tend to occur in microsatellites, which are short, repetitive genomic sequences. Replication within these microsatellites is prone to errors because DNA polymerase frequently slips in regions of repetitive sequences. Slippage of the DNA strand creates insertion–deletion loops in addition to single base pair mismatches. These errors are normally recognized and corrected by the mismatch repair system, but are propagated in the second round of replication if mismatch repair mechanisms are dysfunctional. Both types of error alter the length of the microsatellite sequence in tumor DNA compared to microsatellite sequences of nonneoplastic tissues (Figure 11.3).[27] They occur more commonly in noncoding regions of the genome, but can lead to downstream nonsense mutations if they occur in areas that are transcribed. Single base pair mismatches in the defective daughter strand result in point mutations, whereas insertion–deletion loops cause frameshift mutations.

Frameshift mutations at a few microsatellites are relatively common among colonic carcinomas, including those that are not inherently mismatch repair deficient. In an effort to standardize analysis and avoid overinterpretation of this observation, the National Cancer Institute (NCI) recommended a reference panel of five MSI markers, including two mononucleotide (BAT26 and BAT25) and three dinucleotide (D2S123, D5S346, and D17S250) repeats.[28] They defined cancers with high-frequency MSI (MSI-H) as those that showed instability at two, or more, of the five markers; low-frequency MSI (MSI-L) as those that showed instability at one locus; and those without instability at any marker as microsatellite stable (MSS). Most tumors with defective mismatch repair mechanisms show MSI-H, whereas those with MSS are generally mismatch proficient with rare exception: some tumors with germline-mutated *MSH6* are MSS, as discussed in Chapter 12. The biologic importance of MSI-L in colorectal carcinoma is not established and this category is not used for clinical purposes. However, instability at one locus can indicate the presence of mismatch repair deficiency, and, thus, such cases are now classified as indeterminate, rather than MSI-L. Most laboratories now evaluate a panel of five quasimonomorphic mononucleotide repeat markers (BAT25, BAT26, NR-1, NR-24, MONO-27) in a pentaplex PCR, rather than those proposed by the NCI because the former offers a greater degree of specificity and sensitivity.[29,30]

Immunohistochemical stains for mismatch repair proteins can be used as a reliable surrogate marker of MSI and facilitate germline testing by indicating the likely deficient gene. Mismatch repair proteins are normally expressed by proliferating cells, including mismatch proficient tumors and lymphocytes, so immunohistochemical stains generally show strong nuclear positivity for all four mismatch repair proteins in these populations. Tumors with mismatch repair deficiency show loss of one, or two, markers, and the pattern of expression is a reasonable indicator

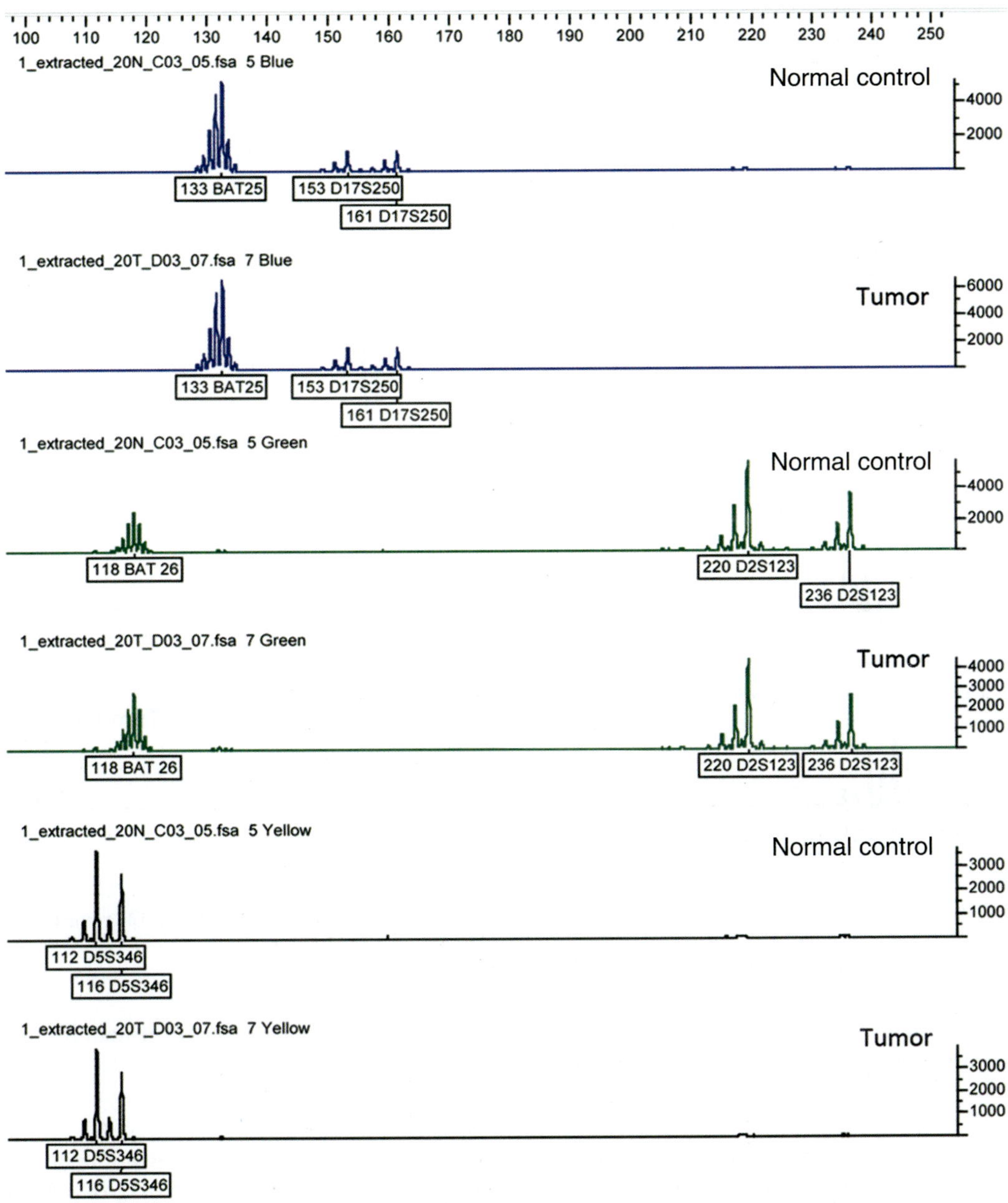


**A**

**FIGURE 11.3:** The Bethesda panel for MSI testing consists of two mononucleotide (BAT25 and BAT26) and three dinucleotide (D2S123, S5S346, D17S250) repeats. MSS tumors show a similar peak number and location compared to nontumor control tissue from the same patient (**A**).

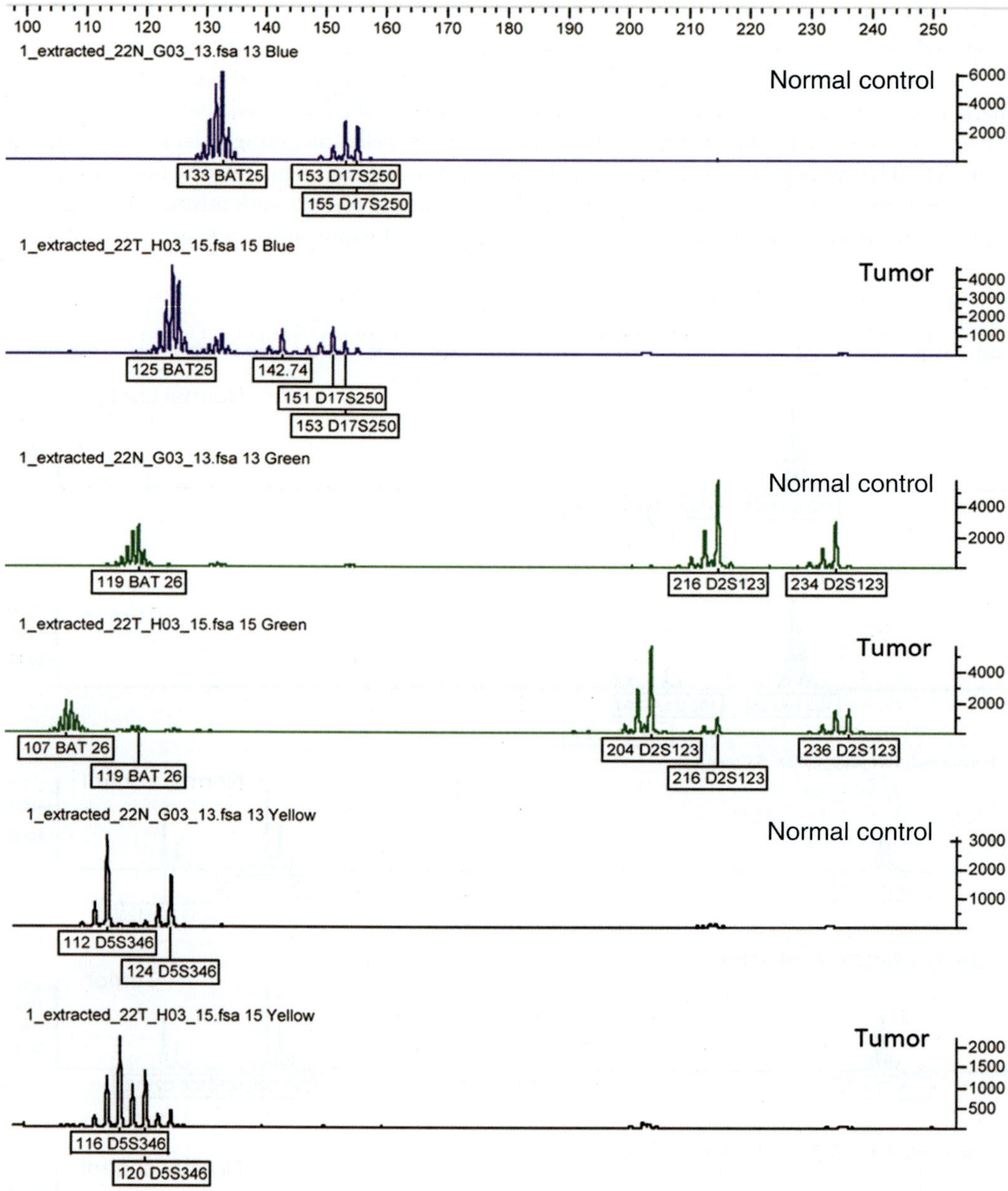


**B**

**FIGURE 11.3:** (*Continued*) A microsatellite unstable tumor shows left-shifted peaks at BAT25 and BAT26 compared to normal control tissues. Location shifts are also present at D17S250, D2S123, and D5S346 (**B**).

of the underlying defective gene (Table 11.1). Interpretation of mismatch repair protein immunohistochemistry and its caveats are discussed in Chapter 12.

## Deviation from the Classic Microsatellite Instability Model

Rare patients have congenital mismatch repair deficiency due to biallelic germline mutations affecting mismatch repair genes, in the form of either homozygosity or compound heterozygosity. Most such cases develop in small populations in which consanguinity occurs relatively frequently, such that the likelihood of biallelic inheritance is increased. Biallelic germline mutations predispose patients to Lynch syndrome–related cancers that develop in late adolescence or early adulthood, which is much sooner than the typical onset of hereditary tumors due to Lynch syndrome. The colorectal

**Table 11.1 Relationships Between Genetic Alteration and Patterns of Mismatch Repair Protein Immunostaining**

| Immunohistochemistry Result | Likely Defective Gene | Microsatellite Status |
|---|---|---|
| Loss of MLH1 and PMS2 | *MLH1* | MSI-H |
| Loss of MSH2 and MSH6 | *MSH2* | MSI-H |
| Isolated loss of PMS2 | *PMS2* | MSI-H |
| Isolated loss of MSH6 | *MSH6* | MSI-H or MSS |

phenotype of patients with biallelic mutations simulates familial adenomatous polyposis in the form of multiple adenomas and carcinomas. Extracolonic manifestations also occur and include a neurofibromatosis-like phenotype with *cafè au lait* spots, leukemia, or lymphoma, as well as cerebral and extracolonic gastrointestinal malignancies.[31] In contrast to Lynch syndrome, which usually results from a single germline mutation affecting *MLH1* or *MSH2*, most patients with congenital mismatch repair deficiency have mutations affecting *PMS2* (66%), followed in frequency by biallelic *MSH6* (21%) mutations.[32] It is possible that defects in *PMS2* and *MSH6* are overrepresented in this group of patients because biallelic inactivation of *MLH1* and *MSH2* is lethal in some cases.

Two additional types of genetic alteration have been recently identified as the genetic bases for some Lynch syndrome cases. The first is heritable epigenetic inactivation of *MLH1*, or *MLH1* constitutional epimutation, in which case the germline defect is promoter methylation of *MLH1*.[33] The second is germline deletion affecting the polyadenylation site located in exon 9 of *EpCAM* (*epithelial cell adhesion molecule*, formerly known as *TACSTD1*) located upstream of *MSH2*. Deletion of this region results in loss of the *EpCAM* stop codon and subsequent CpG methylation in *MSH2* or formation of *EpCAM-MSH2* fusion transcripts, both of which lead to *MSH2* inactivation.[34,35]

## Microsatellite Instability in Sporadic Colorectal Carcinogenesis

Lynch syndrome–related colon cancers and sporadic tumors with MSI are histologically indistinguishable, but the mechanisms by which MSI drives carcinogenesis in these settings are slightly different. Sporadic colorectal cancers with MSI develop *via* somatic *MLH1* promoter methylation and silencing of *MLH1* from transcription.[36–38] Similar to Lynch syndrome–related cancers, these tumors show a predilection for the proximal colon, but they tend to affect older patients, particularly women. At least half of sporadic colonic carcinomas with MSI also contain V600E mutations in *BRAF*, but *KRAS2* and *TP53* are wild type.[39] Activation of Wnt signaling is less important in sporadic cancers with MSI, and, in fact, there is an inverse relationship between the presence of *APC* mutations and MSI in sporadic tumors.[40,41] If *APC* mutations are detected in sporadic tumors with MSI, they are usually frameshift mutations in short nucleotide repeats and likely result from instability.[41] The absence of early *APC* mutations in sporadic cancers with MSI also implies that they may be preceded by a nonadenomatous precursor. This observation has led some investigators to propose that sessile serrated polyps (sessile serrated adenomas) of the abdominal colon represent precursors to sporadic colonic cancers with MSI, as described in Chapter 4.[42,43]

## Other Molecules Involved in Microsatellite Instability Pathway of Colorectal Carcinoma

Mismatch repair deficiency promotes colorectal neoplasia *via* several mechanisms. First, failure to correct base pairing errors that occur during DNA replication leads to multiple base pair changes that ultimately impact protein function and enhance tumorigenicity. Tumors with underlying mismatch repair deficiency also show MSI with expansion or contraction of microsatellite length. Most microsatellites are located in noncoding regions of DNA, and, thus, their alterations have minimal impact on transcription. However, some mononucleotide repeats occur in coding regions, so frameshifts in these regions can cause gene inactivation. For example, *transforming growth factor-β type II receptor* (*TGFβR2*) is an important regulatory gene that inhibits proliferation of colonic epithelium.[44,45] This gene contains two microsatellite sequences in the coding region that negatively affect *TGFβR2* expression when MSI is present. A number of other regulatory genes also contain microsatellites in their coding regions, alterations within which may affect regulation of cell proliferation (e.g., *GRB1, TCF-4, WISP3, activin receptor-2, insulin-like growth factor-2 receptor, axin-2,* and *CDX*), cell cycling and apoptosis (e.g., *BAX, caspase-5, RIZ, BCL-10, PTEN, hG4-1,* and *FAS*), and DNA repair (e.g., *MBD-4, BLM, CHK1, MLH3, RAD50, MSH3,* and *MSH6*).[27,46]

## THE CPG ISLAND METHYLATOR PHENOTYPE

### Overview

Epigenetic alterations, such as DNA hypermethylation, DNA hypomethylation, posttranslational histone modification, and chromatin looping, regulate gene expression. Of these, DNA hypermethylation has been most extensively studied in colorectal carcinoma. DNA methylation is catalyzed by DNA methyltransferases, which add methyl groups to the carbon 5 position of cytosine residues located 5′ to guanine, thereby forming methyl cytosines. These cytosine (C) and guanine (G) dinucleotides are often clustered in CG-rich regions, termed CpG islands, which occur in the promoter regions of up to 50% of mammalian genes. Promoter methylation represses genes from transcription by directly inhibiting transcription factor binding or influencing histone acetylation and blocking access of transcriptional machinery to the gene. Specific promoter sequence methylation occurs physiologically, such as in the case of X chromosome inactivation, but disordered promoter methylation is an important pathologic event in colorectal carcinogenesis. Epigenetic silencing in tumors is biologically equivalent to acquiring an inactivating mutation. This mechanism may account for the first, second, or both hits, in the silencing of important tumor suppressor genes.

### DNA Hypermethylation in Colorectal Carcinoma

Tumors that show DNA hypermethylation at multiple promoters are classified as showing the CpG island methylator phenotype (CIMP). Toyota et al.[47] originally suggested that CIMP may play a role in colorectal carcinogenesis, but characterization of methylation status in colorectal tumors has been challenging because assays and criteria for methylation vary among institutions. Tumor-related DNA hypermethylation is associated with several clinicopathologic features, including increased age, female gender, proximal tumor location, MSI, and wild-type *TP53*.[48] Molecular features, namely, *BRAF* or *KRAS* mutations, segregate with CpG methylation in different sets of genes. Colonic cancers with *BRAF* mutations also show MSI and methylation of *MINT1, MLH1, RIZ1, and TIMP3*, whereas *KRAS* mutations are associated with methylation of several MINT markers.[49] Others have reported higher levels of DNA methylation associated with *BRAF* mutation compared to a lesser degree of methylation in tumors with *KRAS* mutations and essentially no methylation in tumors wild type for both *BRAF* and *KRAS*.[50] Indeed, colorectal carcinomas that show CIMP have emerged as a relatively distinct subset. These tumors tend to occur in the proximal colons of older women and are associated with a history of cigarette smoking.[51] They frequently harbor *BRAF* mutations and show methylation of *MLH1* resulting in MSI. Up to 70% of colonic carcinomas with CIMP show MSI.[52] The mechanisms underlying CIMP are not clear, but may result from increased DNA methyltransferase activity acquired *via* mutation or transcriptional upregulation.[53,54]

## SUMMARY AND CONCLUSIONS

Intensive research and technologic advances have led to discovery of several genetic, epigenetic, and posttranslational regulatory mechanisms that facilitate colorectal carcinogenesis. Recognition of these molecular changes began with the study of patients with heritable cancer syndromes, but efforts have since expanded to encompass sporadic tumors as well. Emerging understanding and dissemination of information have enabled physicians to better identify patients at risk for heritable cancers, such as those with Lynch syndrome, and characterize patients with polyposis disorders who have unconventional genetic changes underlying their diseases. Detection of specific alterations in some tumors has also facilitated development of novel approaches to cancer therapy and prevention. Studies elucidating cellular signal transduction pathways continue to unravel the relationships between proteins that play important roles in cell survival and proliferation, some of which may represent targets for directed medical therapies. Application of these advances to clinical practice is the subject of subsequent chapters in this section.

# References


1. Vogelstein B, Kinzler KW. Cancer genes and the pathways they control. *Nat Med* [Research Support, Non-U.S. Gov't Research Support, U.S. Gov't, P.H.S. Review] 2004;10(8):789–799.
2. Fearon ER, Vogelstein B. A genetic model for colorectal tumorigenesis. *Cell* [Research Support, Non-U.S. Gov't Research Support, U.S. Gov't, P.H.S. Review] 1990;61(5):759–767.
3. Hamilton SR, Liu B, Parsons RE, et al. The molecular basis of Turcot's syndrome. *N Engl J Med* 1995;332(13):839–847.
4. Powell SM, Petersen GM, Krush AJ, et al. Molecular diagnosis of familial adenomatous polyposis. *N Engl J Med* [Research Support, Non-U.S. Gov't Research Support, U.S. Gov't, P.H.S.] 1993;329(27):1982–1987.
5. Leppert M, Burt R, Hughes JP, et al. Genetic analysis of an inherited predisposition to colon cancer in a family with a variable number of adenomatous polyps. *N Engl J Med* 1990;322(13):904–908.
6. Spirio LN, Samowitz W, Robertson J, et al. Alleles of APC modulate the frequency and classes of mutations that lead to colon polyps. *Nat Genet* [Research Support, Non-U.S. Gov't Research Support, U.S. Gov't, Non-P.H.S.] 1998;20(4):385–388.
7. Segditsas S, Rowan AJ, Howarth K, et al. APC and the three-hit hypothesis. *Oncogene* [Research Support, Non-U.S. Gov't] 2009;28(1):146–155.
8. Lamlum H, Ilyas M, Rowan A, et al. The type of somatic mutation at APC in familial adenomatous polyposis is determined by the site of the germline mutation: a new facet to Knudson's "two-hit" hypothesis. *Nat Med* 1999;5(9):1071–1075.
9. Albuquerque C, Breukel C, van der Luijt R, et al. The "just-right" signaling model: *APC* somatic mutations are selected based on a specific level of activation of the beta-catenin signaling cascade. *Hum Mol Genet* [Research Support, Non-U.S. Gov't] 2002;11(13):1549–1560.
10. Lefevre JH, Colas C, Coulet F, et al. MYH biallelic mutation can inactivate the two genetic pathways of colorectal cancer by *APC* or *MLH1* transversions. *Fam Cancer* 2010;9(4):589–594.
11. Powell SM, Zilz N, Beazer-Barclay Y, et al. *APC* mutations occur early during colorectal tumorigenesis. *Nature* 1992;359(6392):235–237.
12. Gregorieff A, Clevers H. Wnt signaling in the intestinal epithelium: from endoderm to cancer. *Genes Dev* [Research Support, Non-U.S. Gov't Review] 2005;19(8):877–890.
13. Kinzler KW, Vogelstein B. Lessons from hereditary colorectal cancer. *Cell* [Research Support, Non-U.S. Gov't Research Support, U.S. Gov't, P.H.S. Review] 1996;87(2):159–170.
14. Roberts DM, Pronobis MI, Poulton JS, et al. Regulation of Wnt signaling by the tumor suppressor *APC* does not require ability to enter the nucleus nor a particular cytoplasmic localization. *Mol Biol Cell* 2012;23(11):2041–2056.
15. Ishidate T, Matsumine A, Toyoshima K, et al. The APC-hDLG complex negatively regulates cell cycle progression from the G0/G1 to S phase. *Oncogene* [Research Support, Non-U.S. Gov't] 2000;19(3):365–372.
16. Qian J, Sarnaik AA, Bonney TM, et al. The *APC* tumor suppressor inhibits DNA replication by directly binding to DNA via its carboxyl terminus. *Gastroenterology* [Research Support, N.I.H., Extramural Research Support, Non-U.S. Gov't] 2008;135(1):152–162.
17. Green RA, Wollman R, Kaplan KB. *APC* and *EB1* function together in mitosis to regulate spindle dynamics and chromosome alignment. *Mol Biol Cell* [Research Support, N.I.H., Extramural Research Support, Non-U.S. Gov't Research Support, U.S. Gov't, P.H.S.] 2005;16(10):4609–4622.
18. Shih IM, Zhou W, Goodman SN, et al. Evidence that genetic instability occurs at an early stage of colorectal tumorigenesis. *Cancer Res* [Research Support, Non-U.S. Gov't Research Support, U.S. Gov't, P.H.S.] 2001;61(3):818–822.

19. Vogelstein B, Fearon ER, Hamilton SR, et al. Genetic alterations during colorectal-tumor development. *N Engl J Med* [Research Support, Non-U.S. Gov't Research Support, U.S. Gov't, P.H.S.] 1988;319(9): 525–532.
20. Woodford-Richens KL, Rowan AJ, Gorman P, et al. SMAD4 mutations in colorectal cancer probably occur before chromosomal instability, but after divergence of the microsatellite instability pathway. *Proc Natl Acad Sci U S A* [Research Support, Non-U.S. Gov't] 2001;98(17):9719–9723.
21. Worthley DL, Whitehall VL, Spring KJ, et al. Colorectal carcinogenesis: road maps to cancer. *World J Gastroenterol* [Research Support, Non-U.S. Gov't Review] 2007;13(28):3784–3791.
22. Mills AA. p53: link to the past, bridge to the future. *Genes Dev* [Comment Comparative Study Review] 2005;19(18):2091–2099.
23. Peltomaki P, Aaltonen LA, Sistonen P, et al. Genetic mapping of a locus predisposing to human colorectal cancer. *Science* [Comment Research Support, Non-U.S. Gov't Research Support, U.S. Gov't, P.H.S.] 1993;260(5109):810–812.
24. Johnson V, Volikos E, Halford SE, et al. Exon 3 beta-catenin mutations are specifically associated with colorectal carcinomas in hereditary non-polyposis colorectal cancer syndrome. *Gut* 2005;54(2):264–267.
25. Muller A, Beckmann C, Westphal G, et al. Prevalence of the mismatch-repair-deficient phenotype in colonic adenomas arising in HNPCC patients: results of a 5-year follow-up study. *Int J Colorectal Dis* [Research Support, Non-U.S. Gov't] 2006;21(7):632–641.
26. Senter L, Clendenning M, Sotamaa K, et al. The clinical phenotype of Lynch syndrome due to germ-line PMS2 mutations. *Gastroenterology* [Multicenter Study Research Support, N.I.H., Extramural Research Support, Non-U.S. Gov't] 2008;135(2):419–428.
27. Boland CR, Goel A. Microsatellite instability in colorectal cancer. *Gastroenterology* [Portraits Research Support, N.I.H., Extramural Review] 2010;138(6):2073–2087.e3.
28. Boland CR, Thibodeau SN, Hamilton SR, et al. A National Cancer Institute Workshop on Microsatellite Instability for cancer detection and familial predisposition: development of international criteria for the determination of microsatellite instability in colorectal cancer. *Cancer Res* [Consensus Development Conference Consensus Development Conference, NIH Review] 1998;58(22):5248–5257.
29. Suraweera N, Duval A, Reperant M, et al. Evaluation of tumor microsatellite instability using five quasimonomorphic mononucleotide repeats and pentaplex PCR. *Gastroenterology* [Research Support, Non-U.S. Gov't] 2002;123(6):1804–1811.
30. Goel A, Nagasaka T, Hamelin R, et al. An optimized pentaplex PCR for detecting DNA mismatch repair-deficient colorectal cancers. *PLoS One* [Research Support, N.I.H., Extramural Research Support, Non-U.S. Gov't] 2010;5(2):e9393.
31. Bandipalliam P. Syndrome of early onset colon cancers, hematologic malignancies and features of neurofibromatosis in HNPCC families with homozygous mismatch repair gene mutations. *Fam Cancer* 2005;4:323–333.
32. Durno CA, Holter S, Sherman PM, et al. The gastrointestinal phenotype of germline biallelic mismatch repair gene mutations. *Am J Gastroenterol* 2010;105(11):2449–2456.
33. Hitchins M, Williams R, Cheong K, et al. MLH1 germline epimutations as a factor in hereditary nonpolyposis colorectal cancer. *Gastroenterology* [Research Support, Non-U.S. Gov't] 2005;129(5): 1392–1399.
34. Ligtenberg MJ, Kuiper RP, Chan TL, et al. Heritable somatic methylation and inactivation of MSH2 in families with Lynch syndrome due to deletion of the 3′ exons of TACSTD1. *Nat Genet* [Research Support, Non-U.S. Gov't] 2009;41(1):112–117.
35. Kovacs ME, Papp J, Szentirmay Z, et al. Deletions removing the last exon of TACSTD1 constitute a distinct class of mutations predisposing to Lynch syndrome. *Hum Mutat* 2009;30:197–203.
36. Kane MF, Loda M, Gaida GM, et al. Methylation of the hMLH1 promoter correlates with lack of expression of hMLH1 in sporadic colon tumors and mismatch repair-defective human tumor cell lines. *Cancer Res* [Research Support, Non-U.S. Gov't Research Support, U.S. Gov't, P.H.S.] 1997;57(5):808–811.
37. Nagasaka T, Koi M, Kloor M, et al. Mutations in both KRAS and BRAF may contribute to the methylator phenotype in colon cancer. *Gastroenterology* [Multicenter Study Research Support, N.I.H., Extramural Research Support, Non-U.S. Gov't] 2008;134(7):1950–1960, 60.e1.
38. Boland CR, Shin SK, Goel A. Promoter methylation in the genesis of gastrointestinal cancer. *Yonsei Med J* [Research Support, N.I.H., Extramural Research Support, Non-U.S. Gov't Review] 2009;50(3): 309–321.

39. Wang L, Cunningham JM, Winters JL, et al. BRAF mutations in colon cancer are not likely attributable to defective DNA mismatch repair. *Cancer Res* [Research Support, U.S. Gov't, P.H.S.] 2003;63(17): 5209–5212.
40. Olschwang S, Hamelin R, Laurent-Puig P, et al. Alternative genetic pathways in colorectal carcinogenesis. *Proc Natl Acad Sci U S A* 1997;94(22):12122–12127.
41. Samowitz WS, Slattery ML, Sweeney C, et al. APC mutations and other genetic and epigenetic changes in colon cancer. *Mol Cancer Res* 2007;5(2):165–170.
42. O'Brien MJ, Yang S, Mack C, et al. Comparison of microsatellite instability, CpG island methylation phenotype, BRAF and KRAS status in serrated polyps and traditional adenomas indicates separate pathways to distinct colorectal carcinoma end points. *Am J Surg Pathol* 2006;30(12):1491–1501.
43. Sheridan TB, Fenton H, Lewin MR, et al. Sessile serrated adenomas with low- and high-grade dysplasia and early carcinomas: an immunohistochemical study of serrated lesions "caught in the act." *Am J Clin Pathol* 2006;126(4):564–571.
44. Markowitz S, Wang J, Myeroff L, et al. Inactivation of the type II TGF-beta receptor in colon cancer cells with microsatellite instability. *Science* [Comment Research Support, Non-U.S. Gov't Research Support, U.S. Gov't, P.H.S.] 1995;268(5215):1336–1338.
45. Wang J, Sun L, Myeroff L, et al. Demonstration that mutation of the type II transforming growth factor beta receptor inactivates its tumor suppressor activity in replication error-positive colon carcinoma cells. *J Biol Chem* [Comparative Study Research Support, U.S. Gov't, Non-P.H.S. Research Support, U.S. Gov't, P.H.S.] 1995;270(37):22044–22049.
46. Duval A, Hamelin R. Mutations at coding repeat sequences in mismatch repair-deficient human cancers: toward a new concept of target genes for instability. *Cancer Res* [Research Support, Non-U.S. Gov't Review] 2002;62(9):2447–2454.
47. Toyota M, Ahuja N, Ohe-Toyota M, et al. CpG island methylator phenotype in colorectal cancer. *Proc Natl Acad Sci U S A* [Research Support, Non-U.S. Gov't Research Support, U.S. Gov't, P.H.S.] 1999;96(15):8681–8686.
48. Samowitz WS. The CpG island methylator phenotype in colorectal cancer. *J Mol Diagn* 2007;9(3): 281–283.
49. Shen L, Toyota M, Kondo Y, et al. Integrated genetic and epigenetic analysis identifies three different subclasses of colon cancer. *Proc Natl Acad Sci U S A* 2007;104(47):18654–18659.
50. Ogino S, Goel A. Molecular classification and correlates in colorectal cancer. *J Mol Diagn* [Research Support, N.I.H., Extramural Research Support, Non-U.S. Gov't Review] 2008;10(1):13–27.
51. Samowitz WS, Albertsen H, Sweeney C, et al. Association of smoking, CpG island methylator phenotype, and V600E BRAF mutations in colon cancer. *J Natl Cancer Inst* [Research Support, N.I.H., Extramural Research Support, Non-U.S. Gov't] 2006;98(23):1731–1738.
52. Funkhouser WK Jr, Lubin IM, Monzon FA, et al. Relevance, pathogenesis, and testing algorithm for mismatch repair-defective colorectal carcinomas: a report of the association for molecular pathology. *J Mol Diagn* 2012;14(2):91–103.
53. Linhart HG, Lin H, Yamada Y, et al. Dnmt3b promotes tumorigenesis in vivo by gene-specific de novo methylation and transcriptional silencing. *Genes Dev* [Research Support, N.I.H., Extramural Research Support, Non-U.S. Gov't] 2007;21(23):3110–3122.
54. Nosho K, Shima K, Irahara N, et al. DNMT3B expression might contribute to CpG island methylator phenotype in colorectal cancer. *Clin Cancer Res* [Research Support, N.I.H., Extramural Research Support, Non-U.S. Gov't] 2009;15(11):3663–3671.

# 12 Practical Issues Related to Ancillary Testing of Colorectal Carcinoma

Wade S. Samowitz

Recent advances in our understanding of colorectal cancer progression have led to discovery of important molecular alterations that are biologically relevant for several reasons. Some changes, such as mutations affecting tumor suppressor genes and DNA mismatch repair genes, underlie heritable cancer syndromes, and thus, evaluation for their presence helps identify patients and their family members with heritable cancer risk. Other molecular abnormalities have therapeutic implications. An increasing number of oncogenic mutations affecting membrane-bound receptors can be exploited, or manipulated, to develop novel interventions, whereas other changes, such as *KRAS* mutations, abrogate the effects of some chemotherapeutic agents. Tumor evaluation for the presence of these alterations is essential to cancer management, and thus, clinicians increasingly demand that ancillary testing be performed on pathology materials. Unfortunately, many clinicians are not fully aware of the limitations of molecular studies, or they inappropriately utilize resources to obtain information that may not be clinically relevant. As a result, pathologists play increasingly important roles as physician scientists and educators regarding the judicious use of molecular assays. The purpose of this chapter is to discuss practical aspects of ancillary testing with focus on caveats unique to the evaluation for mismatch repair deficiency.

## EVALUATION FOR DNA MISMATCH REPAIR DEFICIENCY

### Overview

The Amsterdam criteria are historical guidelines originally set forth to select individuals for germline testing of DNA mismatch repair genes. These criteria primarily identify patients with cancer onset at a young age or a strong family history, but may fail to detect cancer risk in patients who lack a detailed family history. The revised Bethesda criteria not only include recommendations based on family history and age of cancer onset, but they also take into account important histologic features characteristic of microsatellite unstable tumors.[1] Unfortunately, some patients with Lynch syndrome still escape detection by these revised criteria, and thus, many centers now perform universal microsatellite instability (MSI) testing on all colorectal cancers.[2–4] Mismatch repair deficiency is evaluated using two techniques: PCR amplification of a panel of microsatellite repeats and immunohistochemistry for DNA mismatch repair proteins. The Bethesda consensus panel for microsatellite analysis consists of two mononucleotide and three dinucleotide repeats and is widely used to assess for MSI. However, instability in mononucleotide repeats is probably more important than instability in dinucleotide repeats for detection of Lynch syndrome–related tumors.[5,6] Thus, many centers now use a commercially available panel of five mononucleotide repeats, as discussed in Chapter 11.

### Interpretation of Immunohistochemistry for Mismatch Repair Proteins

Immunohistochemistry for mismatch repair proteins, MLH1, MSH2, MSH6, and PMS2, is a fairly good surrogate test for microsatellite status. As with all immunohistochemistry stains, however, immunostain results may be difficult to interpret in some situations. Immunohistochemical staining quality is dependent on a variety of factors, including type of fixative, time interval between removal of the specimen from the patient and fixation, adequacy of tissue fixation, and duration of fixation. The effects of these variables on immunohistochemical staining of colorectal carcinomas have not been studied as systematically as they have been in breast cancer, for example, but they probably affect extent and intensity of staining, which can vary between different areas of a single slide. Fortunately, normal staining of nonneoplastic cells, such as lymphocytes, stromal cells, and colonic crypts, serves as an internal control for DNA mismatch repair protein immunohistochemistry. Only areas of the slide with intact internal control staining are used to evaluate tumor staining, and, in fact, areas that show a lack of internal control staining should be classified as uninterpretable (Figure 12.1). Tumor-infiltrating lymphocytes are a common histologic feature of microsatellite unstable colon cancers and represent a very useful internal control for immunohistochemistry interpretation (Figure 12.2).[7] Mismatch repair protein expression tends to parallel proliferative activity, so cancer cells, germinal centers, and stromal cells in granulation tissue generally show strong nuclear staining. Cells that are not actively proliferating, including surface epithelial cells in the normal colon, show a lack of, or diminished, staining compared to proliferating cells. Thus, it is not uncommon to see negative, or faintly positive, nonproliferative cells, such as lymphoid cells surrounding highly proliferative germinal centers and superficial

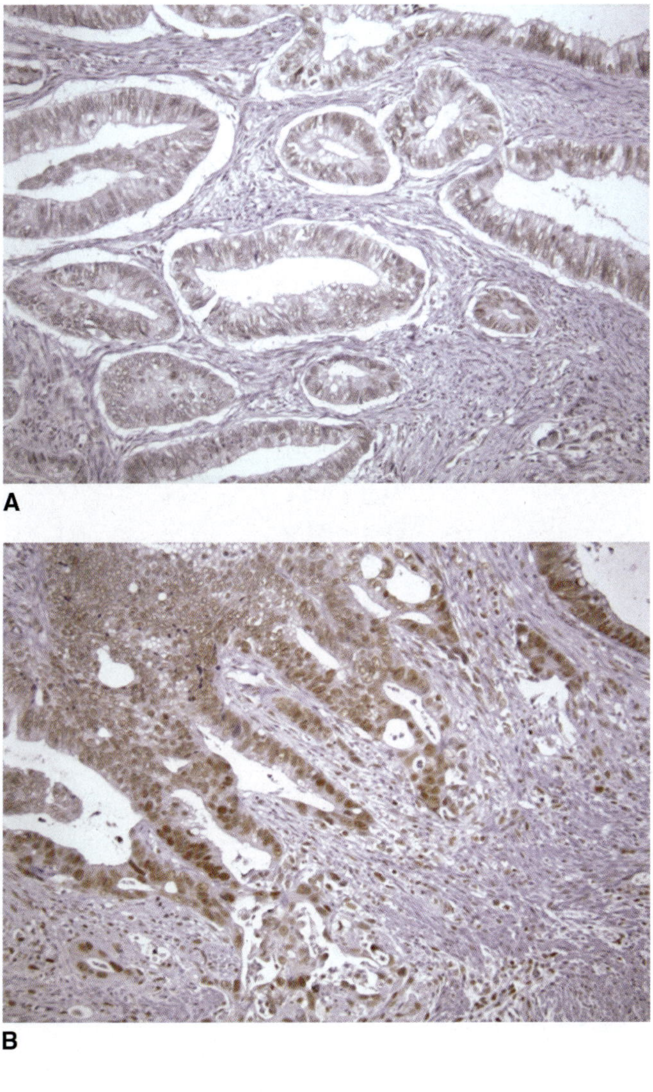

**FIGURE 12.1:** Immunohistochemical staining results for MLH1 vary between areas within a microsatellite stable tumor, as demonstrated by PCR. Both the tumor cell and internal control cell nuclei are negative in one area, leading to an uninterpretable result (**A**). A different area of the same slide shows strong nuclear staining of lymphocytes, which serve as an internal control. The tumor cells show strong nuclear immunostaining reflecting intact MLH1 (**B**).

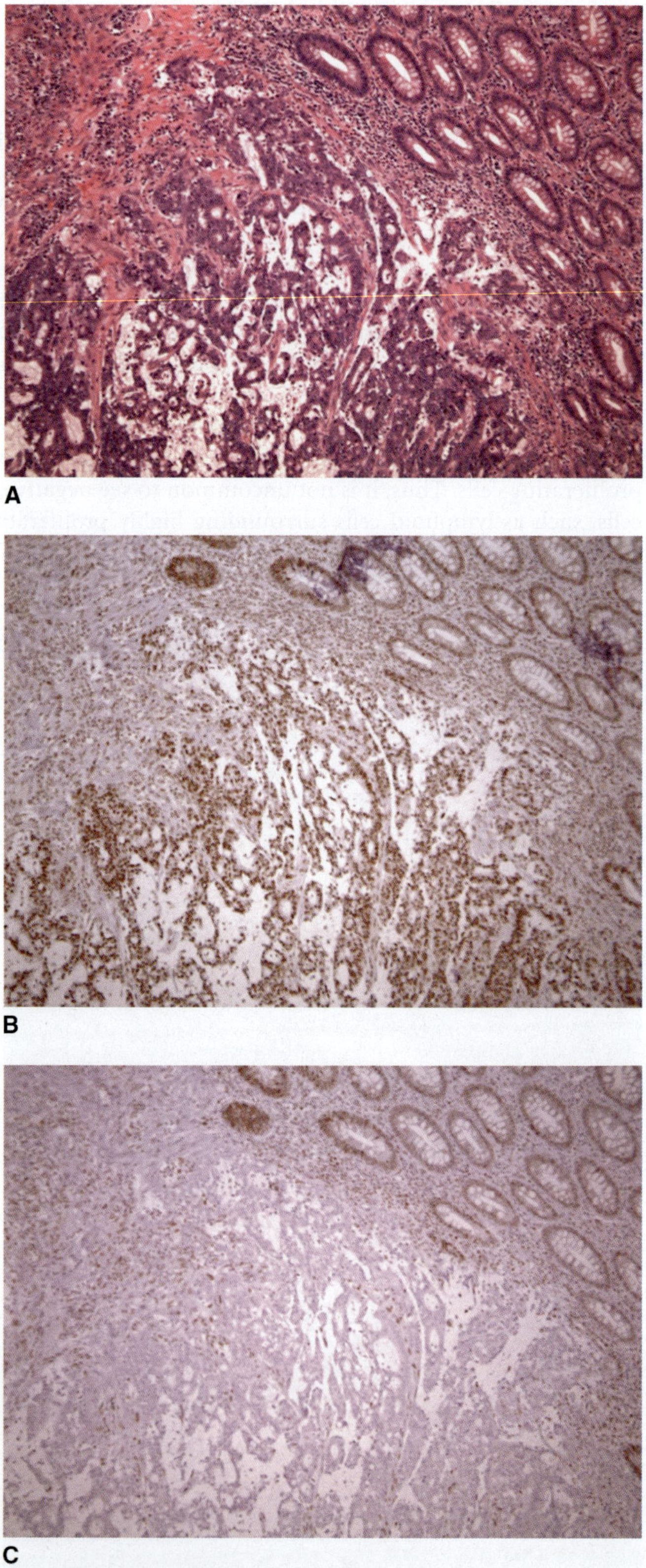

FIGURE 12.2: Tumor-infiltrating lymphocytes are commonly observed in colonic carcinomas with MSI (**A**). An immunostain for MSH2 shows internal control staining of colonic crypts, stromal cells, and lymphocytes, including those in the vicinity of the tumor, as well as preserved staining of tumor cell nuclei (**B**). Loss of staining for MLH1 in the tumor cells is present in association with intact staining of the internal control, reflecting defective function of this protein (**C**).

epithelium of serrated polyps. For this reason, a lack of immunostaining in some, but not all, tumor cells does not necessarily imply the presence of DNA mismatch repair protein deficiency, even if there is intact staining of internal controls.

Finally, it is generally accepted that colon cancers with PCR-proven MSI show complete loss of immunohistochemical staining for one or more antibodies to DNA mismatch repair proteins depending on the nature of the underlying deficiency. This is especially true for sporadic unstable tumors due to acquired *MLH1* methylation because epigenetic silencing of transcription turns off mRNA expression and completely abrogates protein expression. However, we now recognize that some colon cancers due to Lynch syndrome show markedly decreased DNA mismatch repair protein immunoexpression, but the staining reaction is not completely lost.[8] Although overemphasizing the importance of diminished staining intensity may result in "false positives" and unnecessary germline testing, such factors do warrant consideration. We typically recommend evaluation by PCR to help evaluate the significance of markedly decreased staining intensity, especially if the staining reaction is diminished relative to that of the internal control.

Heterodimers formed by DNA mismatch repair proteins (MLH1/PMS2 and MSH2/MSH6) affect interpretation of immunostain results, as discussed in Chapter 11 (Table 11.1). Stability of PMS2 and MSH6 is highly dependent on these complexes, whereas stability of MLH1 and MSH2 is not. Therefore, combined loss of MLH1 and PMS2 immunostaining reflects defective MLH1, and combined loss of MSH2 and MSH6 suggests an abnormality in MSH2. Isolated loss of MSH6 or PMS2 immunostaining usually indicates a defect in MSH6 or PMS2, respectively.[9] However, there are exceptions to these rules. Isolated loss of PMS2 immunostaining can reflect an *MLH1* germline mutation when the mutation results in nonfunctional, but antigenic, MLH1 protein.[10] "Clonal" loss of MSH6 is occasionally encountered in some, but not all, areas of a tumor.[9] This usually occurs in cancers with MSI due to other deficiencies, such as *MLH1* promoter methylation. Underlying MSI in these cancers probably causes instability in coding mononucleotide repeats of *MSH6* through mismatch repair deficiency, leading to inactivation of MSH6 protein.[11]

## Distinction between Sporadic and Hereditary Colorectal Cancers with Microsatellite Instability

The results of DNA mismatch repair protein immunohistochemistry facilitate subsequent evaluation for possible Lynch syndrome (Figure 12.3). Combined loss of MSH2 and MSH6 and isolated loss of MSH6 or PMS2 are most likely indicative of Lynch syndrome.[12] However, the molecular basis for most sporadic colon cancers with MSI is *MLH1* promoter methylation, which results in loss of immunostaining for both MLH1 and PMS2. This pattern of staining is also expected in heritable tumors due to a germline defect in *MLH1*. Sporadic colon cancers with MSI are far more common than those associated with Lynch syndrome, and thus, differentiating sporadic from *MLH1*-deficient Lynch syndrome–related tumors before proceeding to germline testing avoids unnecessary expense for the majority of microsatellite unstable cancers. Fortunately, other molecular features of cancers with MSI can be evaluated to facilitate this distinction. Approximately 50% of sporadic colon cancers with MSI harbor a mutation in *BRAF*, a serine–threonine kinase.[13] The mutation is typically a "hot spot" valine to glutamate substitution at codon 600 (V600E) and has only rarely been reported in unstable tumors associated with Lynch syndrome.[14] Therefore, colon cancers with MSI that harbor the V600E *BRAF* mutation are very likely to be sporadic in nature, and germline evaluation for Lynch syndrome is probably unnecessary. In addition, assessment for *MLH1* promoter methylation can also be used to distinguish between sporadic and hereditary microsatellite unstable tumors.[15] Sporadic colon cancers with MSI develop as a result of *MLH1* promoter methylation, which has only rarely been reported in Lynch syndrome–associated tumors. Rare cancers with a Lynch syndrome phenotype due to germline methylation of the MLH1 promoter are distinguished from sporadic tumors by the presence of *MLH1* promoter methylation in nonneoplastic tissue.[16]

Two important points must be considered when using *BRAF* mutational status and *MLH1* methylation to distinguish sporadic from microsatellite unstable tumors in Lynch syndrome. Although *BRAF* mutations are common among sporadic colorectal cancers with MSI, they

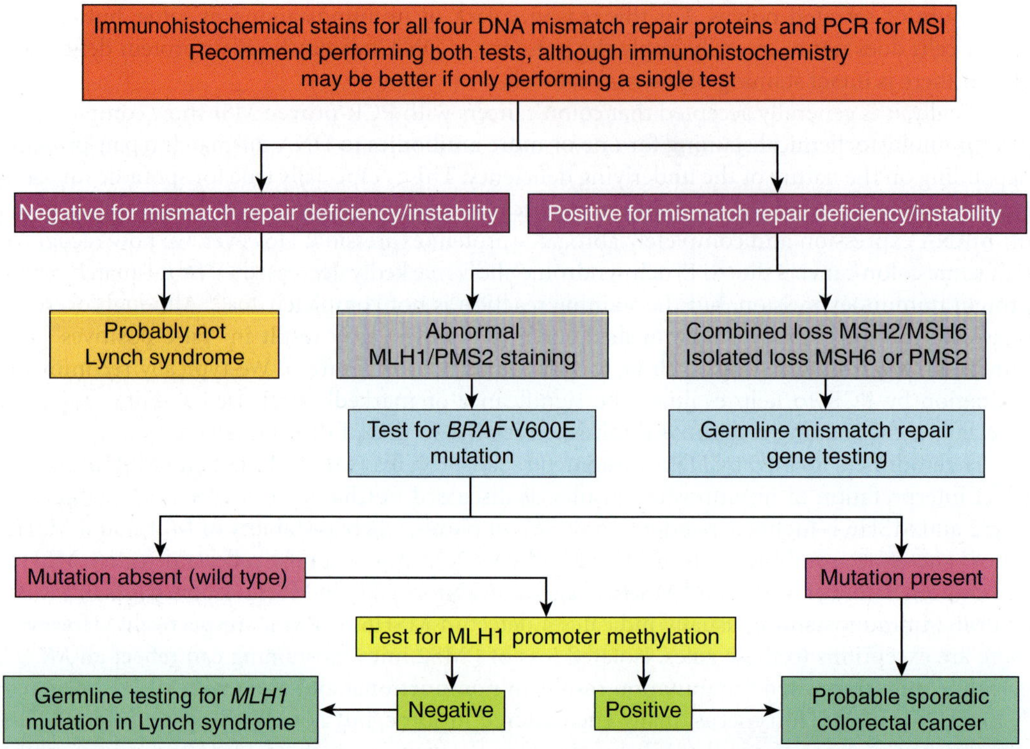


**FIGURE 12.3:** The evaluation of colorectal carcinoma for possible Lynch syndrome is performed using an algorithm. Mismatch proficient cancers are likely unrelated to Lynch syndrome. Combined loss of MSH2 and MSH6, or isolated loss of PMS2 or MSH6 immunostaining, likely reflects Lynch syndrome, which is further evaluated with germline testing of the relevant gene. Combined loss of MLH1 and PMS2 staining, however, could reflect a sporadic tumor with MSI or, less commonly, a heritable cancer due to a germline *MLH1* mutation. *BRAF* mutational analysis followed by assessment for *MLH1* promoter methylation may be performed to distinguish between these scenarios. Detection of either a V600E *BRAF* mutation or *MLH1* promoter methylation is strong evidence of a sporadic colorectal carcinoma, whereas negativity for both assays should prompt germline testing for possible Lynch syndrome. Notably, this algorithm is applicable only to assessment of colorectal carcinomas for Lynch syndrome. Sporadic microsatellite unstable extracolonic carcinomas, such as those of the endometrium, do not harbor *BRAF* mutations.

are infrequently seen in sporadic tumors with MSI from other sites that also give rise to Lynch syndrome–associated tumors, such as the endometrium.[17] Thus, it is unnecessary to evaluate extracolonic tumors with MSI for *BRAF* mutations and reasonable to proceed directly to evaluation for *MLH1* promoter methylation. There are also rare colon cancers in Lynch syndrome that show either *BRAF* mutation or *MLH1* methylation, so clinical suspicion for Lynch syndrome may drive germline evaluation of *MLH1* regardless of the results of these tissue assays.

Finally, patients with biallelic germline mismatch repair gene mutations, such as germline mutations in both *PMS2* genes, are rarely encountered.[18] Mismatch repair protein immunohistochemistry may be difficult to evaluate in a tumor associated with this scenario, since both the tumor and nonneoplastic internal control nuclei typically lack staining for the relevant gene product. Staining results of such tumor may be erroneously classified as "uninterpretable" by immunohistochemistry, if the pathologist assumes that the absence of staining in tumor and control tissues is artifactual in nature. These errors may be avoided if pathologists are aware of the relevant clinical information and the immunophenotypic manifestations of this disorder. As discussed in Chapter 11, patients with biallelic germline mismatch repair gene deficiencies have a fairly distinctive phenotype that simulates the features of familial adenomatous polyposis in some respects. Tumors that develop in this setting do show MSI, so evaluation for both immunohistochemistry and MSI will identify affected individuals. Biallelic inactivation of mismatch repair genes more commonly affects *PMS2* and *MSH6* than *MLH1* and *MSH2*, so lack of staining for one of the former may guide subsequent evaluation.

### Immunohistochemistry versus PCR for Evaluation of Microsatellite Instability

Immunohistochemistry and PCR assays for MSI are complementary tests, and there are advantages and disadvantages to both. Neither assay identifies tumors with mismatch repair deficiency with complete sensitivity and specificity.[9,19] The PCR-based assay is usually straightforward in its interpretation, but it has limitations. Some tumors with germline *MSH6* mutations are microsatellite stable by PCR, so limiting evaluation to a PCR-based assay may fail to identify occasional patients with Lynch syndrome. Microsatellite stability in these cases results from a mild degree of redundancy in the mismatch repair system due to overlapping function between MSH6 and MSH3, and panels enriched in mononucleotide repeats may help correct this problem.[9,20] Microsatellite testing by PCR only shows whether a tumor is stable or unstable, but not which gene, or genes, may be involved; immunohistochemistry must be performed for that purpose. Immunohistochemistry-based tests may be difficult to interpret due to many factors, including variability in formalin fixation, "clonal" MSH6 loss, and uncertainty regarding the significance of decreased, rather than absent, staining. It is also possible for missense mutations that result in substitution of one amino acid for another to create a protein that is not functional, but maintains its antigenicity, thereby producing a false-negative result by immunohistochemistry.

Although immunohistochemistry and PCR are complimentary assays, immunohistochemistry-based assays are generally regarded as more informative tests. The genetic information provided by immunohistochemistry directs subsequent germline evaluation. It is also used to decide whether or not to test a cancer for *BRAF* mutation or *MLH1* methylation in order to distinguish between sporadic and hereditary tumors with MSI. Many institutions screen every colorectal cancer for MSI, and some include endometrial carcinomas in their screening programs.[2,21] It is reasonable to choose one test for universal screening purposes. Most institutions have chosen immunohistochemistry because it is relatively inexpensive and yields more information. A high clinical index of suspicion for Lynch syndrome may prompt both tests, either together or sequentially, to be more certain that instability is not missed.

## SELECTION OF SPECIMENS FOR ANCILLARY TESTING

### Selection of Tumor for Molecular Studies

Colorectal cancers are usually associated with a variety of nonneoplastic elements that are either recruited by the tumor or present in surrounding connective tissue that is infiltrated by the cancer. Formalin-fixed paraffin-embedded blocks of tumor often contain variable amounts of normal mucosa, mucosa–associated lymphoid tissue, lymphoid follicles, other inflammatory cells, desmoplastic stroma, and smooth muscle, as well as the tumor cells (Figure 12.4). Nonneoplastic cells contain wild-type DNA that essentially represents a contaminant to tumor DNA and may affect the results of molecular studies. Inclusion of these nonneoplastic cells in a sample used for molecular analysis dilutes the concentration of tumor DNA such that a molecular abnormality may not be detected in cases with a very high proportion of nonneoplastic cells. Many molecular assays currently employed evaluate for the presence of oncogenic mutations, such as those affecting *KRAS* and *BRAF*. Oncogenic mutations are usually heterozygous (i.e., present in one allele) and are associated with a maximum mutant allele percentage of 50%. In practice, however, one rarely eliminates nonlesional cells entirely, and thus, mutations are generally detected in far less (30% to 40%) of the extracted DNA (Figure 12.5).

The potentially deleterious effect of mixed cell types on molecular analysis requires dissection of tumor away from nonneoplastic cells prior to extraction of nucleic acids. Most laboratories

**FIGURE 12.4:** Tumor-rich areas with few contaminating nonneoplastic cells are ideal for molecular analysis. A *circle* of *red dots* encloses a fairly pure population of tumor cells (**A**) and excludes a lymphoid follicle (*arrow*) at the periphery (**B**). The lymphoid follicle consists of innumerable lymphocytes, all of which contain wild-type DNA that could dilute a mutation signal and lead to a false-negative result (**C**).

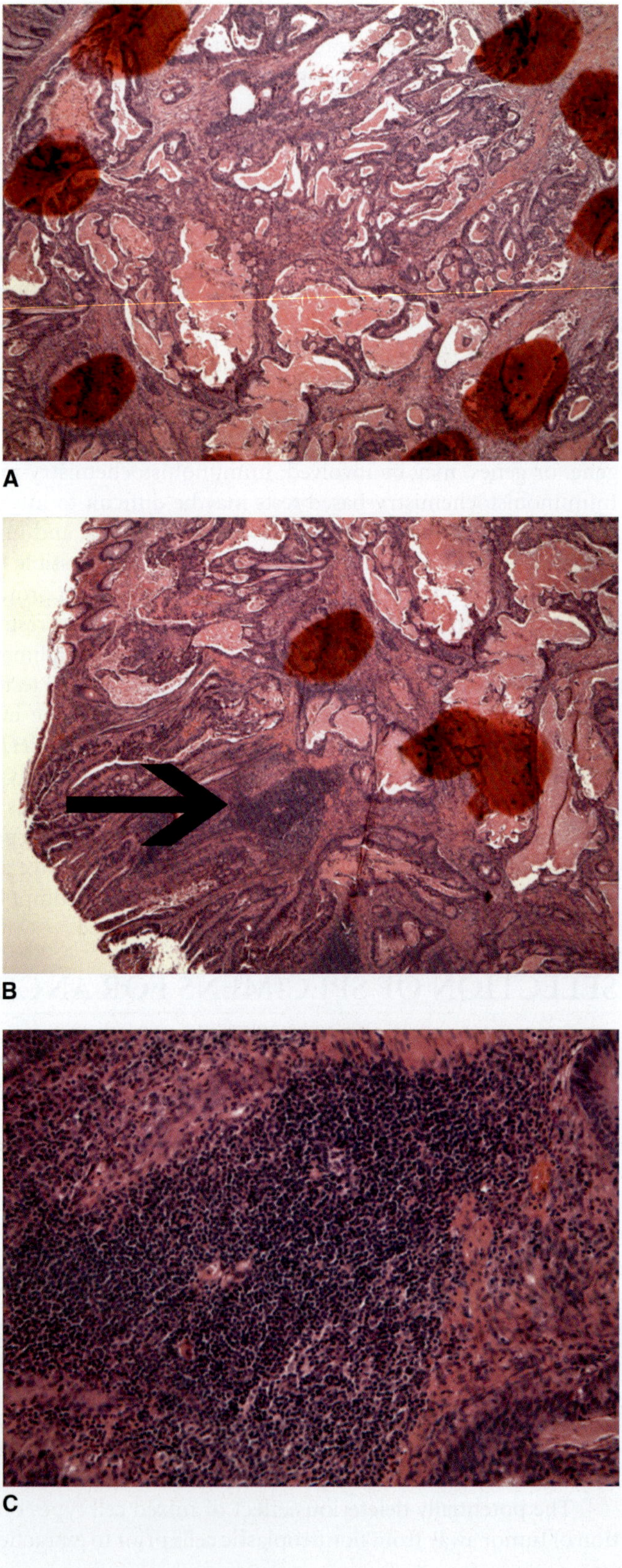

A

B

C

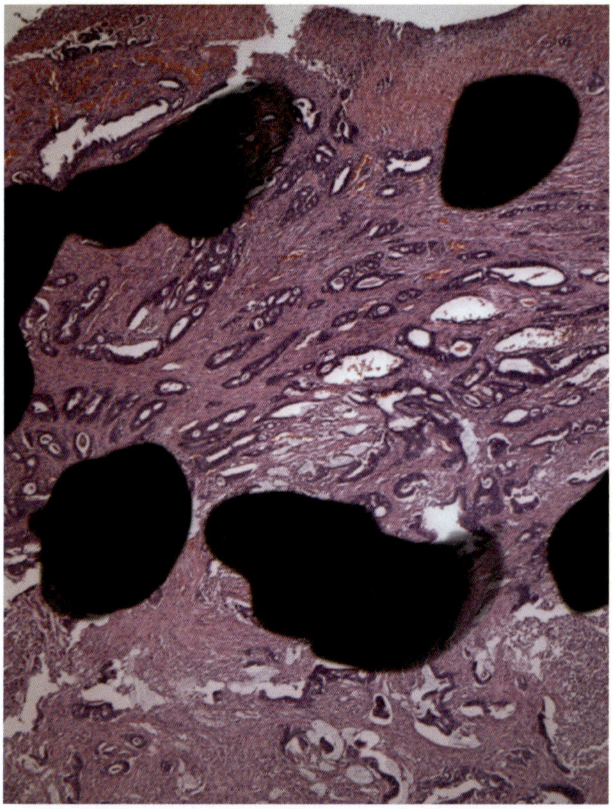

A

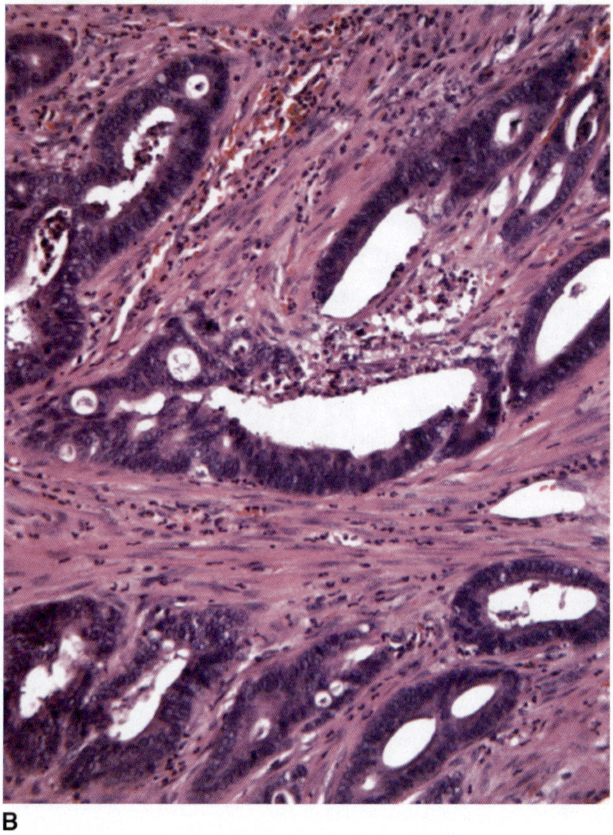

B

FIGURE 12.5: Tumor selection impacts the results of molecular analysis. An area chosen for mutational analysis is surrounded by *black dots* and contains a reasonable volume of tumor (**A**) with a few infiltrating neutrophils (**B**).

**FIGURE 12-5:** (*Continued*) An adjacent area contains a similar volume of tumor that is delineated by a *solid line* (**C**). However, this area also contains a prominent infiltrate of neutrophils, both between and within malignant glands (**D**). Pyrosequencing for *KRAS* revealed the same c.34 G>T, p.Gly12Cys *KRAS* mutation in both regions, although the mutant allele was present in 30% of the DNA extracted from the first region and only 14% of that from the second area. The deviation from 50% in both examples reflects variable dilution of the mutant signal by nonneoplastic cells.

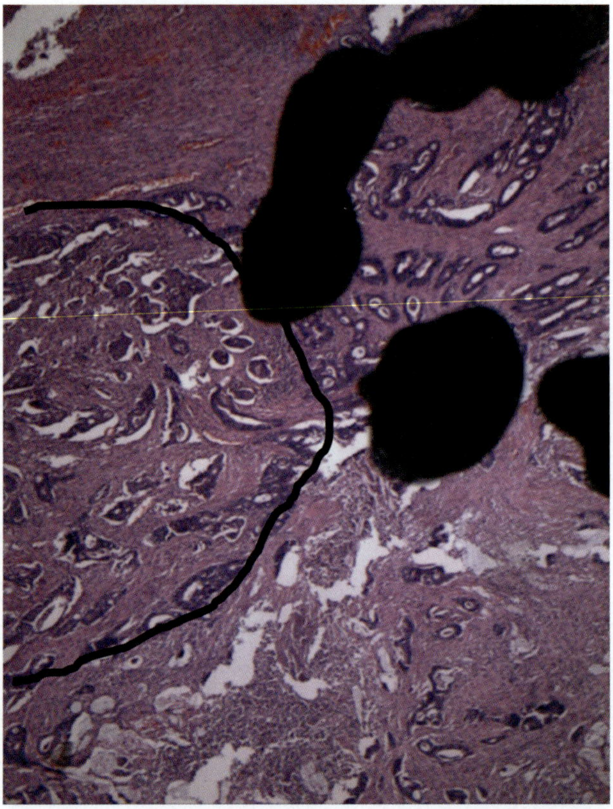

C

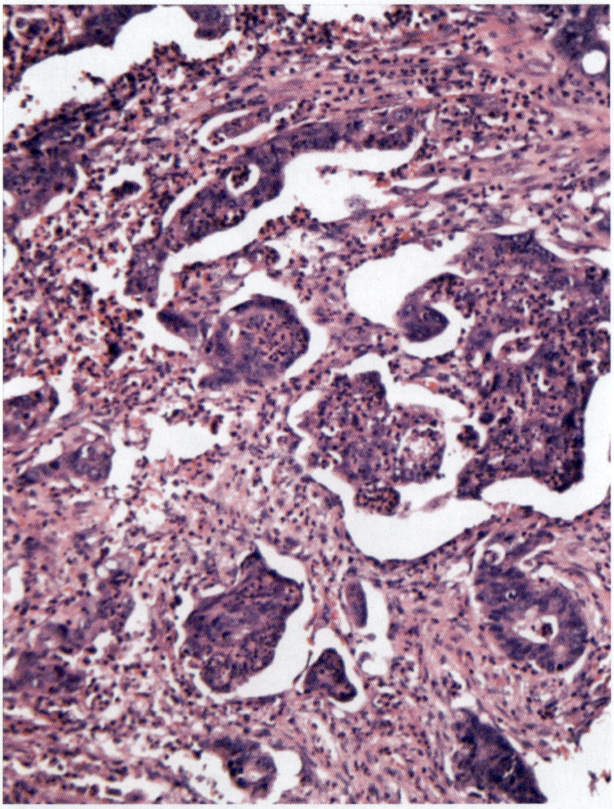

D

use some form of microscope-assisted dissection, in which microscopic assessment identifies an area with a high concentration of tumor that is manually scraped into a tube for DNA extraction. Selection of appropriate materials first requires that a block with a high concentration of tumor and relatively few intermixed nonneoplastic cells be chosen for analysis. This block is not necessarily the one with the most tumor, but, rather, one in which it is easiest to separate the neoplastic from nonneoplastic elements. It is better to choose a block with tumor that is mostly located in one area and nonneoplastic cells in another area than one with a greater volume of tumor intermingled with nonneoplastic elements throughout the sample.

## Neoadjuvantly Treated Cancers

Most human tissue samples evaluated for DNA mismatch repair deficiency are derived from colorectal carcinomas. Material obtained from resections is preferable to that of biopsies because resection specimens generally contain an adequate amount of tumor tissue in the event that molecular studies are desired (e.g., *BRAF*, *MLH1* methylation). Most locally advanced (pT3 or greater) rectal cancers are neoadjuvantly treated with a combination of radiation and chemotherapy prior to surgical resection. Samples obtained from these resection specimens may yield suboptimal amounts of tumor due to a therapeutic effect. Small amounts of residual tumor are often insufficient for molecular studies, and rare tumor cells floating in mucin pools are difficult to evaluate by immunohistochemistry. Notably, diminished MSH6 immunostaining occurs in approximately 25% of microsatellite stable rectal cancers that are preoperatively treated with chemoradiation, and loss of staining in more than 90% of the tumor cells is not infrequent.[22] For these reasons, preoperative biopsy samples are preferable to neoadjuvantly treated rectal cancers when performing ancillary studies.

## Assessment of Colorectal Adenomas for Lynch Syndrome

The adenomatous polyp is the precursor for colorectal cancers in Lynch syndrome, and thus, clinicians may request that DNA mismatch repair deficiency testing be performed on adenomas from patients with a suspected heritable syndrome. MSI in sporadic adenomas is extremely uncommon, so detection of MSI in an adenoma is a very strong evidence for Lynch syndrome. However, most adenomas that develop in patients with Lynch syndrome are microsatellite stable and only develop MSI late in their evolution. The likelihood of detecting MSI in adenomas from patients with Lynch syndrome increases with polyp size and progressive degrees of dysplasia.[23–25] Lynch syndrome–associated adenomas larger than 8 mm are significantly more likely to show mismatch repair deficiency than smaller polyps, although MSI may occur in some very small polyps, including those only 2 mm in size.[25,26] In summary, MSI in an adenoma is very strong evidence for Lynch syndrome, but a lack of MSI in an adenoma is not a reliable criterion for excluding Lynch syndrome. Adenomas are very common in the general population, and thus, a universal screening program that employed MSI testing on adenomas to identify Lynch syndrome patients is unlikely to be cost effective. It is always best to evaluate the most advanced lesion in a particular individual for possible Lynch syndrome; a cancer, if available; or the largest and most high-grade dysplastic adenoma, if cancer is not present. Testing of adenomas should be qualified by a comment indicating that a lack of MSI in an adenoma is not as reliable as the lack of MSI in a carcinoma for excluding Lynch syndrome.

## Assessment of Serrated Colorectal Polyps for Possible Lynch Syndrome

A growing body of evidence suggests that a subset of nondysplastic serrated polyps, namely, sessile serrated polyps, are precursors to sporadic microsatellite unstable cancers, as discussed in Chapters 4 and 11.[27–29] These serrated polyps are variably termed sessile serrated adenoma, sessile serrated polyp, and serrated polyp with abnormal proliferation. The most widely used name for such lesions is sessile serrated adenoma. This label has recently fallen out of favor among many gastrointestinal pathologists and their gastroenterology colleagues because the term "adenoma" is generally considered synonymous with a diagnosis of cytologic dysplasia, yet sessile serrated polyps are not dysplastic. The past decade has also shown us that the diagnosis of sessile serrated polyp is made with a fairly high degree of interobserver variability, which causes confusion in the literature.[30]

Given that the nomenclature of serrated polyps is confusing and the morphologic diagnosis is based on relatively subtle features, it would seem that separating purportedly precancerous serrated polyps from the very common and nonprecancerous hyperplastic polyp would be of great clinical importance. Early studies reported the presence of MSI and CIMP in sessile serrated polyps, thereby strengthening the perceived association between sessile serrated polyps and a subset of sporadic cancers with similar molecular changes. However, we now realize that DNA hypermethylation is much less common in serrated polyps than previously believed. MSI only occurs in regions of the polyp that show overt dysplasia or cancer, both of which are readily apparent upon histologic examination (Figure 12.6).[31] Thus, MSI and dysplasia/carcinoma in these areas are more relevant to sporadic colorectal cancer than Lynch syndrome.

Despite evidence enumerated above, as well as the fact that the typical precancerous lesion of Lynch syndrome is an adenomatous polyp, pathologists occasionally receive requests to evaluate nondysplastic serrated polyps for MSI. The rationale behind these requests is unclear. It is true that occasional serrated polyps from individuals with Lynch syndrome exhibit MSI, but this finding is quite rare given the frequency with which nondysplastic serrated polyps are encountered in routine practice.[25,26] Clinician-driven requests for evaluation of serrated polyps for DNA mismatch repair deficiency are probably due to a combination of factors, including the confusing terminology in the field, the desire to distinguish clinically relevant serrated lesions from those

**FIGURE 12.6:** A serrated polyp contains nondysplastic crypts with a serrated architecture (**left**) and a transition to low-grade dysplasia (**A**).

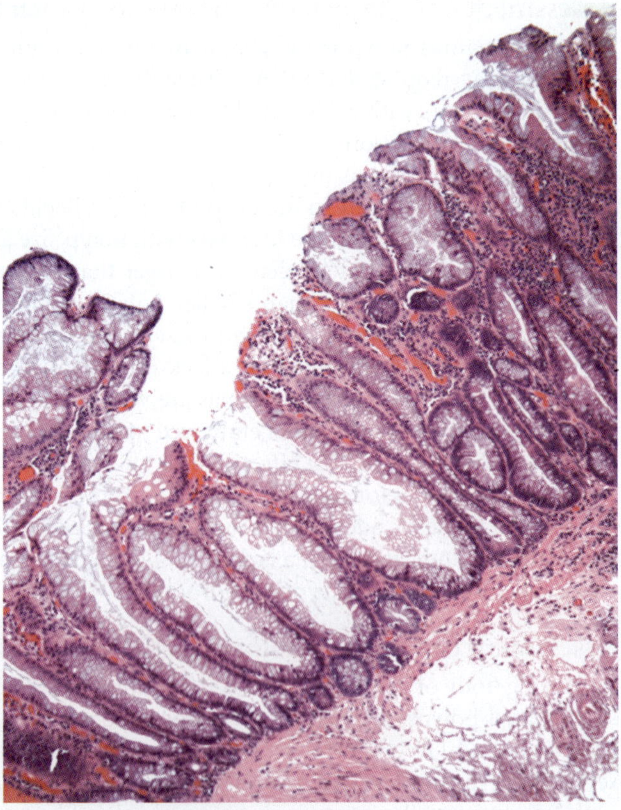

A

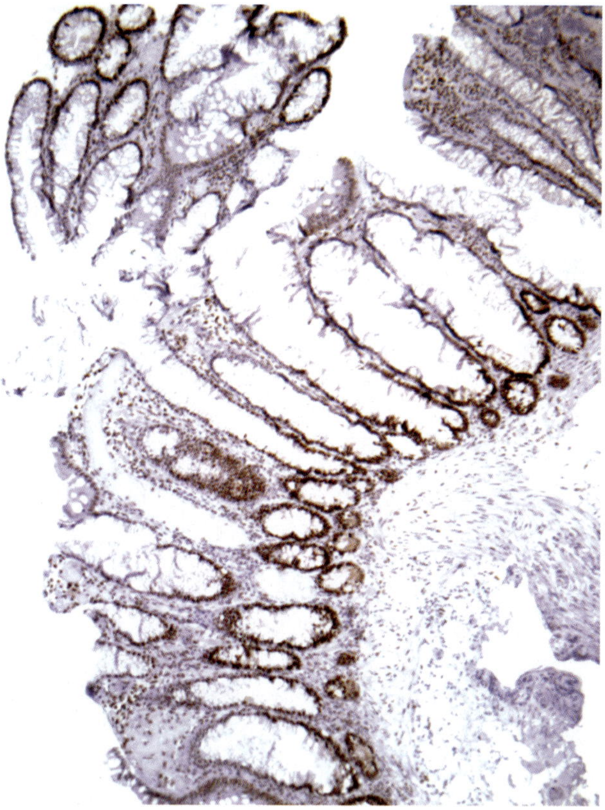

B

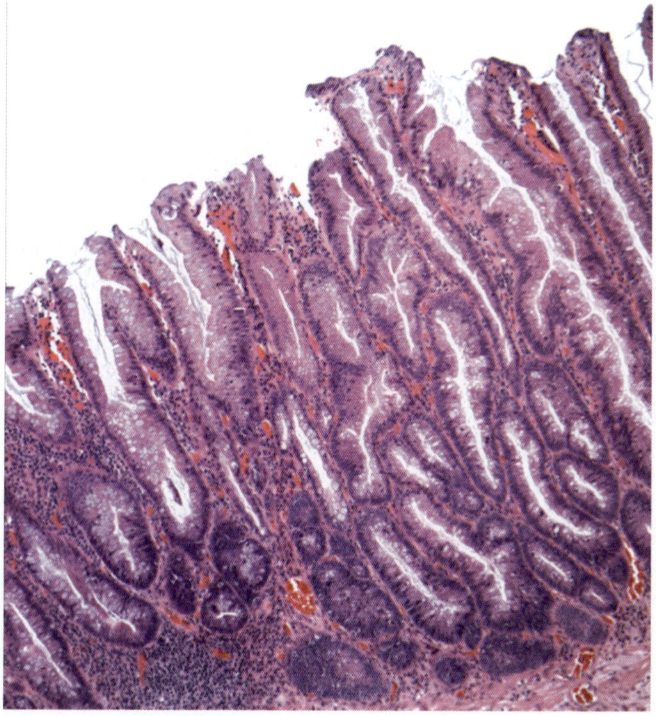

C

**FIGURE 12.6:** (*Continued*) An immunostain for MLH1 shows strong nuclear staining at the crypt bases, but less staining toward the surface in nondysplastic areas (**B**). The area of dysplasia also has a serrated appearance, although the same population of immature cells in the crypts is present at the surface (**C**).

**FIGURE 12.6:** (*Continued*) An immunostain for MLH1 shows loss of staining in areas of dysplasia and preserved internal control staining of a lymphoid follicle (**D**).

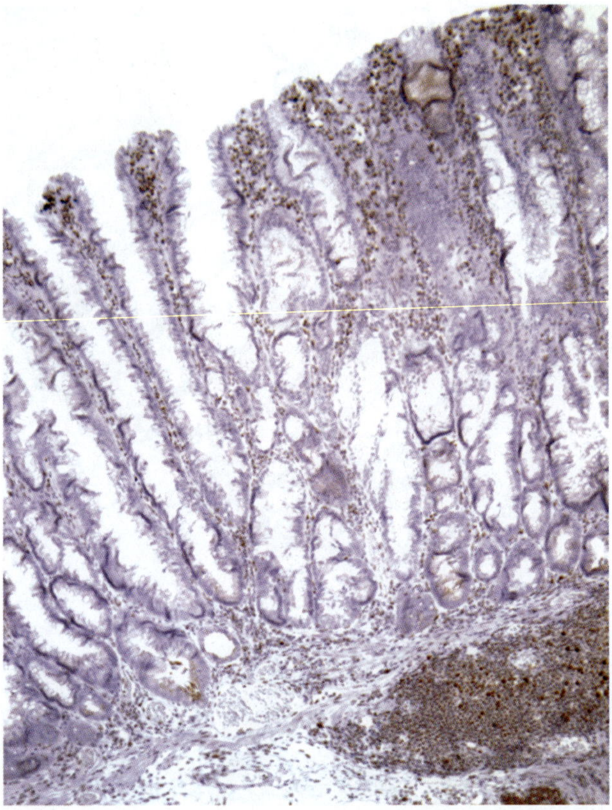

**D**

that are unlikely to progress to carcinoma, and some early mistakes in the literature regarding the molecular features and biologic potential of these lesions, as discussed above. Regardless, evaluation of serrated lesions in the workup of Lynch syndrome is not recommended.

## SUMMARY AND CONCLUSIONS

Ancillary testing of colorectal cancer is an essential part of the workup for Lynch syndrome and the determination of therapy for metastatic tumors. Immunohistochemistry for DNA mismatch repair proteins is an important component of the evaluation for heritable cancer. Not only does it provide information regarding the likelihood of a tumor being associated with Lynch syndrome, but it is also a reliable indicator of the underlying defective gene, or genes. Evaluation of *BRAF* mutational status and *MLH1* promoter methylation helps distinguish between sporadic microsatellite unstable colorectal cancers and those that are due to Lynch syndrome. Analysis is best performed on the most advanced lesion, which is usually an adenocarcinoma. Adenomas may also be evaluated, but not all adenomas from patients with Lynch syndrome exhibit MSI. In other words, a lack of MSI in an adenoma is not as reliable in excluding Lynch syndrome as is the lack of instability in a carcinoma. Immunohistochemical evaluation for DNA mismatch repair protein expression in serrated lesions may be of interest from a biologic standpoint, but does not aid the evaluation for Lynch syndrome. Finally, optimal molecular analysis of colorectal carcinomas requires selection of an appropriate block and some form of microscope-assisted dissection to enrich the sample for tumor and exclude nonneoplastic cells as much as possible. Successful evaluation of these cases is best achieved through close collaboration between surgical pathologists and personnel in the molecular laboratory.

# References

1. Umar A, Boland CR, Terdiman JP, et al. Revised Bethesda Guidelines for hereditary nonpolyposis colorectal cancer (Lynch syndrome) and microsatellite instability. *J Natl Cancer Inst* 2004;96(4):261–268.
2. Hampel H, Frankel WL, Martin E, et al. Screening for the Lynch syndrome (hereditary nonpolyposis colorectal cancer). *N Engl J Med* 2005;352(18):1851–1860.
3. Hampel H, Stephens JA, Pukkala E, et al. Cancer risk in hereditary nonpolyposis colorectal cancer syndrome: later age of onset. *Gastroenterology* 2005;129(2):415–421.
4. Jenkins MA, Hayashi S, O'Shea AM, et al. Pathology features in Bethesda guidelines predict colorectal cancer microsatellite instability: a population-based study. *Gastroenterology* 2007;133(1):48–56.
5. Boland CR, Thibodeau SN, Hamilton SR, et al. A National Cancer Institute Workshop on Microsatellite Instability for cancer detection and familial predisposition: development of international criteria for the determination of microsatellite instability in colorectal cancer. *Cancer Res* 1998;58(22):5248–5257.
6. Berg KD, Glaser CL, Thompson RE, et al. Detection of microsatellite instability by fluorescence multiplex polymerase chain reaction. *J Mol Diagn* 2000;2(1):20–28.
7. Greenson JK, Huang SC, Herron C, et al. Pathologic predictors of microsatellite instability in colorectal cancer. *Am J Surg Pathol* 2009;33(1):126–133.
8. Shia J, Klimstra DS, Nafa K, et al. Value of immunohistochemical detection of DNA mismatch repair proteins in predicting germline mutation in hereditary colorectal neoplasms. *Am J Surg Pathol* 2005;29(1):96–104.
9. Shia J. Immunohistochemistry versus microsatellite instability testing for screening colorectal cancer patients at risk for hereditary nonpolyposis colorectal cancer syndrome: part I. The utility of immunohistochemistry. *J Mol Diagn* 2008;10(4):293–300.
10. Halvarsson B, Lindblom A, Rambech E, et al. The added value of PMS2 immunostaining in the diagnosis of hereditary nonpolyposis colorectal cancer. *Fam Cancer* 2006;5(4):353–358.
11. Samowitz WS, Holden JA, Curtin K, et al. Inverse relationship between microsatellite instability and K-ras and p53 gene alterations in colon cancer. *Am J Pathol* 2001;158(4):1517–1524.
12. Geiersbach KB, Samowitz WS. Microsatellite instability and colorectal cancer. *Arch Pathol Lab Med* 2011;135(10):1269–1277.
13. Samowitz WS, Sweeney C, Herrick J, et al. Poor survival associated with the BRAF V600E mutation in microsatellite-stable colon cancers. *Cancer Res* 2005;65(14):6063–6069.
14. Senter L, Clendenning M, Sotamaa K, et al. The clinical phenotype of Lynch syndrome because of germ-line PMS2 mutations. *Gastroenterology* 2008;135(2):419–428.
15. McGivern A, Wynter CV, Whitehall VL, et al. Promoter hypermethylation frequency and BRAF mutations distinguish hereditary non-polyposis colon cancer from sporadic MSI-H colon cancer. *Fam Cancer* 2004;3(2):101–107.
16. Hitchins MP, Wong JJ, Suthers G, et al. Inheritance of a cancer-associated MLH1 germ-line epimutation. *N Engl J Med* 2007;356(7):697–705.
17. Peterson LM, Kipp BR, Halling KC, et al. Molecular characterization of endometrial cancer: a correlative study assessing microsatellite instability, MLH1 hypermethylation, DNA mismatch repair protein expression, and PTEN, PIK3CA, KRAS, and BRAF mutation analysis. *Int J Gynecol Pathol* 2012;31(3):195–205.
18. Wimmer K, Etzler J. Constitutional mismatch repair-deficiency syndrome: have we so far seen only the tip of an iceberg? *Hum Genet* 2008;124(2):105–122.
19. Zhang L. Immunohistochemistry versus microsatellite instability testing for screening colorectal cancer patients at risk for hereditary nonpolyposis colorectal cancer syndrome: part II. The utility of microsatellite instability testing. *J Mol Diagn* 2008;10(4):301–307.
20. You JF, Buhard O, Ligtenberg MJ, et al. Tumours with loss of MSH6 expression are MSI-H when screened with a pentaplex of five mononucleotide repeats. *Br J Cancer* 2010;103(12):1840–1845.
21. Hampel H, Frankel W, Panescu J, et al. Screening for Lynch syndrome (hereditary nonpolyposis colorectal cancer) among endometrial cancer patients. *Cancer Res* 2006;66(15):7810–7817.
22. Bao F, Panarelli NC, Rennert H, et al. Neoadjuvant therapy induces loss of MSH6 expression in colorectal carcinoma. *Am J Surg Pathol* 2010;34(12):1798–1804.

23. Halvarsson B, Lindblom A, Johansson L, et al. Loss of mismatch repair protein immunostaining in colorectal adenomas from patients with hereditary nonpolyposis colorectal cancer. *Mod Pathol* 2005;18(8):1095–1101.
24. Rijcken FE, Hollema H, Kleibeuker JH. Proximal adenomas in hereditary non-polyposis colorectal cancer are prone to rapid malignant transformation. *Gut* 2002;50(3):382–386.
25. Yurgelun MB, Goel A, Hornick JL, et al. Microsatellite instability and DNA mismatch repair protein deficiency in Lynch syndrome colorectal polyps. *Cancer Prev Res (Phila)* 2012;5(4):574–582.
26. Walsh MD, Buchanan DD, Pearson SA, et al. Immunohistochemical testing of conventional adenomas for loss of expression of mismatch repair proteins in Lynch syndrome mutation carriers: a case series from the Australasian site of the colon cancer family registry. *Mod Pathol* 2012;25(5):722–730.
27. O'Brien MJ, Yang S, Mack C, et al. Comparison of microsatellite instability, CpG island methylation phenotype, BRAF and KRAS status in serrated polyps and traditional adenomas indicates separate pathways to distinct colorectal carcinoma end points. *Am J Surg Pathol* 2006;30(12):1491–1501.
28. Samowitz WS, Slattery ML, Sweeney C, et al. APC mutations and other genetic and epigenetic changes in colon cancer. *Mol Cancer Res* 2007;5(2):165–170.
29. Torlakovic E, Skovlund E, Snover DC, et al. Morphologic reappraisal of serrated colorectal polyps. *Am J Surg Pathol* 2003;27(1):65–81.
30. Farris AB, Misdraji J, Srivastava A, et al. Sessile serrated adenoma: challenging discrimination from other serrated colonic polyps. *Am J Surg Pathol* 2008;32(1):30–35.
31. Sheridan TB, Fenton H, Lewin MR, et al. Sessile serrated adenomas with low- and high-grade dysplasia and early carcinomas: an immunohistochemical study of serrated lesions "caught in the act." *Am J Clin Pathol* 2006;126(4):564–571.

# MicroRNA Expression in Colonic Adenocarcinoma

# 13

Nicole C. Panarelli

MicroRNAs (miRNAs) are 18 to 25 nucleotide noncoding RNA sequences that regulate gene expression by destabilizing transcription and inhibiting translation of target messenger RNAs (mRNAs). They were discovered in *Caenorhabditis elegans* in 1993, and more than 1,000 human miRNA species have since been described (miRBase at http://www.mirbase.org).[1] MicroRNAs have been implicated in the regulation of up to 30% to 60% of human genes, including some that are involved in normal tissue development, inflammation and repair, and carcinogenesis.[2] Data from early human studies indicated that genes encoding miRNAs are often located in close proximity to cancer-associated genomic regions, such as frequently mutated genes and/or common breakpoints, suggesting that they may be altered in neoplasia. In fact, dysregulated miRNAs are detected in a variety of human malignancies. They are found in colon cancer tissue extracts, cell lines, xenografted tumors, and plasma and stool from colon cancer patients.[3–7] Increased or decreased miRNA expression in colon cancer is predictive of cancer-specific survival in some studies, and novel therapies aimed at abrogating their effects are currently under investigation. Thus, these molecules comprise a major class of potentially useful diagnostic and prognostic markers, as well as candidates for future targeted therapies. This chapter discusses current knowledge regarding the role of miRNAs in the development and progression of colonic adenocarcinoma.

## MicroRNA SYNTHESIS, TRANSLATION, AND TRANSCRIPTION

Primary miRNAs (pri-miRNAs) are transcribed in the cell nucleus by RNA polymerase II and processed into hairpin-shaped 60- to 70-nucleotide precursor miRNAs (pre-miRNA) by the Drosha enzyme complex. Pre-miRNAs are then transported to the cytoplasm and further processed by the ribonuclease (RNAse) III enzyme, Dicer, yielding an asymmetric duplex composed of one strand that is loaded into the RNA-induced silencing complex (RISC) and a second strand that is degraded (Figure 13.1).[8]

MicroRNA molecules that bind RISC can potentially bind to either the 3′- or 5′-untranslated region (UTR) of hundreds of different mRNAs by sequence complementarity. The miRNA/RISC apparatus controls gene expression at the translational level by causing bound mRNAs to prematurely dissociate from ribosomes, thereby facilitating degradation of mRNA transcripts (Figure 13.1). MicroRNAs also regulate translation in a RISC-independent fashion. They competitively inhibit mRNAs from binding other molecules that normally regulate protein synthesis, processing, and export.[9] This process is referred to as "decoy activity" and prevents physiologic interactions between translational cofactors and mRNA transcripts, resulting in abnormally increased or decreased levels of target gene products.[10]

MicroRNA-driven transcriptional regulation also occurs, although its mechanisms are less understood. Some data suggest that miRNAs play a role in epigenetic gene silencing. MicroRNA-dependent methylation of target genes can decrease mRNA transcripts in plants that lack Dicer

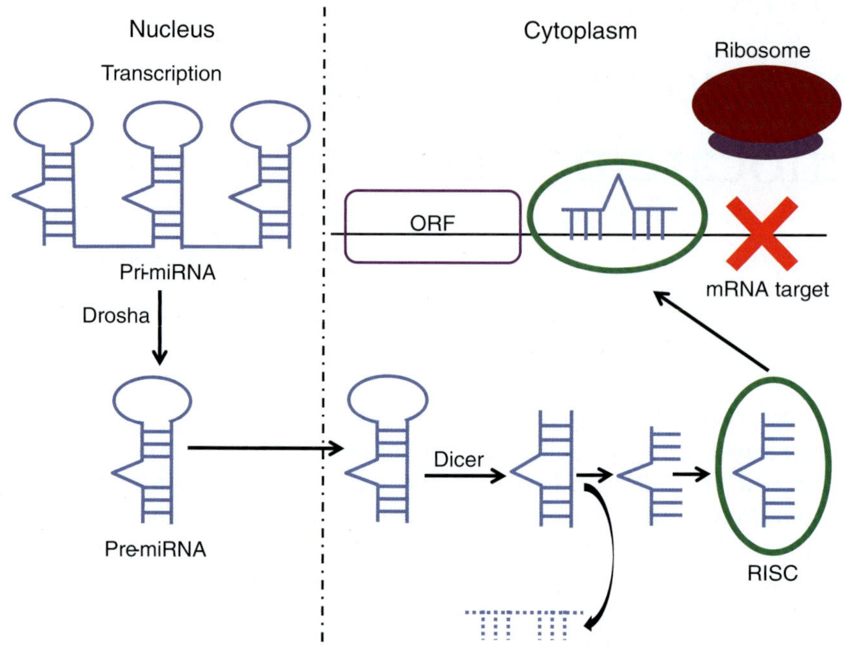


FIGURE 13.1: Primary microRNAs (pri-miRNAs) are transcribed as multimers composed of several hairpin loop structures with imperfect base pairing. These multimers are subsequently cleaved by the Drosha enzyme complex into single hairpin loops and exported to the cytoplasm. The Dicer enzyme complex processes the transcripts into asymmetric duplexes. One strand of nucleic acids is degraded and the other is loaded into the RNA-induced silencing complex (RISC), which represents the functional unit of miRNA-driven translation regulation. Each miRNA–RISC complex can bind to several different mRNA targets by sequence complementarity, thereby preventing ribosomal interaction with the open reading frame (ORF).

activity, and some miRNAs promote epigenetic methylation of cell cycle genes in mammalian cell lines.[11] MicroRNAs also bind directly to DNA within promoter regions, thereby blocking transcription.[12]

Early investigations identified up to 50 miRNA species that were differentially expressed in colonic adenocarcinoma compared to nonneoplastic colonic tissue (Table 13.1).[13,14] Overall, data from several studies indicate that colon cancers commonly show upregulation of miR-31, miR-96, miR-133b, miR-135b, and miR-183.[15] On the other hand, marked downregulation of some species, such as miR-143 and miR-145, suggests that some miRNAs act as tumor suppressors in the colon.[16] The importance of these and additional miRNAs in *in vitro* and *in vivo* studies is discussed below.

## ROLES OF MicroRNAs IN CARCINOGENIC PATHWAYS

Critical genetic and epigenetic events promote the pathogenesis of sporadic and inherited colon cancers. Genetic mutations and alterations in chromatin structure lead to abnormal protein production and dysregulation of cell signaling pathways related to differentiation, proliferation, and survival. MicroRNAs interact with these intracellular mechanisms and promote cancer development through either oncogenic or tumor suppressor effects (Table 13.2).

### APC/β-Catenin/Wnt Signaling

Most colonic adenocarcinomas are derived from preexisting adenomas that progress *via* chromosomal instability, aneuploidy, and loss of heterozygosity.[17] Approximately 80% of sporadic tumors harbor molecular abnormalities in adenomatous polyposis coli (*APC*) or other elements

**Table 13.1** Summary of the Literature Regarding Dysregulation of MicroRNAs in Colon Cancer

| Study | Most Significantly Overexpressed miRNAs in Colorectal Cancer | Most Significantly Underexpressed miRNAs in Colorectal Cancer |
|---|---|---|
| Bandres et al.[15] | miR-31, miR-96, miR-133b, miR-135b, miR-183 | miR-145 |
| Guo et al.[28] | miR-93, miR-92, miR-520h, miR-508, miR-505, miR-449, miR-429, miR-384, miR-373, miR-34c, miR-326, miR-25, miR-224, miR-210, miR-200a, miR-19b, miR-19a, miR-18a, miR-183, miR-182, miR-181b, miR-181a, miR-181c, miR-17-5p, miR-148a, miR-141, miR-130b, miR-128a, miR-106b, miR-106a, miR-let-7d | miR-96, miR-485-5p, miR-422b, miR-342, miR-214, miR-199a, miR-195, miR-150, miR-145, miR-143, miR-133a, miR-126, miR-125b, miR-100 |
| Michael et al.[16] | | miR-143, miR-145 |
| Sarver et al.[45] | miR-135b, miR-96, miR-182, miR-182*, miR-183 | miR-1, miR-133a, miR-30a-3p, miR-30a-5p, miR-20b, miR-363 |
| Schepeler et al.[39] | miR-20a, miR-510, miR-92, miR-513 | miR-145, miR-455, miR-484, miR-101 |
| Schetter et al.[34] | miR-20a, miR-21, miR-106a, miR-181b, miR-203 | |
| Slaby et al.[33] | miR-31, miR-21 | miR-145, miR-143 |
| Volinia et al.[7] | miR-24-1, miR-29b-2, miR-20a, miR-10a, mir-32, miR-203, miR-106a, miR-17-5p, miR-30c, miR-223, miR-126*, miR-128b, miR-21, miR-24-2, miR-99b, miR-155, miR-213, miR-150, miR-107, miR-191, miR-221 | miR-9-3 |
| Wang et al.[14] | miR-106b, miR-135b, miR-18a, miR-18b, miR-196b, miR-19a, miR-224, miR335, miR-424, miR-20a*, miR-301b, miR-734a | miR-378, miR-378* |
| Xi et al.[40] | miR-15b, miR-181b, miR-191, miR-200c | |

of this pathway that promote constitutive activation of Wnt-mediated signaling.[18] In the absence of functional APC, Wnt signaling leads to accumulation of β-catenin in the cytoplasm, which is translocated to the nucleus where it facilitates transcription of protooncogenes, such as *CMYC* and *cyclin D1*.[18] Biallelic *APC* inactivation usually results from mutations, but may also occur due to downregulation by miRNAs. For example, both miR-135a and miR-135b are complementary

**Table 13.2 Regulatory MicroRNA Targets and Function in Colon Cancer**

| Regulatory miRNA | Status in Colon Cancer | Regulatory Function | Net Effect |
|---|---|---|---|
| miR-135a, b | Increased | Inhibits APC translation | Promotes Wnt signaling |
| miR-143 | Decreased | Inhibits *KRAS* translation | Decreased response to EGFR-targeted therapy |
| miR-126 | Decreased | Suppresses p85B regulatory subunit of *PI3K* | Stimulates cell proliferation through the AKT pathway |
| miR-21 | Increased | Inhibits *PDCD4* translation | Increases cell growth and division through TGF-β pathway |
| miR-101 | Decreased | Inhibits COX2 translation | Promotes tumor angiogenesis |
| miR-155 | Increased | Inhibits *MLH1*, *MSH2*, and *MSH6* transcription | Inhibits DNA mismatch repair mechanisms |

to the 3' UTR of *APC* mRNA. Colon cancers with high miR-135a and miR-135b levels also contain fewer APC mRNA transcripts, suggesting that miR-135a and miR-135b regulate Wnt signaling by promoting decay of APC mRNA.[19]

## Ras/Raf/MAPK and PI3K/AKT/mTOR Pathways

Epidermal growth factor receptor (EGFR) is a cell surface tyrosine kinase receptor that is overexpressed in a subset of colonic adenocarcinomas.[20] Increased expression usually results from *EGFR* amplification, but can reflect other poorly characterized alterations. Activation of EGFR-mediated signaling promotes carcinogenesis and cancer progression by stimulating the KRAS/BRAF/MAPK and PI3K/AKT/mTOR pathways, both of which are modulated by miRNAs.[21]

*KRAS* mutations are found in 30% to 40% of colon cancers, and their detection is extremely important from a clinical standpoint. The presence of *KRAS* mutations is strongly predictive of resistance to EGFR inhibitors, such as cetuximab and similar agents.[22] Several miRNA species show different expression levels among *KRAS* wild-type tumors compared to *KRAS*-mutated colon cancers. Colon cancers with *KRAS* mutations typically show increased miR-92a, miR-127-3p, and miR-486-5p and decreased miR-378, miR-143, miR-let-7a, and miR-18a.[23] MicroRNA-92a is a member of the miR-17-92 cluster that promotes cancer cell proliferation, suppresses apoptosis, and facilitates angiogenesis. *KRAS* is also a likely target for miR-143. Transfection of colon cancer cell lines with anti–miR-143 oligonucleotides increases *KRAS* transcript levels, whereas *KRAS* transcripts decrease in cell lines transfected with pre–miR-143.[4,24] These findings suggest that miR-143 downregulation promotes cancer cell growth by disinhibiting *KRAS* translation. Similarly, transfection of both miR-let-7a and miR-18a into colon cancer cell lines reduces *KRAS* expression in a dose-dependent fashion.[25,26]

Phosphatidylinositol 3-kinase mutations are detected in 14% to 18% of colon cancers and predict shorter survival with a diminished response to EGFR-targeted therapy.[27] This gene encodes a protein that activates AKT, a protein kinase involved in the PI3K/AKT/mTOR pathway that triggers downstream responses related to cell growth, proliferation, and cell motility. Restoration of miR-126, a species that is minimally expressed, or absent, in colon cancer, impedes cancer cell growth by targeting the p85B subunit of PI3K.[28] Thus, loss of miR-126 probably removes a critical checkpoint in the PI3K/AKT/mTOR pathway and facilitates tumor growth.

### Cyclooxygenase-2

Cyclooxygenase-2 (COX-2) is a proangiogenic factor that is overexpressed in 40% of colonic adenomas and 80% of colonic adenocarcinomas. Its expression is associated with decreased apoptosis, increased tumor cell invasion, and development of metastases.[29] Data from mouse models and human colon cancer cell line studies indicate that miR-101 is a key regulator of COX-2 expression. This miRNA is complementary to the 3' UTR of *COX-2* transcripts and downregulates *COX-2* expression through mRNA decay.[30,31] There is an inverse relationship between miR-101 expression and COX-2 levels in both primary colon cancers and metastatic tumor deposits in the liver.[30]

## THE PROGNOSTIC VALUE OF MicroRNAs IN COLONIC ADENOCARCINOMA

Some miRNAs are dysregulated in a wide variety of human malignancies and their expression correlates with clinical and pathologic parameters. For example, miR-21 is aberrantly expressed in colon cancer, and its high expression predicts shorter disease-free survival among patients with stage II disease.[7,32] Increased miR-21 expression in the primary tumor is also associated with regional lymph node and distant metastases.[33,34] Although its specific targets are not known, miR-21 likely regulates inflammatory mediators and cell cycle regulators. High miR-21 expression is associated with increased levels of interleukin (IL)-6, a proinflammatory cytokine, and lower levels of IL-12a, which facilitates T cell–mediated host responses to tumors.[34] Presumably, IL-6 upregulates miR-21 expression, which then negatively regulates IL-12a, leading to decreased immune-mediated host defense to cancer. Programmed cell death 4 (*PDCD4*) is a recently described tumor suppressor gene with a 3'UTR that is a specific conserved target of miR-21. The protein product of this gene has proapoptotic and antiproliferative properties, and its levels inversely correlate with rising miR-21 levels in colonic adenomas and carcinomas.[35]

MicroRNA-31 is upregulated in colonic adenocarcinoma and several other solid tumors.[15,36] High miR-31 levels are identified in locally advanced primary colon cancers and are associated with high-grade histology.[15,33,37] More than 100 genes have been implicated as putative targets of miR-31. Its effects on cell migration are more readily observed in colon cancer cell lines with wild-type *p53*, suggesting that miR-31 may potentiate carcinogenesis *via* dysregulation of p53-mediated cell proliferation (miRBASE, http://microrna.sanger.ac.uk).[38] MicroRNA-31 also plays a role in inflammatory bowel disease (IBD)–related neoplasia, as detailed below.

Other dysregulated miRNAs are also associated with clinical behavior and pathologic features among colon cancers. Shorter survival is observed in patients whose tumors show increased miR-320, miR-498, and miR-200c, as well as those with decreased levels of miR-106a expression.[39–41] MicroRNA-137 expression is higher in colon cancer patients with regional lymph node metastases than in those with node-negative disease.[42] Differences in expression of mir-20a, miR-145, miR-181b, and miR-203 have also been reported among younger colon cancer patients compared to patients greater than 40 years of age.[43]

## MicroRNA EXPRESSION IN MICROSATELLITE INSTABILITY-HIGH CARCINOMAS

Approximately 15% of colonic adenocarcinomas show a high frequency of microsatellite instability-high (MSI-H) due to defective mismatch repair mechanisms. Sporadic MSI-H colon cancers usually result from epigenetic silencing of *MLH1*, an important mismatch repair gene, whereas patients with hereditary MSI-H cancers (i.e., Lynch syndrome) harbor germline mutations in at least one of the mismatch repair genes (e.g., *MLH1*, *MSH2*, *MSH6*, *PMS2*). Colon

**Table 13.3 MicroRNA Expression in Microsatellite Stable and Microsatellite Unstable Colorectal Cancer**

| Study | MSS Colorectal Cancers | | MSI-H Colorectal Cancers | |
|---|---|---|---|---|
| | *Overexpressed* | *Underexpressed* | *Overexpressed* | *Underexpressed* |
| Schepeler et al.[39] | miR-20a, miR-510, miR-92, miR-513 | miR-142-3p, miR-212, miR-miR-146b, miR-217 | miR-492, miR-20a, miR-432*, miR-21 | miR-145, miR-455, miR-484, miR-101 |
| Sarver et al.[45] | | miR-552, miR-592, miR-181c, miR-196b | miR-625, miR-31 | |
| Lanza et al.[44] | miR-215, miR-192, miR-191, miR-203, miR-32, miR-17, miR-25, miR-106a, miR-92-1, miR-92-2, miR-93-1, miR-20 | | miR-223, miR-155 | |
| Earle et al.[46] | miR-196a | | miR-155, miR-223, miR-31, miR-26b | |

cancers with MSI-H show characteristic features. They are often located proximal to the splenic flexure and display heterogeneous, medullary, or mucinous morphology with numerous intratumoral lymphocytes. These tumors also show miRNA alterations that are different from microsatellite stable (MSS) colon cancers (Table 13.3). Mismatch proficient tumors usually show increased miR-17-5p, miR-20, miR-25, miR-92-1, miR-92-2, miR-93-1, miR-106a miR-1, miR-133a, miR-328, and miR-9, but decreased miR-142-3p, miR-212, miR-151, and miR-144 compared to MSI-H cancers.[44,45] Indeed, high miR-142-3p, miR-212, miR-151, and miR-144 distinguish MSS cancers from those that are MSI-H with 81% specificity and 92% sensitivity.[39] Some miRNA species that are increased in MSI-H tumors likely drive oncogenesis by depressing mismatch repair mechanisms.[44,46] For example, colon cancer cell lines transfected with pre–miR-155 show decreased *MLH1*, *MSH2*, and *MSH6* transcripts.[47]

## THERAPEUTIC IMPLICATIONS

Some miRNA species are attractive therapeutic targets because they are relatively tissue specific. Data from several lines of evidence indicate that targeting miRNAs impacts tumor growth. Proliferation of colon cancer cells is inhibited by successful targeting and inactivation of miRNAs that are overexpressed, whereas reconstitution of underexpressed miRNAs diminishes tumor growth.[48,49]

Overexpressed miRNAs are potential targets for therapeutic inhibition with antisense oligonucleotides that act as competitive inhibitors. These small molecules abrogate the function of miRNAs by annealing to them, blocking their interaction with target mRNAs, and promoting their degradation (Figure 13.2A).[50] MicroRNA sponges are synthetic polynucleotides containing multiple tandem sequences that are complementary to specific miRNAs. They act as decoy transcripts to sequester miRNA–RISC complexes and prevent their binding to mRNA transcripts (Figure 13.2B).[51] MicroRNA masks complement mRNA transcripts and are used in a similar fashion. Binding of the miRNA mask to messenger transcripts prevents attachment of the miRNA–RISC, thereby inhibiting mRNA degradation (Figure 13.2C).[52] Both miRNA sponges

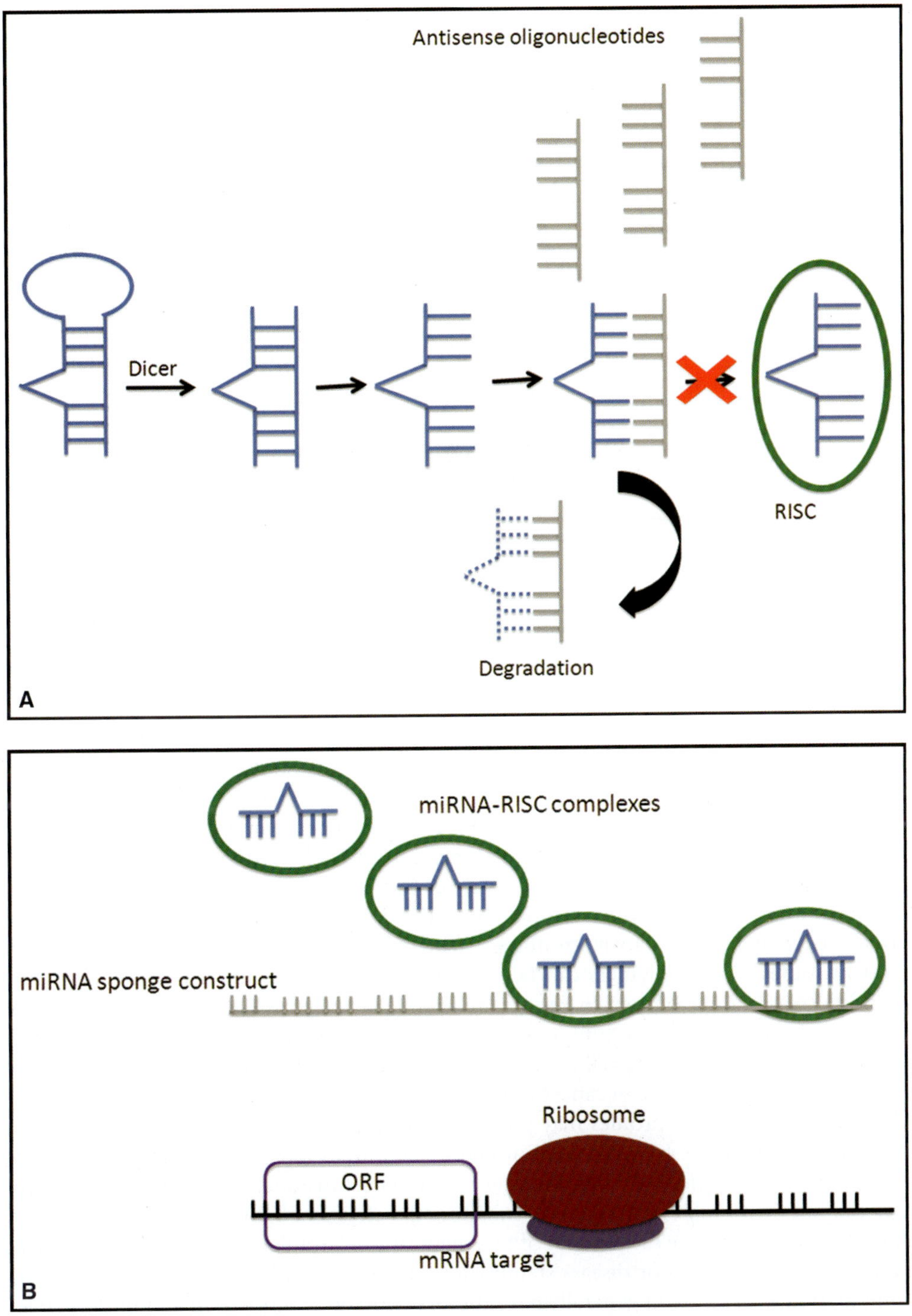


FIGURE 13.2: Therapeutic strategies targeting overexpressed miRNAs. Antisense oligonucleotides competitively inhibit miRNAs by binding them and preventing their incorporation into the RISC complex. Oligonucleotide-bound miRNAs are subsequently degraded (**A**). MicroRNA sponges consist of oligonucleotide repeats that are complementary to specific miRNAs. Binding to miRNAs permits access of ribosomes to the ORF (**B**).

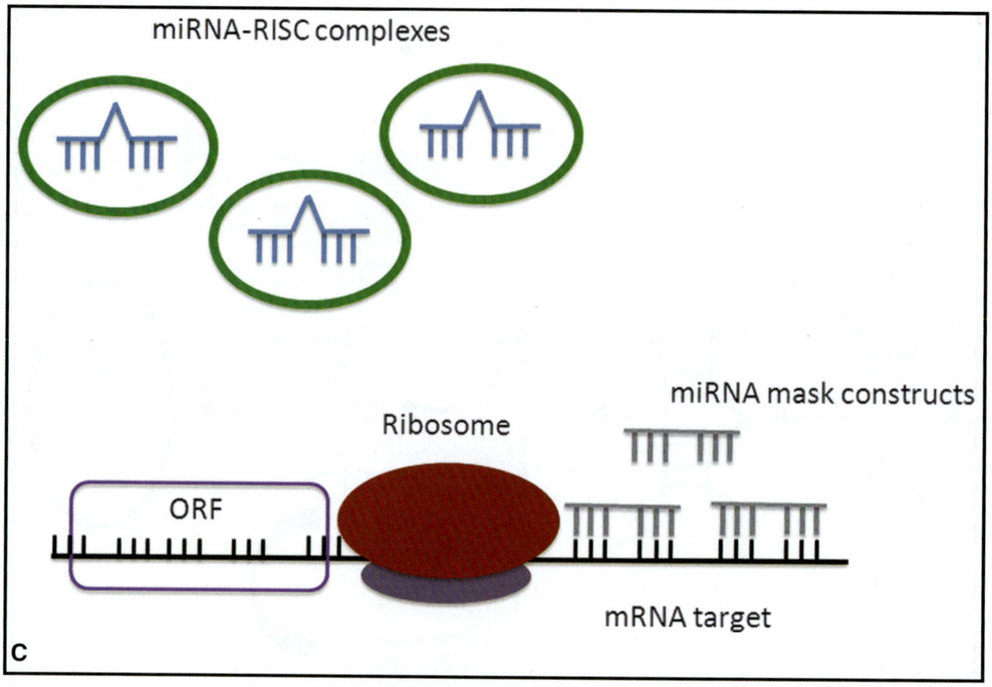


FIGURE 13.2: (*Continued*) MicroRNA mask constructs are homologous to miRNAs and bind directly to mRNA targets, thereby preventing RISC–mRNA interaction. These oligonucleotides do not interfere with ribosome–ORF interaction (**C**).

and masks have been recently developed, and their efficacy has not been tested in colon cancers cell lines.

Treatment strategies employing miRNA replacement depend on creating synthetic miRNA mimics that are modified by methylation or elongation and delivered to cancer cell lines *via* one of several techniques. Adenovirus-associated vectors that encode miRNAs can be effectively transduced into tumor cells and induce tumor cell death with minimal toxicity.[53] Polyethylenimines are branched polymers that form complexes with nucleic acids and enter cells *via* clathrin-dependent routes. These polymers can be used to deliver specific miRNAs to deficient tumor cells and decrease tumor burden in xenografted models.[54] MicroRNAs can also be mixed with liposomes to facilitate entry into tumor cells. Cationic liposomes form complexes with negatively charged miRNAs and permeate cell membranes. Delivery of miR-143 with this technique exerts substantial suppressive effects on cancer cell growth.[49]

MicroRNA expression profiles may predict chemosensitivity of colon cancers. In vitro and retrospective studies have shown correlations between miRNA levels and likelihood of therapeutic response to 5-fluorouracil among colon cancer patients. Introduction of anti–miR-31 to colon cancer cell lines with high miR-31 levels enhances the effects of 5-fluorouracil, suggesting that high miR-31 levels decrease the potency of this medication.[38] Similarly, patients who experienced remission, partial response, or disease stability after treatment with oral 5-fluorouracil alone or in combination with cisplatin generally have tumors with lower miR-let-7g and miR-181b levels than those with tumor progression.[55] Colon cancer cells with normal miR-131 levels show a better response to 5-fluourouracil than those with decreased miR-143 levels.[56] High miR-21 levels are associated with decreased survival among patients with stage II or stage III colorectal cancer who receive 5-fluorouracil.[34]

Methotrexate is an antimetabolite that is used for colon cancer treatment in some patients. Resistance to this agent is associated with decreased miR-224 levels, but increased miR-215 expression, suggesting that miRNAs could represent markers of chemosensitivity and facilitate therapy selection.[57–59]

## MicroRNAs AS MINIMALLY INVASIVE BIOMARKERS OF COLON CANCER

MicroRNAs are small enough to resist RNase activity, yet they are also relatively stable. Thus miRNAs are potentially useful targets of noninvasive disease monitoring assays, such as plasma and stool analyses.[3] Colon cancer patients have detectable cancer miRNAs in their plasma that can be used to monitor therapeutic response of the primary tumor as well as development of advanced disease. Both miR-17 and miR-92 are increased in plasma from colon cancer patients, but plasma levels fall following complete surgical resection.[4] Plasma miR-141 levels are significantly higher in patients with stage IV colon cancer compared to those with localized disease, and thus, this marker may have utility in the stage assessment of colon cancer patients.[60] MicroRNA-21 and miR-92 are detectable in stool samples from colon cancer patients at the time of diagnosis and fall to undetectable levels after tumor resection.[5] Current techniques for detecting specific plasma and stool miRNAs lack adequate sensitivity and specificity for monitoring colon cancer patients, but improved miRNA assays may play a role in the future surveillance of cancer patients.

## MicroRNAs IN INFLAMMATORY BOWEL DISEASE

A variety of miRNAs have been identified in patients with ulcerative colitis and Crohn disease, but only miR-31 is specifically associated with IBD-related neoplasia. Tissue biopsies containing uninflamed mucosa, chronic active colitis, dysplastic mucosa, and carcinoma from IBD patients show progressively increased miR-31 levels. Although miR-31 levels are higher in many cancers compared to nontumor tissues, they are generally higher in IBD-associated tumors than sporadic carcinomas.[38,61] MicroRNA-31 downregulates factor inhibiting HIF-1 (*FIH-1*), which is an angiogenesis inhibitor. Presumably, high miR-31 levels facilitate vascularization of colonic adenocarcinomas by suppressing inhibitors of angiogenesis.[61]

## SUMMARY AND CONCLUSIONS

MicroRNAs comprise a newly recognized class of molecules that can promote carcinogenesis in some situations. Specific miRNA species affect cancer development by modulating gene expression and influencing signaling pathways. Others represent potential therapeutic targets, either through restoration of silenced miRNAs or inhibition of overexpressed species. Monitoring plasma and stool miRNA levels may facilitate assessment of disease progression and screening of high-risk patients. Future investigations of miRNA dysregulation will likely enhance understanding of colon cancer pathogenesis and lead to development of miRNA-based diagnostic and therapeutic strategies.

## ACKNOWLEDGMENTS

The author thanks Debra Beneck, M.D., for her critical review of this chapter.

# References

1. Lee RC, Feinbaum RL, Ambros V. The *C. elegans* heterochronic gene lin-4 encodes small RNAs with antisense complementarity to lin-14. *Cell* 1993;75:843–854.
2. Friedman RC, Farh KK, Burge CB, et al. Most mammalian mRNAs are conserved targets of microRNAs. *Genome Res* 2009;19(1):92–105.
3. Mitchell PS, Parkin RK, Kroh EM, et al. Circulating microRNAs as stable blood-based markers for cancer detection. *Proc Natl Acad Sci U S A* 2008;105(30):10513–10518.

4. Ng EK, Chong WW, Jin H, et al. Differential expression of microRNAs in plasma of patients with colorectal cancer: a potential marker for colorectal cancer screening. *Gut* 2009;58(10):1375–1381.
5. Wu CW, Ng SS, Dong YJ, et al. Detection of miR-92a and miR-21 in stool samples as potential screening biomarkers for colorectal cancer and polyps. *Gut* 2012;61(5):739–745.
6. Kalimutho M, Di Cecilia S, Del Vecchio Blanco G, et al. Epigenetically silenced miR-34b/c as a novel faecal-based screening marker for colorectal cancer. *Br J Cancer* 2011;104(11):1770–1778.
7. Volinia S, Calin GA, Liu CG, et al. A microRNA expression signature of human solid tumors defines cancer gene targets. *Proc Natl Acad Sci U S A* 2006;103(7):2257–2261.
8. Zhang W, Dahlberg JE, Tam W. MicroRNAs in tumorigenesis: a primer. *Am J Pathol* 2007;171:728–738.
9. Eiring AM, Harb JG, Neviani P, et al. miR-328 functions as an RNA decoy to modulate hnRNP E2 regulation of mRNA translation in leukemic blasts. *Cell* 2010;140(5):652–665.
10. Beitzinger M, Meister G. Preview. MicroRNAs: from decay to decoy. *Cell* 2010;140(5):612–614.
11. Kim DH, Saetrom P, Snove O Jr, et al. MicroRNA-directed transcriptional gene silencing in mammalian cells. *Proc Natl Acad Sci U S A* 2008;105(42):16230–16235.
12. Gonzalez S, Pisano DG, Serrano M. Mechanistic principles of chromatin remodeling guided by siRNAs and miRNAs. *Cell Cycle* 2008;7(16):2601–2608.
13. Cummins JM, He Y, Leary RJ, et al. The colorectal microRNAome. *Proc Natl Acad Sci U S A* 2006;103(10):3687–3692.
14. Wang YX, Zhang XY, Zhang BF, et al. Initial study of microRNA expression of profiles of colonic cancer without lymph node metastasis. *J Dig Dis* 2010;11:50–54.
15. Bandres E, Cubedo E, Agirre X, et al. Identification by real-time PCR of 13 mature microRNAs differentially expressed in colorectal cancer and non-tumoral tissues. *Mol Cancer* 2006;5:29–39.
16. Michael MZ, O'Connor SM, van Holst Pellekaan NG, et al. Reduced accumulation of specific microRNAs in colorectal neoplasia. *Mol Cancer Res* 2003;1:882–891.
17. Hermsen M, Postma C, Baak J, et al. Colorectal adenoma to carcinoma progression follows multiple pathways of chromosomal instability. *Gastroenterology* 2002;123(4):1109–1119.
18. Fearon ER. Molecular genetics of colorectal cancer. *Annu Rev Pathol Mech Dis* 2011;6:479–507.
19. Nagel R, leSage C, Diosdado B, et al. Regulation of the adenomatous polyposis coli gene by the miR-135 family on colorectal cancer. *Cancer Res* 2008;68(14):5795–5802.
20. McKay J, Murray L, Curran S, et al. Epidermal growth factor receptor (EGFR) in colorectal tumours and lymph node metastases. *Eur J Cancer* 2002;38(17):2258–2264.
21. Krasinskas AM. EGFR signaling in colorectal carcinoma. *Pathol Res Int* 2011;2011:932932.
22. Karapetis C, Khambata-Ford S, Jonker D, et al. K-ras mutations and benefit from cetuximab in advanced colorectal cancer. *N Engl J Med* 2008;359(17):1757–1765.
23. Mosakhani N, Sarhadi VK, Borze I, et al. MicroRNA profiling differentiates colorectal cancer according to KRAS status. *Genes Chromosomes Cancer* 2012;51(1):1–9.
24. Chen X, Guo X, Zhang H, et al. Role of miR-143 in targeting KRAS in colorectal tumorigenesis. *Oncogene* 2009;28(10):1385–1392.
25. Akao Y, Nakagawa Y, Naoe T. let-7 microRNA functions as a potential growth suppressor in human colon cancer cells. *Biol Pharm Bull* 2006;29(5):903–906.
26. Tsang WP, Kwok TT. The miR-18a* microRNA functions as a potential tumor suppressor by targeting on K-Ras. *Carcinogenesis* 2009;30(6):953–959.
27. Ogino S, Nosho K, Kirkner G, et al. PIK3CA mutation is associated with poor prognosis among patients with curatively resected colon cancer. *J Clin Oncol* 2009;27(9):1477–1484.
28. Guo C, Sah FJ, Beard L, et al. The non-coding RNA, miR-126, suppresses growth of neoplastic cells by targeting phosphatidylinositol 3-kinase signaling and is frequently lost in colon cancers. *Genes Chromosomes Cancer* 2008;47(11):939–946.
29. Strillacci A, Griffoni C, Spisni E, et al. RNA interference as a key to knockdown overexpressed cyclooxygenase-2 gene in tumour cells. *Br J Cancer* 2006;94(9):1300–1310.
30. Strillacci A, Griffoni C, Sansone P, et al. MiR-101 downregulation is involved in cyclooxygenase-2 overexpression in human colon cancer cells. *Exp Cell Res* 2009;315(8):1439–1447.
31. Chakrabarty A, Tranguch S, Daikoku T, et al. MicroRNA regulation of cyclooxygenase-2 during embryo implantation. *Proc Natl Acad Sci U S A* 2007;104(38):15144–15149.
32. Nielsen BS, Jorgensen S, Fog JU, et al. High levels of microRNA-21 in the stroma of colorectal cancers predict short disease-free survival in stage II colon cancer patients. *Clin Exp Metastasis* 2011;28(1):27–38.

33. Slaby O, Svoboda M, Fabian P, et al. Altered expression of miR-21, miR-31, miR-143 and miR-145 is related to clinicopathologic features of colorectal cancer. *Oncology* 2007;72:397–402.
34. Schetter AJ, Nguyen GH, Bowman ED, et al. Association of inflammation-related and microRNA gene expression with cancer specific mortality of colon adenocarcinoma. *Clin Cancer Res* 2009;15(18): 5878–5887.
35. Waters LC, Strong SL, Ferlemann E, et al. Structure of the tandem MA-3 region of Pdcd4 protein and characterization of its interactions with eIF4A and eIF4G: molecular mechanisms of a tumor suppressor. *J Biol Chem* 2011;286(19):17270–17280.
36. Stuelten CH, Salomon DS. miR-31 in cancer: location matters. *Cell Cycle* 2010;9(23):4608–4609.
37. Wang CJ, Zhou ZG, Wang L, et al. Clinicopathological significance of microRNA-31, -143 and -145 expression in colorectal cancer. *Dis Markers* 2009;26(1):27–34.
38. Wang CJ, Stratmann J, Zhou ZG, et al. Suppression of microRNA-31 increases sensitivity to 5-FU at an early stage, and affects cell migration and invasion in HCT-116 colon cancer cells. *BMC Cancer* 2010;10:616.
39. Schepeler T, Reinert JT, Ostenfeld MS, et al. Diagnostic and prognostic microRNAs in stage II colon cancer. *Cancer Res* 2008;63(15):6416–6424.
40. Xi Y, Formentini A, Chien M, et al. Prognostic values if microRNAs in colorectal cancer. *Biomark Insights* 2006;1:113–121.
41. Diaz R, Silva J, Garcia JM, et al. Deregulated expression of miR-106a predicts survival in human colon cancer patients. *Genes Chromosomes Cancer* 2008;47(9):794–802.
42. Huang ZM, Yang J, Shen XY, et al. MicroRNA expression profile in non-cancerous colonic tissue associated with lymph node metastasis of colon cancer. *J Dig Dis* 2009;10(3):188–194.
43. Yantiss RK, Goodarzi M, Zhou XK, et al. Clinical, pathologic, and molecular features of early-onset colorectal carcinoma. *Am J Surg Pathol* 2009;33(4):572–582.
44. Lanza G, Ferracin M, Gafa R, et al. mRNA/microRNA gene expression profile in microsatellite unstable colorectal cancer. *Mol Cancer* 2007;6:54–65.
45. Sarver AL, French AJ, Borralho PM, et al. Human colon cancer profiles show differential microRNA expression depending on mismatch repair status and are characteristic of undifferentiated proliferative states. *BMC Cancer* 2009;9:401–416.
46. Earle JS, Luthra R, Romans A, et al. Association of microRNA expression with microsatellite instability status in colorectal adenocarcinoma. *J Mol Diagn* 2010;12(4):433–440.
47. Valeri N, Gasparini P, Braconi C, et al. MicroRNA-21 induces resistance to 5-fluorouracil by down-regulating human DNA MutS homolog 2 (hMSH2). *Proc Natl Acad Sci U S A* 2010;107(49):21098–21103.
48. Borralho PM, Simoes AE, Gomes SE, et al. miR-143 overexpression impairs growth of human colon carcinoma xenografts in mice with induction of apoptosis and inhibition of proliferation. *PLoS One* 2011;6(8):e23787.
49. Akao Y, Nakagawa Y, Hirata I, et al. Role of anti-oncomirs miR-143 and -145 in human colorectal tumors. *Cancer Gene Ther* 2010;17(6):398–408.
50. Krutzfeldt J, Rajewsky N, Braich R, et al. Silencing of microRNAs in vivo with "antagomirs." *Nature* 2005;438:685–689.
51. Ebert MS, Neilson JR, Sharp PA. MicroRNA sponges: competitive inhibitors of small RNAs in mammalian cells. *Nat Methods* 2007;4(9):721–726.
52. Choi WY, Giraldez AJ, Schier AF. Target protectors reveal dampening and balancing of Nodal agonist and antagonist by miR-430. *Science* 2007;318(5848):271–274.
53. Kota J, Chivukula RR, O-Donnell KA, et al. Therapeutic delivery of miR-26a inhibits cancer cell proliferation and induces tumor-specific apoptosis. *Cell* 2009;137(6):1005–1017.
54. Ibrahim AF, Weirauch U, Thomas M, et al. MicroRNA replacement therapy for miR-145 and miR-33a is efficacious in a model of colon carcinoma. *Cancer Res* 2011;71(15):5214–5224.
55. Nakajima G, Hayashi K, Xi Y, et al. Non-coding microRNAs hsa-let-7g and hsa-miR-181b are associated with chemoresponse to S-1 in colon cancer. *Cancer Genomics Proteomics* 2006;3(5):317–324.
56. Borralho PM, Kren BT, Castro RE, et al. MicroRNA-143 reduces viability and increases sensitivity to 5-fluorouracil in HCT116 human colorectal cancer cells. *FEBS J* 2009;276(22):6689–6700.
57. Morales C, Ribas M, Aiza G, et al. Genetic determinants of methotrexate responsiveness and resistance in colon cancer cells. *Oncogene* 2005;24(45):6842–6847.

58. Mencia N, Selga E, Noe V, et al. Underexpression of miR-224 in methotrexate resistant human colon cancer cells. *Biochem Pharmacol* 2011;82(11):1572–1582.
59. Song B, Wang Y, Titmus MA, et al. Molecular mechanism of chemoresistance by miR-215 in osteosarcoma and colon cancer cells. *Mol Cancer* 2010;9:96.
60. Cheng H, Zhang L, Cogdell DE, et al. Circulating plasma MiR-141 is a novel biomarker for metastatic colon cancer and predicts poor prognosis. *PLoS One* 2011;6(3):e17745.
61. Olaru AV, Selaru FM, Mori Y, et al. Dynamic changes in the expression of MicroRNA-31 during inflammatory bowel disease-associated neoplastic transformation. *Inflamm Bowel Dis* 2011;17(1):221–231.

# Noninvasive Biomarkers and Early Detection of Colorectal Cancer

# 14

Carl V. Crawford, Jr.
Rhonda K. Yantiss

The risk of colorectal cancer begins to increase after the age of 50 years and doubles with each successive decade of life. Screening and surveillance programs that decrease cancer risk are aimed at removing precancerous polyps (adenomas) and early-stage carcinomas before they develop potential to metastasize.[1] The United States Preventive Services Task Force and the American Cancer Society recommend screening of average-risk individuals by one of the following methods: colonoscopy every 10 years; flexible sigmoidoscopy, double-contrast barium enema, or virtual colonoscopy every five years with fecal occult blood test every three years; or annual fecal occult blood test.[2] Colonoscopy remains the gold standard for colorectal cancer screening, but is limited by several barriers. No more than two-thirds of eligible individuals undergo screening as recommended. Colonoscopy is uncomfortable, is expensive, requires a bowel preparation, is not without risks, and may not always detect precancerous lesions. Thus, noninvasive screening tests for colorectal cancer, such as biomarker analysis, may be advantageous in some respects. Compared to colonoscopy, noninvasive assays are easier to administer, more economical, and potentially distributable to a mass population. Positive results could, in theory, trigger colonoscopic examinations in patients who require them, but decrease the overall number of patients who undergo colonoscopy while continuing to detect early-stage disease.

As discussed in Chapter 11, colorectal cancer develops *via* three major mechanisms: chromosomal instability, microsatellite instability (MSI), and the CpG island methylator phenotype (CIMP). Advances in genomics, proteomics, and metabolomics have shed light on complex mechanisms of carcinogenesis and identified molecular alterations inherent in these pathways. Molecular changes, such as loss of heterozygosity, MSI, and DNA hypermethylation, represent potential targets of biomarker analysis. The National Cancer Institute defines a biomarker as a biologic molecule found in blood, other body fluids, and tissues that is a sign of a normal or disease state and may be used to detect disease or monitor response to therapy. The signature molecule should be differentially expressed in normal, high-risk, and tumor tissue. Its assay must provide acceptable predictive accuracy for risk with sufficient sensitivity and specificity to be clinically useful. Potential biomarkers of colorectal carcinoma are detected in stool and serum samples, reflecting cellular material shed into the gut lumen and small numbers of circulating tumor cells, respectively. The purpose of the chapter is to discuss the evolving field of noninvasive screening and surveillance methods for detection of colorectal carcinoma and, specifically, biomarkers that are currently available in the clinical setting (Table 14.1).

## FECAL OCCULT BLOOD TESTS

Several available assays evaluate stool samples for occult blood, and they vary with respect to cost, sensitivity, and specificity.[3] These include guaiac, heme-porphyrin, and immunochemical fecal occult blood tests. The premise for fecal occult blood testing is based on the notion that

Table 14.1 Commercially Available Biomarker Assays Used in Early Detection of Colorectal Carcinoma and Monitoring of Disease

| Commercial Test | Sample | Abnormality | Detection Method | Sensitivity | Specificity |
|---|---|---|---|---|---|
| Fecal occult blood | Stool | | | | |
| Guaiac | Stool | Pseudoperoxidase | Color indicator | 13%, 88%–94%[a] | 87%–93% |
| Heme-porphyrin | Stool | Porphyrins | Fluorescence | 71% | 88%–92% |
| Immunohisto-chemistry | Stool | Antigens | Immunohisto-chemistry | 94% | 96% |
| PreGen Plus | Stool | Mutations, MSI | Real-time PCR | 52% | 94% |
| Septin 9 | Plasma | Methylation | Real-time PCR | 72% | 90% |
| CEA | Plasma | Elevations | ELISA | 64% | 90% |
| ColonSentry | Blood | Elevated RNA | Quantitative real-time-PCR | 72% | 70% |

[a]Sensitivity with one test is 13%, whereas that of multiple tests is much higher. Some guaiac-based stool assays have improved sensitivity compared to others.

cancers disrupt the mucosal barrier, thereby allowing blood to ooze into the colonic lumen. Occult blood is by no means specific for colorectal cancer; diet, nonsteroidal anti-inflammatory drugs, trauma, and bleeding from the upper gastrointestinal tract all have potential to yield false-positive results. The guaiac-based assay utilizes gum guaiac from resin of the Guaiacum tree as an indicator reagent. Pseudoperoxidase present in hemoglobin converts guaiac to a blue color in a reaction catalyzed by hydrogen peroxide. Guaiac-based assays have high specificity (95%) and are inexpensive, but show low (30%) specificity and must be followed by colonic examination when they yield a positive result. The heme-porphyrin test quantifies porphyrins derived from hemoglobin present in the stool. This reaction requires reducing conditions and low pH to remove iron from nonfluorescent heme and convert it to fluorescent porphyrin that can be measured. Heme-porphyrin assays are not affected by exogenous peroxidases that can lead to false positives in a colorimetric reaction, such as the guaiac test. Their main limitations include higher cost than guaiac assays and high false-positive rates secondary to bleeding from other parts of the gastrointestinal tract. Fecal immunochemical tests for occult blood are based on antigenic recognition of intact human hemoglobin, which circumvents problems of cross-reactivity with nonhuman hemoglobin, albumin, and other blood components, as well as animal-based peroxidases. They tend to be more specific for lower gastrointestinal bleeding. Guaiac-based tests detect clinically significant lesions with a sensitivity of 7.2% compared to 23% to 48% for commercially available immunohistochemical tests when compared to colonoscopy.[4]

## GENETIC ALTERATIONS AS BIOMARKERS OF COLORECTAL CARCINOMA

### Alterations in APC/β-Catenin/Wnt Signaling

As discussed in Chapter 11, *adenomatous polyposis coli* (*APC*) is a tumor suppressor gene that interacts with β-catenin and glycogen synthase kinase-3β to regulate β-catenin signaling. Loss of APC results in cytoplasmic accumulation of β-catenin and activation of the Wingless (Wnt) pathway, leading to persistent cell proliferation (Figure 11.2). Biallelic *APC* inactivation is detected in most conventional adenomas and more than 60% of sporadic colorectal cancers. Unfortunately, evaluation of stool and serum for *APC* mutations has not yielded optimistic results. Slightly more than 50% of patients with colorectal adenomas or carcinoma have detectable *APC* mutations in their stool, but mutations are also found in 2% of healthy patients.[5]

## Mutations in *KRAS*

Approximately 30% of colorectal cancers contain oncogenic *KRAS* mutations.[6] The *RAS* gene family encodes small GTPases involved in cellular signal transduction that drive cell growth and differentiation. Mutated *KRAS* produces a constitutively activated protein that results in persistent activation of signaling, thereby promoting cell growth. Unfortunately, only 50% of tumors with mutated *KRAS* show detectable *KRAS* mutations in DNA extracted from stool samples.[7] Overall, mutations in *KRAS* are found in approximately 10% to 27% of stool samples from colorectal cancer patients and may also be detected in patients without cancer.[8] The low sensitivity and specificity of this biomarker precludes its use in clinical practice. However, *KRAS* mutational status is an important pharmacologic biomarker of response to epidermal growth factor inhibitors used in the treatment of metastatic colorectal cancer, namely, cetuximab, as discussed in Chapter 16.

## Alterations in *TP53*

*TP53* encodes a tumor suppressor protein that is responsible for angiogenesis, cell cycle progression, genomic integrity, and apoptosis. Loss of TP53 function occurs late in colorectal carcinogenesis and may be detected in large adenomas with high-grade dysplasia. Alterations in *TP53* result from loss of heterozygosity or GC to AT transitions at CpG dinucleotide hot spots along the gene.[9] Inactivating *TP53* mutations are detected in approximately one-third of colorectal cancers and are more frequent in rectal than proximal colon tumors, as well as those with poor prognostic features, such as venous and lymphovascular invasion.[10] Slightly more than 50% of stool samples from colorectal cancer patients contain *TP53*-mutated DNA.[7] Stool assays for *TP53* may prove to be prognostically useful since mutated *TP53* correlates with a better clinical outcome among patients with advanced colorectal cancer treated with cetuximab. However, it is not a suitable biomarker for colorectal screening in the general population.[11]

Mutations in *TP53* result in cellular accumulation of TP53, which may induce development of autoantibodies to this protein. Slightly more than 25% of colorectal cancer patients have abnormally elevated TP53 antibody titers, which correlate with high histologic grade and vascular invasion, as well as decreased overall and disease-free survival.[12] Autoantibody titers that disappear after colorectal cancer surgery are highly associated with curability by surgical resection, whereas persistently elevated TP53 antibody titers predict recurrent disease.[13]

## Loss of Heterozygosity

Loss of heterozygosity reflects losses of large amounts of genetic material and is characteristic of colorectal cancers with chromosomal instability. Tumor suppressor genes on 18q, such as *Deleted in Colorectal Cancer* (*DCC*) and *Deleted in Pancreatic Carcinoma, locus 4* (*DPC4*), as well as those regulating the TGF-β1 pathway often show loss of heterozygosity. Losses of *DCC* and *DPC4* reportedly show an aggressive phenotype that may warrant adjuvant chemotherapy among patients who would otherwise receive surgery alone, such as those with stage II colorectal cancer.[14,15] However, prospective data are inadequate to support widespread testing for alterations in either of these genes.[16]

## Defects in Mismatch Repair Genes and Microsatellite Instability

Deficient DNA mismatch repair protein function underlies colorectal cancers related to Lynch syndrome as well as sporadic tumors with MSI, as discussed in Chapters 11 and 12. MSI is not seen in DNA from the normal colon, but is found in more than 90% of colorectal cancers that develop in patients with Lynch syndrome as well as 15% of sporadic tumors.[17] The presence of MSI in colorectal tumor tissue may be used as a biomarker of Lynch syndrome in the appropriate clinical setting, but the utility of stool and/or serum analysis for detection of Lynch syndrome is limited. Most assays for MSI utilize big adenine tract-26 (BAT-26), a quasimonomorphic repeat of 26 deoxyadenosines localized to an intron of *MSH2*. Although MSI detection in stool samples is highly specific and sensitive for the presence of a colorectal cancer with MSI, the infrequency of this tumor subtype precludes BAT-26 stool assays from clinical utility as a general screening tool.[7] Only 6% of stool samples from colorectal cancer patients contain DNA with MSI, and most of these reflect sporadic tumors with DNA hypermethylation rather than Lynch syndrome, as described in Chapters 11 and 12.

### Human Telomerase Reverse Transcription

Telomeres are linear chromosome ends composed of hexameric repeats and associated proteins. They are essential for chromosomal integrity, but cannot be replicated by DNA polymerases in the absence of telomerase. Cells that lack telomerase activity lose telomeric DNA with each round of cell division, and shortened telomeres signal onset of cellular senescence. Insertion of *Human Telomerase Reverse Transcriptase* (*hTERT*) increases telomerase levels in cells that lack this important enzyme.[18] Increased telomerase activity occurs in approximately 90% of colorectal tumors, reflecting increased expression of *hTERT*. Serum levels of hTERT mRNA are higher in colorectal cancer patients than in healthy individuals and show high sensitivity (98%) and specificity (64%) for cancer detection.[19]

## EPIGENETIC ALTERATIONS AS BIOMARKERS OF COLORECTAL CANCER

### DNA Hypermethylation and the CpG Island Methylator Phenotype

Methylation of CpG islands in gene promoters and alterations in histone proteins are the primary mechanisms by which silencing of tumor suppressor genes occurs without mutations. Aberrant DNA methylation occurs to a limited degree in normal mucosa, but substantial hypermethylation promotes colorectal carcinogenesis in a subset of tumors, as described in Chapters 11 and 12.[20] Histone modifications that affect chromatin structure also play an important role in gene silencing and tumor suppressor modulation in colorectal cancer.[20]

Hypermethylation of specific cancer-related genes can be detected in both blood and stool extracts from patients with colorectal cancer. One commercially available plasma-based assay targets *septin 9*, which encodes a GTPase and displays frequent promoter hypermethylation in colorectal cancer.[21] Detection of methylated *septin 9* in plasma reflects the presence of colorectal cancer with a high degree of sensitivity (72%) and specificity (90%) compared to available assays for other markers.[22] Stool and serum assays for methylated genes, including *MLH1* and *N-Myc Downregulated Gene 4* (*NDRG4*), distinguish colorectal cancer patients from controls with sensitivities and specificities ranging from 53% to 72% and 89% to 100%, respectively.[22,23] Stool methylation assays also show promise as tools to detect precancerous lesions. Methylation of *MGMT*, *MLH-1*, and *CDKN2A* is associated with tubulovillous and villous adenomas, rather than tubular adenomas, and is more common among larger polyps.[24]

Other methylated genes that are less commonly detected in stool from colorectal cancer patients include *Secreted Frizzled-Related Protein 2* (*SFRP2*), *Secreted Frizzled-Related Protein 1* (*SFRP1*), *GATA4*, *GATA5*, *Hypermethylated In Cancer 1* (*HIC 1*), *Oncostatin M Receptor–β* (*OSMR*), and *Tissue Factor Pathway Inhibitor 2* (*TFPI2*). *Secreted Frizzled-Related Protein 2* is a tumor suppressor gene that normally inhibits the Wnt signaling pathway. Hypermethylation of its cysteine residues results in activation of APC/Wnt/β-catenin signaling and is found in 77%

to 90% of stool samples from colorectal cancer patients (Figure 11.2). However, it can also be found in stools from patients with adenomas, hyperplastic polyps, and ulcerative colitis, so its specificity is relatively low (54%).[25] Methylation and inactivation of transcription factors *GATA4* and *GATA5* occurs in approximately 70% to 80% of colorectal cancers and is detected in stool DNA with low sensitivity (51%), but high specificity (93%).[26] *Hypermethylated In Cancer 1* is also an aberrantly methylated tumor suppressor gene that is detected in 42% of fecal DNA samples from colorectal cancer patients as well as nearly one-third of those from patients with adenomas.[27] *Tissue Factor Pathway Inhibitor 2* inhibits factor Xa and factor IIa in the coagulation cascade and shows reasonably high sensitivity (68%) and specificity (100%) for colorectal cancer when detected in stool samples.[28] Some of these biomarkers may prove to be useful components of stool-based panel assays in the future, but do not show adequate sensitivity as isolated biomarkers.

### Loss of Imprinting

Genomic imprinting is an epigenetic method of regulating gene expression, such that certain alleles from only one parent are expressed. Imprinted alleles are silenced *via* methylation leaving only nonimprinted alleles inherited from the other parent to be transcribed. *Insulin-Like Growth Factor II* (*IGF2*) is an important imprinted gene that is overexpressed in colorectal cancer. Normal cells express only the paternal copy of *IGF2*; whereas the maternal copy is imprinted and is not transcribed. Colorectal cancers, however, show increased expression of the maternal allele due to hypomethylation. Loss of differentially methylated regions present in *IGF2*. Loss of *IGF2* imprinting is detectable in peripheral blood samples from patients with a family and personal history of colorectal cancer. Levels are approximately five times higher in patients with a family history of colorectal cancer and 22 times higher in patients with current, or prior, colorectal cancer compared to patients without these risk factors.[29]

### Alterations in MicroRNA

MicroRNAs (miRNA) are highly conserved regulatory sequences of noncoding RNA that modulate gene expression at the posttranscriptional level, as described in Chapter 13. Aberrant expression of some miRNA species results in dysregulation of gene expression, either by suppressing translation of tumor suppressor genes or promoting translation of oncogenes. Abnormally expressed miRNAs can be detected in plasma of colorectal cancer patients. For example, colorectal cancer patients have markedly elevated plasma miR-29a and miR-92a levels compared to those of healthy controls with high sensitivity (83%) and specificity (85%). These same plasma markers are also sensitive (73%) and specific (80%) for detecting advanced adenomas, as defined by large size, villous architecture, or high-grade dysplasia.[30] Stool assays for miR-21 and miR-92a distinguish patients with colorectal cancer from healthy controls with 72% sensitivity and 73% specificity and also identify patients with adenomas with 56% sensitivity.[31] Hypermethylation of miR-34b/c and miR-148a occurs in nearly 98% of primary colorectal cancers and is detectable in 75% of fecal specimens from colorectal cancer patients.[32] Expression of other species, such as miR-320 and miR-498, correlates with a strong probability of recurrence-free survival. These preliminary data suggest that miRNAs will soon emerge as an important group of biomarkers amenable to stool and blood-based assays.

## GLYCOPROTEINS AS BIOMARKERS OF COLORECTAL CARCINOMA

Glycosylation of proteins and lipids plays an important role in cell–cell and cell–substrate interactions, bacterial adhesion, membrane organization, cell immunogenicity, and protein targeting. Glycan structure depends on cell type, developmental stage, and differentiation and is altered in several types of cancer. Modification of cellular glycosylation is a phenotypic change affecting the outer aspects of glycans and leading to expression of tumor-associated carbohydrate antigens.

## Carcinoembryonic Antigen

Carcinoembryonic antigen (CEA) is a glycoprotein involved in cell adhesion that is localized to epithelial cell membranes in normal adult intestine as well as carcinomas with an intestinal phenotype. Serum CEA levels represent a useful biomarker of colorectal carcinoma, being present in more than half of colorectal cancer patients.[33] They may be particularly helpful when monitoring patients in apparent clinical remission who have elevated preoperative serum levels. However, serum CEA levels also occur in heavy smokers without colorectal carcinoma, diabetes mellitus, ulcerative colitis, pancreatitis, cirrhosis, and carcinomas of the pancreas, stomach, lung, and breast. Serum CEA levels, in conjunction with clinical evaluation, detects recurrent colorectal cancer with a sensitivity and specificity of 64% and 90%, respectively.[34]

Serial CEA measurements over time are frequently used to detect disease recurrence among patients with colorectal cancer. The American Society of Clinical Oncology recommends that serum CEA levels be obtained prior to surgical resection in order to facilitate cancer staging and subsequent management. Postoperative serum CEA levels are obtained from patients with stage II and III disease every three months for at least three years.[16] This protein is the only soluble biomarker that is approved by the Food and Drug Administration as a diagnostic serum biomarker and is the marker of choice for monitoring response of metastatic colorectal cancer to systemic therapy. Unfortunately, its relatively low sensitivity and specificity preclude its use as a screening biomarker in patients without a history of cancer.

## Carbohydrate Antigen 19-9 (CA 19-9) and Other Carbohydrate Antigens

Carbohydrate antigens (CA) are membrane-bound glycoproteins that may be increased in sera from patients with colorectal cancer. Serum CA 19-9 levels are increased in 65% of colorectal cancer patients and elevated CA 195 levels are detected in nearly 71% of colorectal cancer patients.[33] Serum levels are not affected by age, gender, alcohol consumption, or tobacco use, yet show similar sensitivity and specificity for colorectal cancer compared to CEA.[35] Although serum CA 19-9 and CA 195 levels may facilitate postoperative surveillance to detect disease recurrence, neither marker is specific for colorectal cancer. Both are far more common in pancreatic carcinomas (>90% and 100%, respectively) and frequently detected in patients with gastric cancer (42% and 50%, respectively).[33]

Sialyl Lewis X antigen is a ligand for cell adhesion molecules, such as endothelial cell leukocyte adhesion molecule-1, that usually attaches to glycans on cell surfaces and plays an important role in leukocyte tethering and rolling. Changes in its glycosylation may affect ligand binding and facilitate metastasis. Increased expression of sialyl Lewis X is associated with advanced disease, a high incidence of recurrence, and decreased survival among colorectal cancer patients.[36] Other carbohydrate antigens, including CA 50, CA 195, CA 242, CA M25, CA M26, CA M43, CA 72-4, and PA 8-15, have been examined as potential serum biomarkers for detection of colon cancer. None of these antigens are in current clinical use due to their low sensitivities and specificities, as well as their appearances in serum at different stages of disease.[37,38]

## Carcinoembryonic Gene Member 2

Carcinoembryonic gene member 2 is an immunoglobulin-like domain bound to epithelial cell membranes through a glycosyl phosphatidylinositol anchor. It is expressed on colorectal adenocarcinomas and can be detected in sera from approximately 59% of colorectal cancer patients.[39] Serum levels of this marker increase among patients with tumors of advanced stage and show overall sensitivities for cancer detection ranging from 32% to 69%.[6]

## PROTEOMICS IN DETECTION OF COLORECTAL CANCER

Emerging proteomic technologies have shown that protein expression profiles of colorectal cancer and normal colonic mucosa are clustered in separate and distinct patterns.[40] Several recently described proteins are increased in serum samples of colorectal cancer patients compared to healthy controls and, thus, represent potentially useful biomarkers. Transferrin, α–1-antitrypsin, and complement C3a desArg levels are detected in sera from colorectal cancer patients with 95% sensitivity and 91% specificity.[41] Nicotinamide *N*-methyltransferase is an enzyme that transfers one-carbon groups and participates in posttranscriptional protein modification. Proteasome activator complex subunit 3 promotes degradation of TP53, thereby limiting its accumulation, and collapsin response mediator protein-2 is a cytosolic phosphoprotein that regulates cellular differentiation. Serum levels of all three proteins show sensitivities and specificities comparable to those of CEA in detection of colorectal cancer.[37,42]

### Matrix Metalloproteinases

Matrix metalloproteinases are zinc-dependent endopeptidases that degrade extracellular matrix proteins and participate in a variety of other cellular functions. These proteins and their inhibitors play important roles in tumor invasion and metastases, and thus, it is not surprising that patients with colorectal cancer have altered serum levels of these molecules. Several matrix metalloproteinases, including matrix metalloproteinase-1, metalloproteinase-3, metalloproteinase-7, and metalloproteinase-9, as well as tissue inhibitor of metalloproteinase-1, are elevated in sera from colorectal cancer patients compared to sera of healthy subjects and degrees of elevation correlate with progressively advanced disease.[43] Elevated serum matrix metalloproteinase-1 levels among colorectal cancer patients are associated with a 51% disease-free survival, compared to 81% for low levels of this marker, and expression of this enzyme, an independent prognostic factor in colorectal cancer.[44] Serum matrix metalloproteinase-9 has a sensitivity of 79% and specificity of 70% in detection of colorectal cancer.[45]

## COMMERCIALLY AVAILABLE BIOMARKER PANELS

Several stool and serum assays improve detection of *de novo* and recurrent colorectal cancer. Most data evaluating these panels are extracted from studies involving relatively small numbers of patients and have not been independently validated in larger populations. They tend to employ combinations of various markers previously mentioned and show similar sensitivities and specificities. Two biomarker panels have recently become widely available. PreGen Plus is a commercially available stool-based assay that analyzes 21 point mutations, including three on *KRAS*, ten on *APC*, and eight on *TP53*, as well as MSI at BAT-26. It also includes a DNA integrity assay, as defined by the presence of long form, unfragmented DNA (L-DNA). Reported sensitivities of the assay for colorectal cancer and adenoma with high-grade dysplasia are 52% and 33%, compared to only 13% for fecal occult blood test, and its overall specificity is approximately 94%.[46] ColonSentry is the first commercially available blood-based assay for colorectal cancer. It comprises a panel of seven genes (*ANXA3, CLEC4D, LMNB1, PRRG4, TNFAIP6, and VN1*) identified from an original group of 196 gene expression profiles. The assay reliably detects colorectal cancer with reasonably high sensitivity (72%) and specificity (70%).[47]

## SUMMARY AND CONCLUSIONS

Colorectal cancer is a heterogeneous disease with respect to mechanisms of development, disease progression, survival, and response to chemotherapeutic agents, and thus, biomarker assays aimed at detecting colorectal carcinoma must be designed to address its complexity. The fecal occult blood tests are the least expensive biomarker assays for detection of colorectal cancer and the only biomarker tests approved by Food and Drug Administration for screening of the general population. Stool-based DNA tests generally have low positive predictive value and are currently less cost-effective than colonoscopic screening for colorectal cancer, although it is a potentially cost-effective means of limiting the number of diagnostic colonoscopies performed for cancer prevention. Most blood-based assays for single markers have low performance characteristics, but combination biomarker panels may overcome this limitation. Personalized biomarker panels aimed at detecting tumor-specific mutations, methylated genes, and proteins in blood and/or stool will likely complement, or even replace, invasive procedures in the surveillance of colorectal cancer patients and may potentially individualize treatment strategies for cancer patients in the future.

# References


1. Siegel R, Naishadham D, Jemal A. Cancer statistics, 2012. *CA Cancer J Clin* 2012;62(1):10–29.
2. Qaseem A, Denberg TD, Hopkins RH Jr, et al. Screening for colorectal cancer: a guidance statement from the American College of Physicians. *Ann Intern Med* 2012;156(5):378–386.
3. Van Dam J, Bond JH, Sivak MV Jr. Fecal occult blood screening for colorectal cancer. *Arch Intern Med* 1995;155(22):2389–2402.
4. Wong CK, Fedorak RN, Prosser CI, et al. The sensitivity and specificity of guaiac and immunochemical fecal occult blood tests for the detection of advanced colonic adenomas and cancer. *Int J Colorectal Dis* 2012;27(12):1657–1664.
5. Traverso G, Shuber A, Levin B, et al. Detection of APC mutations in fecal DNA from patients with colorectal tumors. *N Engl J Med* 2002;346(5):311–320.
6. Srivastava S, Verma M, Henson DE. Biomarkers for early detection of colon cancer. *Clin Cancer Res* 2001;7(5):1118–1126.
7. Dong SM, Traverso G, Johnson C, et al. Detecting colorectal cancer in stool with the use of multiple genetic targets. *J Natl Cancer Inst* 2001;93(11):858–865.
8. Notarnicola M, Cavallini A, Cardone R, et al. K-ras and p53 mutations in DNA extracted from colonic epithelial cells exfoliated in faeces of patients with colorectal cancer. *Dig Liver Dis* 2000;32(2): 131–136.
9. Petitjean A, Mathe E, Kato S, et al. Impact of mutant p53 functional properties on TP53 mutation patterns and tumor phenotype: lessons from recent developments in the IARC TP53 database. *Hum Mutat* 2007;28(6):622–629.
10. Iacopetta B, Russo A, Bazan V, et al. Functional categories of TP53 mutation in colorectal cancer: results of an international collaborative study. *Ann Oncol* 2006;17(5):842–847.
11. Oden-Gangloff A, Di Fiore F, Bibeau F, et al. TP53 mutations predict disease control in metastatic colorectal cancer treated with cetuximab-based chemotherapy. *Br J Cancer* 2009;100(8):1330–1335.
12. Houbiers JG, van der Burg SH, van de Watering LM, et al. Antibodies against p53 are associated with poor prognosis of colorectal cancer. *Br J Cancer* 1995;72(3):637–641.
13. Takeda A, Shimada H, Nakajima K, et al. Monitoring of p53 autoantibodies after resection of colorectal cancer: relationship to operative curability. *Eur J Surg* 2001;167(1):50–53.
14. Shibata D, Reale MA, Lavin P, et al. The DCC protein and prognosis in colorectal cancer. *N Engl J Med* 1996;335(23):1727–1732.
15. Thiagalingam S, Lengauer C, Leach FS, et al. Evaluation of candidate tumour suppressor genes on chromosome 18 in colorectal cancers. *Nat Genet* 1996;13(3):343–346.
16. Locker GY, Hamilton S, Harris J, et al. ASCO 2006 update of recommendations for the use of tumor markers in gastrointestinal cancer. *J Clin Oncol* 2006;24(33):5313–5327.
17. Davies RJ, Miller R, Coleman N. Colorectal cancer screening: prospects for molecular stool analysis. *Nat Rev Cancer* 2005;5(3):199–209.
18. Ulaner GA, Hu JF, Vu TH, et al. Telomerase activity in human development is regulated by human telomerase reverse transcriptase (hTERT) transcription and by alternate splicing of hTERT transcripts. *Cancer Res* 1998;58(18):4168–4172.

19. Lledo SM, Garcia-Granero E, Dasi F, et al. Real time quantification in plasma of human telomerase reverse transcriptase (hTERT) mRNA in patients with colorectal cancer. *Colorectal Dis* 2004;6(4):236–242.
20. Lao VV, Grady WM. Epigenetics and colorectal cancer. *Nat Rev Gastroenterol Hepatol* 2011;8(12): 686–700.
21. Grutzmann R, Molnar B, Pilarsky C, et al. Sensitive detection of colorectal cancer in peripheral blood by septin 9 DNA methylation assay. *PLoS One* 2008;3(11):e3759.
22. Newton KF, Newman W, Hill J. Review of biomarkers in colorectal cancer. *Colorectal Dis* 2012;14(1): 3–17.
23. Melotte V, Lentjes MH, van den Bosch SM, et al. N-Myc downstream-regulated gene 4 (NDRG4): a candidate tumor suppressor gene and potential biomarker for colorectal cancer. *J Natl Cancer Inst* 2009;101(13):916–927.
24. Petko Z, Ghiassi M, Shuber A, et al. Aberrantly methylated CDKN2A, MGMT, and MLH1 in colon polyps and in fecal DNA from patients with colorectal polyps. *Clin Cancer Res* 2005;11(3):1203–1209.
25. Tang D, Liu J, Wang DR, et al. Diagnostic and prognostic value of the methylation status of secreted frizzled-related protein 2 in colorectal cancer. *Clin Invest Med* 2011;34(2):E88–E95.
26. Hellebrekers DM, Lentjes MH, van den Bosch SM, et al. GATA4 and GATA5 are potential tumor suppressors and biomarkers in colorectal cancer. *Clin Cancer Res* 2009;15(12):3990–3997.
27. Lenhard K, Bommer GT, Asutay S, et al. Analysis of promoter methylation in stool: a novel method for the detection of colorectal cancer. *Clin Gastroenterol Hepatol* 2005;3(2):142–149.
28. Zhang J, Yang S, Xie Y, et al. Detection of methylated tissue factor pathway inhibitor 2 and human long DNA in fecal samples of patients with colorectal cancer in China. *Cancer Epidemiol* 2012;36(1): 73–77.
29. Cui H, Cruz-Correa M, Giardiello FM, et al. Loss of IGF2 imprinting: a potential marker of colorectal cancer risk. *Science* 2003;299(5613):1753–1755.
30. Huang Z, Huang D, Ni S, et al. Plasma microRNAs are promising novel biomarkers for early detection of colorectal cancer. *Int J Cancer* 2010;127(1):118–126.
31. Wu CW, Ng SS, Dong YJ, et al. Detection of miR-92a and miR-21 in stool samples as potential screening biomarkers for colorectal cancer and polyps. *Gut* [Controlled Clinical Trial Research Support, Non-U.S. Gov't] 2012;61(5):739–745.
32. Kalimutho M, Di Cecilia S, Del Vecchio Blanco G, et al. Epigenetically silenced miR-34b/c as a novel faecal-based screening marker for colorectal cancer. *Br J Cancer* 2011;104(11):1770–1778.
33. Kornek G, Depisch D, Temsch EM, et al. Comparative analysis of cancer-associated antigen CA-195, CA 19-9 and carcinoembryonic antigen in diagnosis, follow-up and monitoring of response to chemotherapy in patients with gastrointestinal cancer. *J Cancer Res Clin Oncol* 1991;117(5):493–496.
34. Tan E, Gouvas N, Nicholls RJ, et al. Diagnostic precision of carcinoembryonic antigen in the detection of recurrence of colorectal cancer. *Surg Oncol* 2009;18(1):15–24.
35. Verdi CJ, Ahmann FR, Schifman RB, et al. Comparative evaluation of serum CA 195 and carcinoembryonic antigen in metastatic carcinoma. *Cancer* 1993;71(11):3625–3632.
36. Nakamori S, Kameyama M, Imaoka S, et al. Increased expression of sialyl Lewis x antigen correlates with poor survival in patients with colorectal carcinoma: clinicopathological and immunohistochemical study. *Cancer Res* 1993;53(15):3632–3637.
37. Kim HJ, Yu MH, Kim H, et al. Noninvasive molecular biomarkers for the detection of colorectal cancer. *BMB Rep* 2008;41(10):685–692.
38. Carpelan-Holmstrom M, Louhimo J, Stenman UH, et al. CEA, CA 242, CA 19-9, CA 72-4 and hCGbeta in the diagnosis of recurrent colorectal cancer. *Tumour Biol* 2004;25(5–6):228–234.
39. Douard R, Le Maire V, Wind P, et al. Carcinoembryonic gene member 2 mRNA expression as a marker to detect circulating enterocytes in the blood of colorectal cancer patients. *Surgery* 2001;129(5): 587–594.
40. O'Dwyer D, Ralton LD, O'Shea A, et al. The proteomics of colorectal cancer: identification of a protein signature associated with prognosis. *PLoS One* 2011;6(11):e27718.
41. Ward DG, Suggett N, Cheng Y, et al. Identification of serum biomarkers for colon cancer by proteomic analysis. *Br J Cancer* 2006;94(12):1898–1905.
42. Wu CC, Chen HC, Chen SJ, et al. Identification of collapsin response mediator protein-2 as a potential marker of colorectal carcinoma by comparative analysis of cancer cell secretomes. *Proteomics* 2008;8(2):316–332.

43. Dragutinovic VV, Radonjic NV, Petronijevic ND, et al. Matrix metalloproteinase-2 (MMP-2) and -9 (MMP-9) in preoperative serum as independent prognostic markers in patients with colorectal cancer. *Mol Cell Biochem* 2011;355(1–2):173–178.
44. Tahara K, Mimori K, Iinuma H, et al. Serum matrix-metalloproteinase-1 is a bona fide prognostic marker for colorectal cancer. *Ann Surg Oncol* 2010;17(12):3362–3369.
45. Wilson S, Damery S, Stocken DD, et al. Serum matrix metalloproteinase 9 and colorectal neoplasia: a community-based evaluation of a potential diagnostic test. *Br J Cancer* 2012;106(8):1431–1438.
46. Imperiale TF, Ransohoff DF, Itzkowitz SH, et al. Fecal DNA versus fecal occult blood for colorectal-cancer screening in an average-risk population. *N Engl J Med* 2004;351(26):2704–2714.
47. Marshall KW, Mohr S, Khettabi FE, et al. A blood-based biomarker panel for stratifying current risk for colorectal cancer. *Int J Cancer* [Multicenter Study Research Support, Non-U.S. Gov't] 2010;126(5): 1177–1186.

SECTION

# V

# Advances in the Management of Colorectal Carcinoma

# Emerging Endoscopic Techniques in the Management of IBD-related Neoplasia

# 15

▶ Nicole C. Panarelli
▶ Ellen J. Scherl
▶ Rhonda K. Yantiss

Endoscopic examination plays a critical role in diagnosis, management, and treatment of inflammatory bowel disease. One of its most important applications in this patient group is surveillance for development of dysplasia and carcinoma. Patients with inflammatory bowel disease have an increased lifetime risk of colorectal adenocarcinoma, which is usually preceded by onset of dysplasia. Factors most strongly associated with increased cancer risk in this patient population include prolonged (>10 years) disease duration, pancolitis, family history of colorectal cancer, and concurrent primary sclerosing cholangitis.[1–3] Unfortunately, early neoplastic changes in the colonic mucosa may be difficult to identify endoscopically, and thus, enhancing techniques that improve dysplasia detection are needed. This chapter discusses emerging endoscopic techniques and their potential roles in the management of inflammatory bowel disease.

## CLASSIFICATION OF DYSPLASIA

Inflammatory bowel disease–related neoplasia is broadly classified as elevated dysplasia and flat dysplasia. Elevated lesions, or dysplasia-associated lesions or masses (DALMs), are further subclassified based on their resemblance, or lack thereof, to colonic adenomas (Figure 15.1). Adenoma-like DALMs are circumscribed lesions, similar to sporadic colorectal adenomas. Nonadenoma-like DALMs appear as plaques, strictures, or ill-defined, broad-based nodules. Flat dysplasia is much less common, accounting for less than 5% of inflammatory bowel disease–related dysplasias. It is, by definition, endoscopically inapparent and discovered by random surveillance biopsies.[4]

Both raised and flat dysplasias are histologically classified as low or high grade using criteria that parallel those applied to sporadic adenomas, as discussed in Chapter 4. Briefly, low-grade dysplasia shows crypts lined by epithelial cells with elongated, hyperchromatic, pseudostratified nuclei that do not mature at the luminal surface (Figure 15.2A). High-grade dysplasia contains cell with round, stratified nuclei that show severe atypia and contain prominent nucleoli. Most high-grade dysplasias also display architectural complexity with cribriform and interanastomosing glands (Figure 15.2B). Lesions that show some degree of cytologic atypia but do not meet criteria for low-grade dysplasia may be classified as indefinite for dysplasia. This situation is typically encountered when cytologic atypia is present in the crypts, but not the surface epithelium, or when cytologic changes resembling those of dysplasia occur in combination with active inflammation (Figure 15.3).

Accurate gross and histologic classification of inflammatory bowel disease–associated dysplasia is important because treatment recommendations vary depending on the endoscopic appearance of the lesion and severity of dysplasia (Figure 15.4). The natural history of low-grade dysplasia in inflammatory bowel disease is variable; 5% to 50% of cases are associated with cancer development.[5,6] Unifocal low-grade dysplasia in nonadenoma-like DALMs or flat mucosa may be managed with either surveillance colonoscopy or proctocolectomy. Multifocal non adenoma-like DALMS

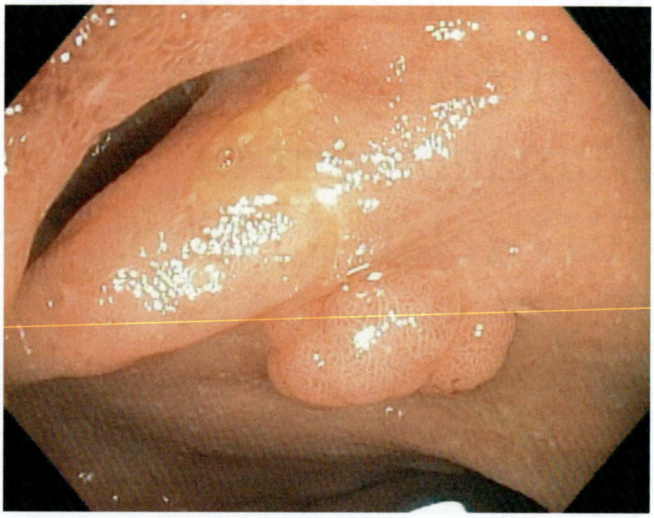

**FIGURE 15.1:** An adenoma-like DALM (*white light*) appears as a sessile polyp in the right colon. Biopsies of the surrounding nonpolypoid mucosa showed chronic colitis.

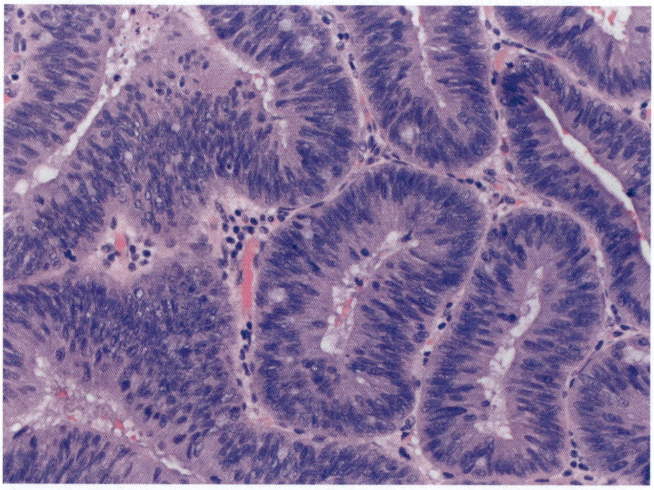

**A**

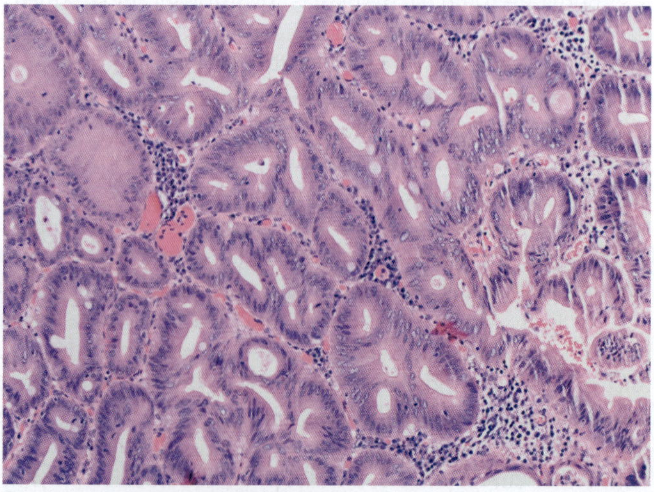

**B**

**FIGURE 15.2:** Crypts of a low-grade dysplastic lesion contain epithelial cells that lack surface maturation and contain elongated, hyperchromatic nuclei (**A**). Fused glands fill the lamina propria of a high-grade dysplastic lesion. Crypt epithelial cells lack orientation to the basement membrane and apoptotic debris is readily identified. The nuclei contain prominent nucleoli and numerous mitotic figures are present (**B**).

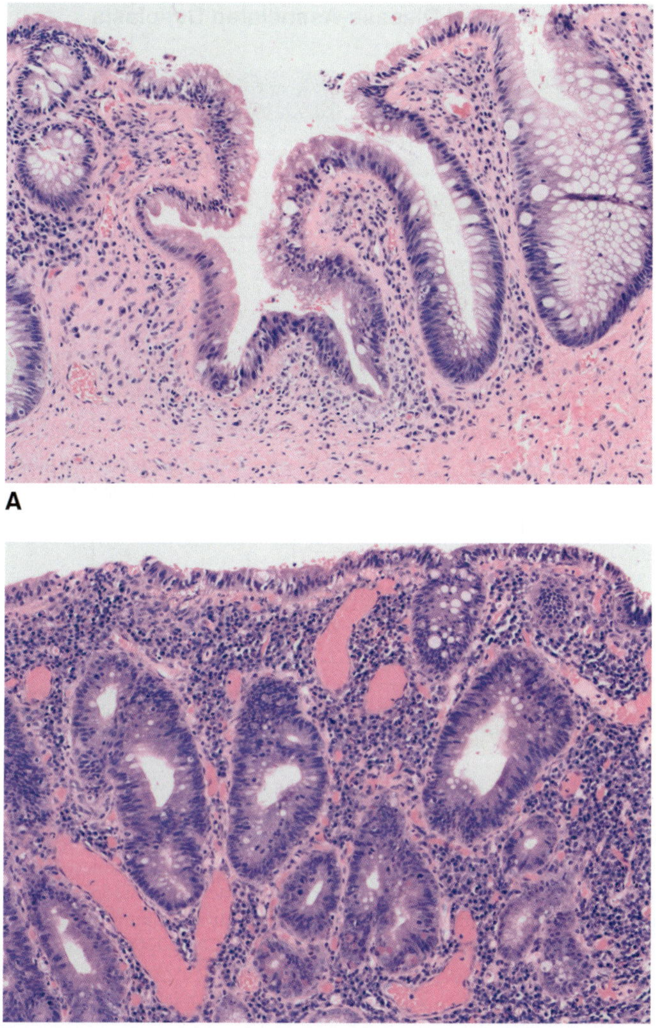

A

B

FIGURE 15.3: A diagnosis of indefinite for dysplasia may be rendered when cytologic atypia of crypt epithelium occurs in the presence of surface maturation (**A**) or when epithelial cell atypia is present in all regions of the mucosa that contain active inflammation (**B**).

and flat dysplasia are indications for colectomy owing to the high incidence of synchronous and metachronous adenocarcinoma in these situations.[2] In contrast to flat dysplasia and nonadenoma-like DALMs, adenoma-like DALMs can be managed with complete endoscopic resection, similarly to sporadic adenomas, irrespective of dysplasia grade.[7] Patients with adenoma-like DALMs are followed according to standard surveillance guidelines, provided that biopsies of the surrounding mucosa are negative for dysplasia and no dysplasia is found elsewhere in the colon.[4]

## CURRENT SURVEILLANCE GUIDELINES

Patients with ulcerative colitis undergo endoscopic surveillance at intervals that are determined based on the extent and duration of disease. Comprehensive colonoscopic examinations of the entire colon are performed at 1- to 2-year intervals. Examinations typically begin 8 to 10 years after onset of disease among patients with pancolitis or after 15 to 20 years among patients with disease limited to the distal colon. Suggested protocols call for random four-quadrant biopsies every 10 cm of colonic mucosa, producing at least 33 biopsies per procedure. Any mucosal irregularities are also sampled.[3,8] This approach is both costly and time-consuming but has not been proven to reduce the risk of carcinoma development among patients with inflammatory bowel disease.[9]

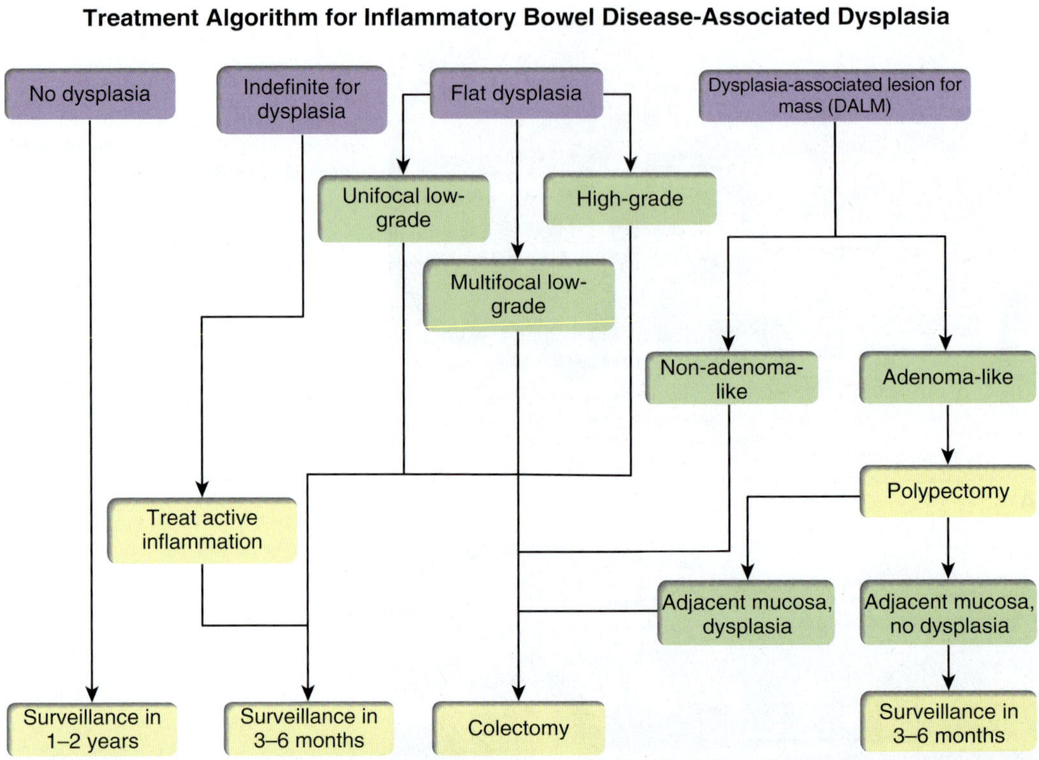


FIGURE 15.4: Patients without dysplasia may undergo surveillance colonoscopy at 1–2 years, whereas detection of dysplasia prompts more rigorous evaluation. Flat dysplasia is often treated with colectomy, particularly when it is multifocal, although some patients with flat low-grade dysplasia may undergo surveillance at a short interval (3–6 months). Adenoma-like DALMs are increasingly treated with polypectomy and continued surveillance, even if the lesion contains high-grade dysplasia. Nonadenoma-like DALMs require colectomy. Patients with biopsies interpreted to be indefinite for dysplasia should be treated for inflammation and undergo repeat examination at a short interval (3–6 months).

# ENDOSCOPIC TECHNIQUES USED IN EVALUATION OF DYSPLASIA

Surveillance of patients with inflammatory bowel disease is largely performed using white light (conventional) colonoscopy. Most colonoscopes contain magnifying lenses that enlarge white light images up to 150 times and reveal distinct patterns of surface colonic crypt openings that correlate with the presence of histologic dysplasia (Figure 15.5).[10] Unfortunately, white light fails to detect a substantial number of colitis-associated dysplasias.[2] Other endoscopic techniques have been recently developed with the hope to increase the sensitivity and specificity of endoscopic evaluation but decrease the number of biopsies required for dysplasia detection. These techniques are broadly grouped into chromoendoscopic methods and optical biopsy technologies, as discussed further below.

## Chromoendoscopy

Chromoendoscopy employs dyes, selected wavelengths of light, or digitally reconstructed images to improve identification and characterization of mucosal abnormalities. Dye-based chromoendoscopy and narrowband imaging represent the most extensively studied and widely available advanced endoscopic techniques for inflammatory bowel disease surveillance.

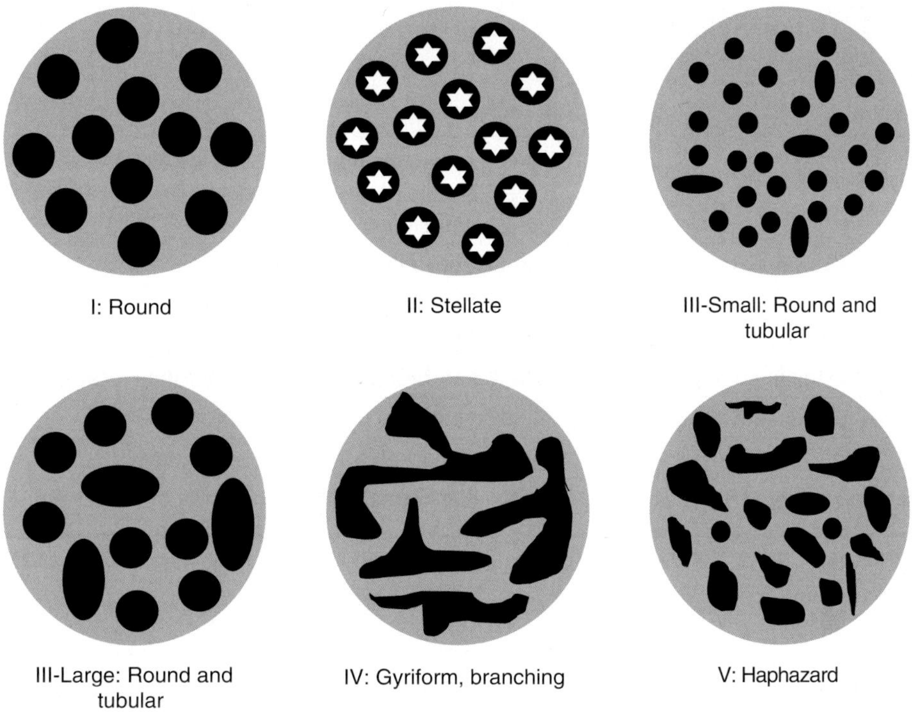


FIGURE 15.5: Crypt patterns are used to classify lesions by chromoendoscopic findings based on the Kudo classification. Normal crypts are round, similar to each other, and evenly spaced in the mucosa (*I*). Stellate, regularly distributed crypts are observed in hyperplastic polyps and regenerative mucosa (*II*). Combinations of small round and tubular crypts (*III-small*) or large round and tubular crypts (*III-large*) are typical of dysplastic lesions, whereas branched (*IV*) or haphazardly arranged crypts (*V*) are worrisome for carcinoma.[10]

## *Dye-based Chromoendoscopy*

Dye solutions, such as methylene blue and indigo carmine, enhance details of the mucosal surface. These solutions are painted or sprayed over the entire mucosal surface and preferentially absorbed by normal mucosa but spare areas of inflammation and neoplasia. The contrast unmasks subtle mucosal abnormalities and enables endoscopists to target their biopsies to dye-negative areas.[11,12] Dye-based chromoendoscopy can be used in combination with magnifying colonoscopy to distinguish reactive surface pit patterns from those suspicious for dysplasia, as illustrated in Figure 15.5.

Dye-based chromoendoscopy improves dysplasia detection by three- to sixfold compared to white light colonoscopy and only increases the procedure time by approximately 10 minutes.[11,13–21] Chromoendoscopy-targeted biopsy protocols also require fewer biopsies than standard nontargeted biopsy protocols. In fact, dysplasia can be detected at rates comparable to white light colonoscopy with far fewer biopsies.[15] However, chromoendoscopy does not entirely eliminate the need for random biopsies. Adequate coating of the mucosal surface with dye may be difficult to achieve, particularly if gastroenterologists have limited experience with the technique. Interobserver variability also limits the generalized use of stain-guided biopsies. Current recommendations for dye-based chromoendoscopy surveillance protocols advocate a combination of stain-guided and nontargeted biopsies (Table 15.1).[12] This technique has been largely replaced by other visualization methods that do not require the use of dyes.

## *Narrowband Imaging*

Narrowband imaging is a form of optical chromoendoscopy that visualizes the mucosal microvasculature by narrowing the red-green-blue bands of white light while increasing the

**Table 15.1 Surface Guidelines for Chromoendoscopy in Inflammatory Bowel Disease**

| Criterion | Definition |
|---|---|
| **S**trict patient selection | Histologically proven inflammatory bowel disease<br>At least 8 years of disease duration<br>Clinical remission |
| **U**nmask mucosal surfaces | Thorough bowel preparation<br>Remove remaining mucus, if necessary |
| **R**educe peristaltic waves | Use spasmolytic agents, if necessary |
| **F**ull-length staining of the colon | Perform panchromoendoscopy rather than local staining |
| **A**ugment detection with dyes | Employ methylene blue or indigo carmine |
| **C**rypt architectural analysis | Classify pit pattern according to the Kudo criteria[10] |
| **E**ndoscopic targeted biopsies | Biopsy all abnormal areas, particularly pit patterns III–V |

Data from Kiesslich R, Neurath MF. Chromoendoscopy: an evolving standard in surveillance for ulcerative colitis. *Inflamm Bowel Dis* 2004;10:695–696.

relative intensity of the blue band. Differences in light absorption by hemoglobin between nonneoplastic and neoplastic tissues allow analysis of capillary patterns.[22] Narrowband imaging produces a characteristically tortuous capillary pattern in dysplastic mucosa that is distinct from the honeycomb or villous capillary patterns associated with nonneoplastic mucosa (Figure 15.6).[23] The technique is used in conjunction with magnifying colonoscopy to allow simultaneous analysis of the lesional appearance, mucosal microvasculature, and pit pattern (Figure 15.7).

Narrowband imaging reliably distinguishes nondysplastic from dysplastic polyps when used for screening colonoscopy, but data regarding its utility for detecting dysplasia in inflammatory bowel disease are conflicting.[24] Some studies show similar rates of dysplasia detection among patients undergoing narrowband imaging compared to those undergoing dye-based chromoendoscopy, whereas others find dye-based chromoendoscopy to be superior to both white light colonoscopy and narrowband imaging.[25,26] Many endoscopists who are comfortable with the technique prefer narrowband imaging to dye-based chromoendoscopy because modern colonoscopes are now equipped with filters that allow one to switch easily between white light and narrowband imaging, thereby avoiding messy dye solutions that require extra catheters and are difficult to apply to targeted areas.

### *Computed Virtual Chromoendoscopy*

Computed virtual chromoendoscopy is an experimental technology utilizing digitally reconstructed images that project the mucosal appearance as if it were illuminated by selected wavelengths. Limited data indicate that computed virtual endoscopy is at least as sensitive as dye-based chromoendoscopy for identification of dysplasia in the setting of inflammatory bowel disease, but its use is not currently recommended for inflammatory bowel disease surveillance.[27]

## Optical Biopsy Technologies

Optical biopsy technologies exploit light–tissue interactions to reveal histologic tissue features *in situ*. These techniques, including confocal laser endomicroscopy, optical coherence tomography, multiphoton microscopy, and fluorescence endoscopy, may be used to direct biopsies to abnormal areas of the mucosa. No single optical biopsy method displays comprehensive

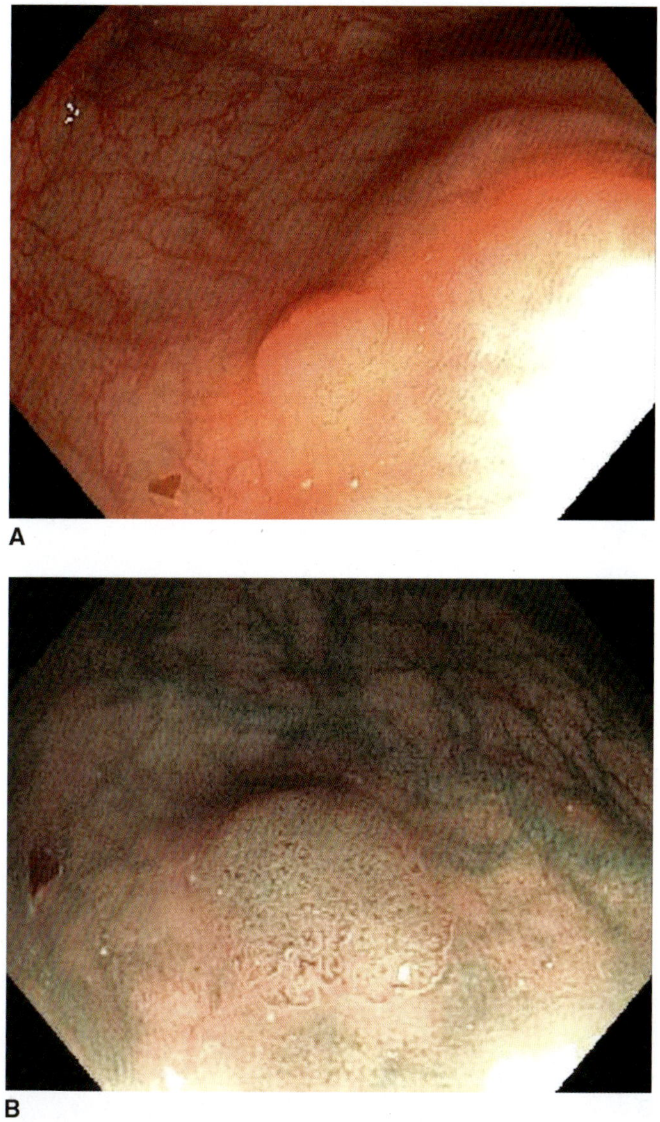

FIGURE 15.6: Narrowband imaging augments white light colonoscopy in patients with inflammatory bowel disease who undergo dysplasia surveillance. An endoscopically subtle polypoid excrescence lacks the normal vascular pattern of the colonic mucosa (**A**). Narrowband imaging enhances the appearance of the polyp and highlights an abnormal pit pattern typical of dysplasia (**B**). Better visualization of this adenoma-like DALM lesion facilitates its complete removal. (Photographs courtesy of Dr. Vinita E. Jacob, Weill Cornell Medical College, New York, NY.)

architectural and cytologic tissue characteristics, but all offer an opportunity for instantaneous evaluation of tissue substructure. Presumably, these techniques could stratify mucosal abnormalities into reactive lesions and those worrisome for dysplasia, thereby providing endoscopists with the opportunity to selectively biopsy only those abnormalities that are suspicious for neoplasms.

### *Confocal Laser Endomicroscopy*

Confocal laser endomicroscopy is the only optical biopsy technology currently used in clinical practice. Tissue illumination with blue laser light follows topical or systemic administration of

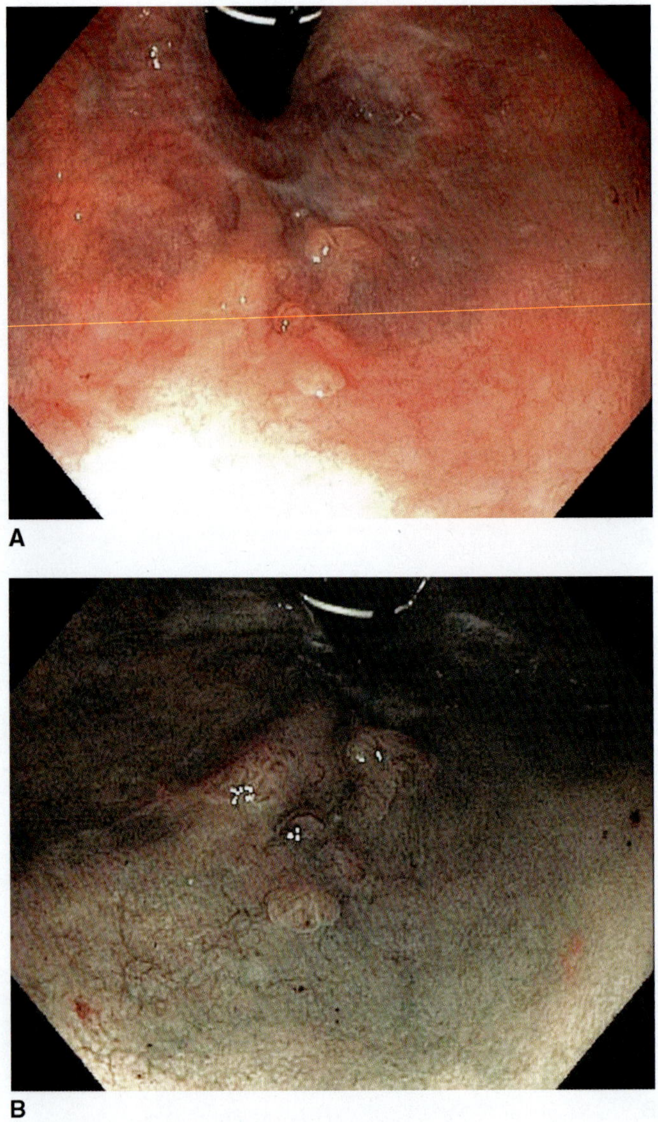

**FIGURE 15.7:** Narrowband imaging better demonstrates the extent of a nonadenoma-like DALM compared to white light endoscopy. A subtle mucosal irregularity is detected during colonoscopic examination of a patient with long-standing inflammatory bowel disease (**A**). Narrowband imaging demonstrates the fuller extent of the lesion as well as abnormal pit and vascular patterns (**B**). (Photograph courtesy of Dr. Vinita E. Jacob, Weill Cornell Medical College, New York, NY.)

a fluorescent agent, allowing visualization of cellular and subcellular structures.[28] Assessment of resultant images is based on a combination of crypt architecture, cellular composition of the crypts, and vascular pattern (Table 15.2).[29] Some systemically administered fluorescence agents, such as fluorescein sodium, allow visualization of cell types, connective tissue, and vascular architecture but do not stain nuclei. Topically applied acriflavine stains nuclei but is poorly absorbed by the cytoplasm.[30] Protocols may combine both agents in order to maximize visible tissue detail.

Limited data suggest that confocal laser endomicroscopy detects dysplasia with 98% accuracy.[31] However, it is not appropriate for examination of the entire colon because the available devices have minute fields of view (240 to 600 μm) that render comprehensive surveillance impractical. The technique is better used to characterize abnormal areas identified by other

**Table 15.2 Classification of Crypt Architecture and Microvasculature by Confocal Laser Endomicroscopy**

| Class Grouping | Vessel Architecture | Crypt Architecture |
|---|---|---|
| Normal | Honeycomb pattern of capillaries surrounding crypt openings | Round crypts of regular size and distribution<br>Homogeneous layer of surface epithelial cells, including goblet cells |
| Regenerative | Honeycomb pattern maintained<br>Increased number of capillaries | Aggregation of round crypts<br>Stellate crypts<br>Reduced goblet cells |
| Neoplastic | Dilated vessels with irregular distribution<br>Leakage of fluorescent agent | Tubular, villous, or irregular architecture<br>Loss of goblet cells |

Data from van den Broek FJ, Fockens P, van Eeden S, et al. Endoscopic tri-modal imaging for surveillance in ulcerative colitis: randomised comparison of high-resolution endoscopy and autofluorescence imaging for neoplasia detection; and evaluation of narrow-band imaging for classification of lesions. *Gut* 2008;57:1083–1089.

colonoscopic techniques. For example, the combination of chromoendoscopy followed by confocal laser endomicroscopy detects nearly five times more dysplastic lesions than white light colonoscopy while simultaneously reducing the number of biopsy specimens by half.[20] Experimental data also suggest that confocal laser endomicroscopy distinguishes endoscopically resectable dysplastic lesions from those that require surgical resection for complete removal.[32] Thus, this technique may enable gastroenterologists to identify and definitively manage adenoma-like DALMs in one session, prior to histologic assessment. Limitations of confocal laser endomicroscopy include a substantial increase in procedure length and technical constraints, such as suboptimal image quality and a high degree of interobserver variability.[33]

### *Optical Coherence Tomography*

Optical coherence tomography utilizes images formed by light reflected back from illuminated tissue and provides imaging of the colonic wall to depths of up to 3 mm.[34] The technique distinguishes adenomas from hyperplastic polyps and normal mucosa in screening colonoscopies and allows endoscopists to assess the depth of chronic inflammation in patients with inflammatory bowel disease.[35,36] Although this technique may aid subclassification of inflammatory bowel disease, the image resolution of available probes is insufficient to distinguish reactive from dysplastic changes in inflammatory bowel disease.

### *Multiphoton Microscopy*

Multiphoton microscopy relies on tissue absorption of low-energy photons to produce distinct optical signals from different tissue components. This imaging modality allows visualization of the tissue to a depth of 0.5 mm below the mucosal surface. Multiphoton microscopy may offer advantages over other optical biopsy technologies because it does not rely on absorption of exogenous contrast agents and produces higher-resolution images than confocal laser endomicroscopy and optical coherence tomography.[35] It has been used experimentally in mouse and human tissues to diagnose inflammatory disease and sporadic adenomas, but data regarding it utility for identifying inflammatory bowel disease–associated dysplasia are not yet available.[37]

### *Fluorescence Endoscopy*

Fluorescence endoscopy detects neoplasia by revealing differences in endogenous production of protoporphyrin IX, a fluorophore, between neoplastic and nonneoplastic epithelial cells.

Endoscopists use orally or locally administered 5-aminolevulinic acid to induce protoporphyrin IX production, which emits a weak autofluorescent signal in nonneoplastic epithelial cells and a much stronger signal in dysplastic lesions.[36] Early studies applying this technology in patients with ulcerative colitis show sensitivities in excess of 85% for detecting dysplastic lesions.[38] There are no available data comparing the utility of fluorescence endoscopy with other advanced endoscopic techniques for dysplasia detection in patients with inflammatory bowel disease.

## SUMMARY AND CONCLUSIONS

Most inflammatory bowel disease–related colorectal cancers are preceded by noninvasive dysplastic lesions that are amenable to endoscopic detection and, in some cases, removal. Thus, efficient and accurate detection of dysplasia is important to the subsequent management of patients with inflammatory bowel disease. Recent advances in endoscopic imaging techniques have improved endoscopic detection of inflammatory bowel disease–related dysplasia, and some of these may eventually replace white light colonoscopy. Generalized implementation of advanced endoscopic techniques is currently limited by lack of standardized criteria for evaluation, inadequate experience with these technologies in most centers, and technical shortcomings related to specific systems. Nonetheless, ongoing refinement of these methods and increased familiarity with their use promise to improve rates of dysplasia detection in inflammatory bowel disease patients while reducing the number of biopsies required for adequate surveillance.

# References

1. Friedman S, Rubin PH, Bodian C, et al. Screening and surveillance colonoscopy in chronic Crohn's colitis. *Gastroenterology* 2001;120:820–826.
2. Bernstein CN, Shanahan F, Weinstein WM. Are we telling patients the truth about surveillance colonoscopy in ulcerative colitis? *Lancet* 1994;343:71–74.
3. Itzkowitz SH, Present DH. Consensus conference: colorectal cancer screening and surveillance in inflammatory bowel disease. *Inflamm Bowel Dis* 2005;11:314–321.
4. Farraye FA, Odze RD, Eaden J, et al. AGA medical position statement on the diagnosis and management of colorectal neoplasia in inflammatory bowel disease. *Gastroenterology* 2010;138:738–745.
5. Befrits R, Ljung T, Jaramillo E, et al. Low-grade dysplasia in extensive, long-standing inflammatory bowel disease: a follow-up study. *Dis Colon Rectum* 2002;45:615–620.
6. Ullman TA, Loftus EV Jr, Kakar S, et al. The fate of low grade dysplasia in ulcerative colitis. *Am J Gastroenterol* 2002;97:922–927.
7. Odze RD, Farraye FA, Hecht JL, et al. Long-term follow-up after polypectomy treatment for adenoma-like dysplastic lesions in ulcerative colitis. *Clin Gastroenterol Hepatol* 2004;2:534–541.
8. Ullman TA. Colonoscopic surveillance in inflammatory bowel disease. *Curr Opin Gastroenterol* 2005;21:585–588.
9. Rutter MD, Saunders BP, Wilkinson KH, et al. Thirty-year analysis of a colonoscopic surveillance program for neoplasia in ulcerative colitis. *Gastroenterology* 2006;130:1030–1038.
10. Kudo S, Tamura S, Nakajima T, et al. Diagnosis of colorectal tumorous lesions by magnifying endoscopy. *Gastrointest Endosc* 1996;44:8–14.
11. Kiesslich R, Neurath MF. Chromoendoscopy in inflammatory bowel disease. *Gastroenterol Clin North Am* 2012;41:291–302.
12. Kiesslich R, Neurath MF. Chromoendoscopy: an evolving standard in surveillance for ulcerative colitis. *Inflamm Bowel Dis* 2004;10:695–696.

13. Kiesslich R, Fritsch J, Holtmann M, et al. Methylene blue-aided chromoendoscopy for the detection of intraepithelial neoplasia and colon cancer in ulcerative colitis. *Gastroenterology* 2003;124:880–888.
14. Marion JF, Waye JD, Present DH, et al. Chromoendoscopy-targeted biopsies are superior to standard colonoscopic surveillance for detecting dysplasia in inflammatory bowel disease patients: a prospective endoscopic trial. *Am J Gastroenterol* 2008;103:2342–2349.
15. Rutter MD, Saunders BP, Schofield G, et al. Pancolonic indigo carmine dye spraying for the detection of dysplasia in ulcerative colitis. *Gut* 2004;53:256–260.
16. Hlavaty T, Huorka M, Koller T, et al. Colorectal cancer screening in patients with ulcerative and Crohn's colitis with use of colonoscopy, chromoendoscopy and confocal endomicroscopy. *Eur J Gastroenterol Hepatol* 2011;23:680–689.
17. Gunther U, Kusch D, Heller F, et al. Surveillance colonoscopy in patients with inflammatory bowel disease: comparison of random biopsy vs. targeted biopsy protocols. *Int J Colorectal Dis* 2011;26:667–672.
18. Rutter M, Bernstein C, Matsumoto T, et al. Endoscopic appearance of dysplasia in ulcerative colitis and the role of staining. *Endoscopy* 2004;36:1109–1114.
19. Hurlstone DP, Sanders DS, Lobo AJ, et al. Indigo carmine-assisted high-magnification chromoscopic colonoscopy for the detection and characterisation of intraepithelial neoplasia in ulcerative colitis: a prospective evaluation. *Endoscopy* 2005;37:1186–1192.
20. Kiesslich R, Goetz M, Lammersdorf K, et al. Chromoscopy-guided endomicroscopy increases the diagnostic yield of intraepithelial neoplasia in ulcerative colitis. *Gastroenterology* 2007;132:874–882.
21. Matsumoto T, Nakamura S, Jo Y, et al. Chromoscopy might improve diagnostic accuracy in cancer surveillance for ulcerative colitis. *Am J Gastroenterol* 2003;98:1827–1833.
22. Emura F, Saito Y, Ikematsu H. Narrow-band imaging optical chromocolonoscopy: advantages and limitations. *World J Gastroenterol* 2008;14:4867–4872.
23. Esaki M, Kubokura N, Kudo T, et al. Endoscopic findings under narrow band imaging colonoscopy in ulcerative colitis. *Dig Endosc* 2011;23(suppl 1):140–142.
24. Uraoka T, Higashi R, Saito Y, et al. Impact of narrow-band imaging in screening colonoscopy. *Dig Endosc* 2010;22(suppl 1):S54–S56.
25. Pellise M, Lopez-Ceron M, Rodriguez de Miguel C, et al. Narrow-band imaging as an alternative to chromoendoscopy for the detection of dysplasia in long-standing inflammatory bowel disease: a prospective, randomized, crossover study. *Gastrointest Endosc* 2011;74:840–848.
26. van den Broek FJ, Fockens P, van Eeden S, et al. Endoscopic tri-modal imaging for surveillance in ulcerative colitis: randomised comparison of high-resolution endoscopy and autofluorescence imaging for neoplasia detection; and evaluation of narrow-band imaging for classification of lesions. *Gut* 2008;57:1083–1089.
27. Hoffman A, Kagel C, Goetz M, et al. Recognition and characterization of small colonic neoplasia with high-definition colonoscopy using i-Scan is as precise as chromoendoscopy. *Dig Liver Dis* 2010;42:45–50.
28. Salvatori F, Siciliano S, Maione F, et al. Confocal laser endomicroscopy in the study of colonic mucosa in IBD patients: a review. *Gastroenterol Res Prac* 2012;2012:525098.
29. Kiesslich R, Burg J, Vieth M, et al. Confocal laser endoscopy for diagnosing intraepithelial neoplasias and colorectal cancer in vivo. *Gastroenterology* 2004;127:706–713.
30. Neumann H, Monkemuller K, Gunther C, et al. Advanced endoscopic imaging for diagnosis of Crohn's disease. *Gastroenterol Res Prac* 2012;2012:301541.
31. Sanduleanu S, Driessen A, Gomez-Garcia E, et al. In vivo diagnosis and classification of colorectal neoplasia by chromoendoscopy-guided confocal laser endomicroscopy. *Clin Gastroenterol Hepatol* 2010;8:371–378.
32. De Palma GD, Staibano S, Siciliano S, et al. In-vivo characterization of DALM in ulcerative colitis with high-resolution probe-based confocal laser endomicroscopy. *World J Gastroenterol* 2011;17:677–680.
33. van den Broek FJ, van Es JA, van Eeden S, et al. Pilot study of probe-based confocal laser endomicroscopy during colonoscopic surveillance of patients with longstanding ulcerative colitis. *Endoscopy* 2011;43:116–122.
34. Adler DC, Zhou C, Tsai TH, et al. Three-dimensional endomicroscopy of the human colon using optical coherence tomography. *Opt Express* 2009;17:784–796.

35. Pfau PR, Sivak MV Jr, Chak A, et al. Criteria for the diagnosis of dysplasia by endoscopic optical coherence tomography. *Gastrointest Endosc* 2003;58:196–202.
36. Shen B, Zuccaro G Jr, Gramlich TL, et al. In vivo colonoscopic optical coherence tomography for transmural inflammation in inflammatory bowel disease. *Clin Gastroenterol Hepatol* 2004;2: 1080–1087.
37. Makino T, Jain M, Montrose DC, et al. Multiphoton tomographic imaging: a potential optical biopsy tool for detecting gastrointestinal inflammation and neoplasia. *Cancer Prev Res (Phila)* 2012;5: 1280–1290.
38. Messmann H, Endlicher E, Freunek G, et al. Fluorescence endoscopy for the detection of low and high grade dysplasia in ulcerative colitis using systemic or local 5-aminolaevulinic acid sensitisation. *Gut* 2003;52:1003–1007.

# Targeted Therapies for the Treatment of Advanced Colorectal Carcinoma

16

Allyson J. Ocean
Romae Palmer
Manish A. Shah

Colorectal cancer is the second most common malignancy in the United States and the third most common cancer worldwide. Approximately 143,000 individuals were diagnosed with colorectal cancer in the United States in 2012 and 51,000 died of the disease.[1] Nearly 80% of tumors are limited to the colorectum and/or regional lymph nodes at the time of diagnosis and, thus, are potentially amenable to surgical resection with a chance for cure. The 5-year relative survival rates are 58% to 97% following surgery for disease limited to the colorectum without regional lymph node metastases but drop to 30% to 70% for stage III disease, in which case lower survival rates inversely correlate with the extent of regional lymphadenopathy. Twenty percent of patients present with distant metastatic disease (stage IV) which is associated with a 10% 5-year survival rate. Long-term survival is mostly limited to patients with disease amenable to resection of metastatic deposits.[2,3] Treatment advances include the development of novel biologic therapeutic agents and their increased application to advanced tumors, as well as an increased proclivity toward surgical resection of tumor deposits in distant metastatic sites. These approaches may be used in combination to maximize survival and minimize morbidity of colorectal cancer patients. Emerging techniques have identified molecular markers of colorectal cancer that represent potential drug targets, thereby allowing physicians to tailor specific therapies and personalize patient treatment. The purpose of this chapter is to provide information regarding important treatment aspects in colorectal cancer with a focus on the most recent advances in chemotherapy, particularly targeted therapies.

## CYTOTOXIC THERAPIES FOR MANAGEMENT OF COLORECTAL CANCER

The Food and Drug Administration has approved nine drugs for the treatment of colorectal cancer. Four of these are cytotoxic chemotherapy agents: 5-fluorouracil (5-FU), oxaliplatin, irinotecan, and capecitabine. Bevacizumab, cetuximab, panitumumab, and ziv-aflibercept are approved for treatment of advanced colorectal cancer when used in combination with conventional chemotherapy, whereas cetuximab, panitumumab, and regorafenib are approved as single agents in the treatment of this disease.

### 5-Fluorouracil

The pyrimidine analog 5-FU is an antimetabolite that works *via* noncompetitive inhibition of thymidylate synthase. Folinic acid (leucovorin) is usually given in combination with 5-FU to enhance its cytotoxicity by increasing the formation of ternary complexes with thymidylate synthase.[4] The specific metabolites of fluorouridine triphosphate and fluorodeoxyuridine monophosphate are incorporated into RNA and DNA, respectively, through ribosylation and phosphorylation. Five-fluorouracil is an S phase–specific drug that induces cell cycle arrest and apoptosis that is administered as a continuous infusion.[5] It is usually administered in combination with other cytotoxic chemotherapy, such as oxaliplatin (i.e., 5-FU, leucovorin, and oxaliplatin [FOLFOX] regimen) or irinotecan (i.e., 5-FU, leucovorin, and irinotecan [FOLFIRI] regimen), although it may also be administered as a single intravenous agent or directly infused into the liver or peritoneal cavity.

## Oxaliplatin

Oxaliplatin is a third-generation platinum analog that covalently binds DNA and kills tumor cells in all stages of the cell cycle. This agent binds DNA through intra- and interstrand cross-links that inhibit DNA synthesis and functionality. Platinum analogs also bind to both cytoplasmic and nuclear proteins, thereby enhancing their cytotoxic effects. The major route of platinum elimination is renal excretion, and thus, clearance correlates with glomerular filtration rate. Peripheral neuropathy is a major toxicity of oxaliplatin and manifests as an acute and/or chronic injury. Acute neurologic toxicity is reversible and often triggered by exposure to cold temperatures. It presents as transient paresthesia, dysesthesia, or hypoesthesia in the hands, feet, perioral skin, or laryngopharyngeal space. Chronic neurologic toxicity develops after cumulative doses and manifests as persistent, sometimes irreversible, neuropathy and/or deficits in proprioception that interfere with activities of daily living.

Oxaliplatin was initially used as a component of second-line therapy.[6] However, emerging data suggest that the combination of oxaliplatin and 5-FU is superior to 5-FU and leucovorin with respect to tumor response rate, progression-free survival, and overall survival as a first-line therapy for advanced colorectal cancers and metastatic disease.[7,8] Oxaliplatin is inactive as a single agent and should be administered only in combination with other chemotherapeutic agents, such as 5-FU or irinotecan. Either combination may be administered with bevacizumab or epidermal growth factor inhibitors.

## Irinotecan

Irinotecan is a derivative of camptothecin that is isolated from the *Camptotheca acuminate* tree. It is a topoisomerase I inhibitor and S phase–specific agent that binds to the topoisomerase I–DNA complex. Irinotecan is the water-soluble precursor of the lipophilic metabolite SN-38, which is approximately 1,000 times more potent than irinotecan as an inhibitor of topoisomerase I. Irinotecan is active as monotherapy for patients with advanced colorectal carcinoma, although it is more effective in combination with 5-FU and targeted agents, such as bevacizumab, cetuximab, and panitumumab.

Addition of irinotecan to 5-FU and leucovorin improves tumor response and survival compared to 5-FU and leucovorin alone.[9–11] Different administration schedules (weekly, every 2 or 3 weeks) result in similar therapeutic outcomes. The most severe dose-limiting toxicity is diarrhea, which may be debilitating, although myelosuppression may also occur. Early use of loperamide decreases the severity of diarrhea and is essential to prevent treatment-related morbidity and mortality. Administration on a 3-week schedule is associated with significantly less severe diarrhea than more frequent doses.[12]

## Capecitabine

Capecitabine is an orally administered fluoropyrimidine carbamate that is absorbed through the gastrointestinal tract and converted to 5-FU *via* three sequential enzymatic reactions, the last of which involves thymidine phosphorylase. This enzyme is present at consistently higher levels in tumor cells compared with nonmalignant tissue, thereby enhancing selectivity of this agent for tumor cells and improving its tolerability among patients compared to 5-FU.[13] Capecitabine monotherapy is similarly effective as a first-line treatment of metastatic colorectal cancer compared to 5-FU and leucovorin.[14,15] Capecitabine can be combined with oxaliplatin (XELOX) to achieve similar efficacy and tolerability compared to other 5-FU/oxaliplatin combinations and may be used as a convenient alternative to the latter.[16–18]

# TARGETED AGENTS IN METASTATIC COLORECTAL CANCER

## Vascular Endothelial Growth Factor

Angiogenesis is essential for the advancement of tumor growth, supplying nutrients and oxygen and removing of waste products, but it is also a key factor in promoting cell migration and development of distant metastases.[19] Vascular endothelial growth factor (VEGF) is a diffusible glycoprotein expressed by both endothelial cells and tumor cells that plays a pivotal role in regulating angiogenesis.[20,21] There are several different isoforms of the receptor: VEGF-A, VEGF-B, VEGF-C, VEGF-D, and VEGF-E. VEGF-A is the most potent stimulator of angiogenesis and binds to two related tyrosine kinase receptors: VEGFR-1 and VEGFR-2.[20,21] Binding of a VEGF isoform to one, or both, of its receptors results in activation of a cell type–dependent signaling cascade leading to neovascularization, mitogenesis, and suppression of apoptosis (Figure 16.1). Inhibition of VEGF reduces the rates of tumor growth, metastases, tumor vascularity, and the permeability of tumor microvessels.[22] Expression of VEGF correlates with development of colorectal cancer metastases and early recurrence.[23]

## Bevacizumab

Antiangiogenic agents have a high binding affinity to VEGF and interfere with binding of VEGF-A to VEGFR-1 and VEGFR-2, thereby inhibiting VEGF-mediated intracellular signaling.[24] Bevacizumab is a monoclonal antibody with high affinity for VEGF-A. It sequesters VEGF-A and prevents its binding to VEGFR, thereby preventing endothelial cell signaling.[19] Bevacizumab has minimal efficacy as a single agent and is most commonly administered in combination with cytotoxic chemotherapy. Enhanced antitumor activity presumably results from bevacizumab-mediated inhibition of tumor neoangiogenesis, tumor growth, and the development of new metastasis. These effects reduce intratumoral hydrostatic pressure, thereby promoting delivery of cytotoxic chemotherapy to tumor cells.[25]

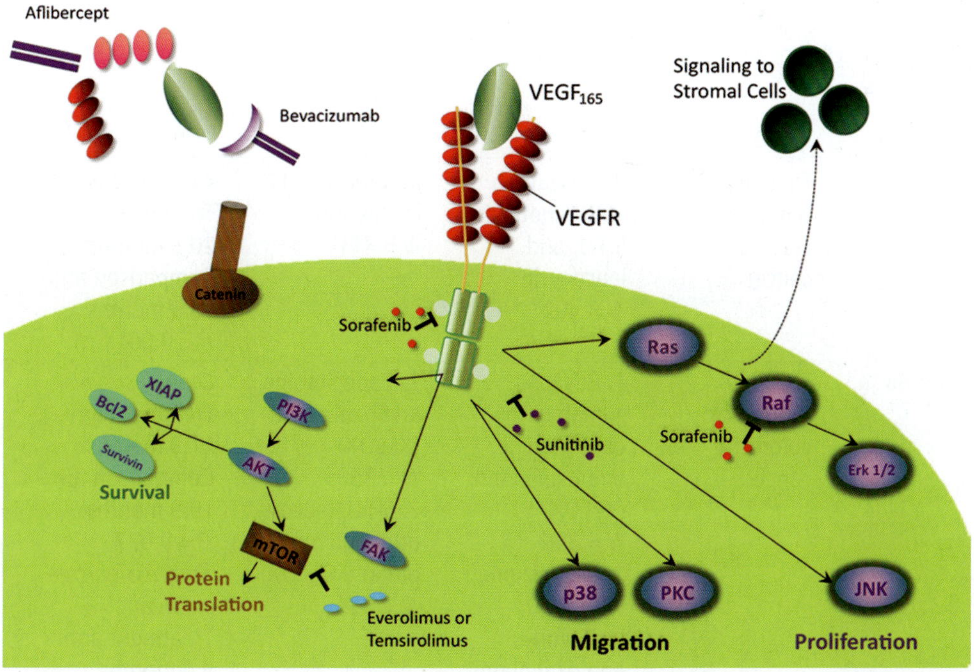


FIGURE 16.1: Binding of a VEGF isoform to VEGFR leads to dimerization and phosphorylation of intracellular domains that, in turn, activate multiple intracellular signaling cascades, thereby promoting endothelial cell proliferation, migration, and survival. Molecular therapies, such as aflibercept and bevacizumab, inhibit cell signaling by binding extracellular domains, whereas sorafenib, sunitinib, everolimus, and temsirolimus act on specific intracellular targets.

Data from several studies clearly demonstrate the efficacy of bevacizumab in the treatment of stage IV colorectal cancer, although it is not associated with substantial benefit when used to treat patients with stages II and III colorectal cancer (Table 16.1).[21,26–30] Bevacizumab may be combined with infusional FOLFIRI to improve overall survival of patients with stage IV colorectal cancer and increases the median time to progression of disease.[12,30] Bevacizumab improves the efficacy of FOLFOX in the second-line treatment of patients with distant metastases and increases median overall survival time to 12.9 months compared to 10.8 months when FOLFOX is used alone.[29] Tumor response rates are substantially higher among patients receiving bevacizumab in combination with cytotoxic chemotherapy (44.8%) compared to those receiving cytotoxic therapy alone (34.8%).[30] The demonstrable added benefit of bevacizumab led the Food and Drug Administration to approve it for use in combination with intravenous 5-FU–based chemotherapy as first-line treatment of stage IV colorectal carcinoma.[31] In fact, it is now standard of care to administer bevacizumab with cytotoxic chemotherapy as first-line therapy for patients with stage IV colorectal carcinoma as well as a second-line agent regardless of whether or not patients received prior antiangiogenic therapy.

## Bevacizumab beyond Progression

Recent research initiatives have focused on the potential benefit of inhibiting angiogenesis through multiple lines of chemotherapy. Data from the Bevacizumab Regimens: Investigation of Treatment Effects and Safety (BRITE) study suggest that patients with stage IV colorectal cancer may benefit from continuation of bevacizumab and cytotoxic chemotherapy despite progression of disease, rather than cessation of bevacizumab once disease progression is detected.[26] Similar findings have been described in randomized trials evaluating the benefit of continued bevacizumab with second-line chemotherapy in patients with stage IV colorectal cancer who progressed while receiving bevacizumab as a first-line agent. However, the impact of bevacizumab on

**Table 16.1** Pivotal Trials Evaluating Bevacizumab in the Treatment of Advanced Colorectal Cancer

| Trial Name | Study Design | Treatment Arm | Comparison Arm | Primary End Point |
|---|---|---|---|---|
| Hurwitz et al. | First line Metastatic colorectal cancer | Bevacizumab with irinotecan, 5-FU, and leucovorin $N = 402$ | Irinotecan, 5-FU, leucovorin $N = 411$ | *Overall survival* Treatment arm: 20.3 months Comparison arm: 15.6 months $P < 0.001$ |
| NO16966 | First line Metastatic colorectal cancer | 1. Bevacizumab with capecitabine and oxaliplatin (XELOX) $N = 350$ 2. Bevacizumab with 5-FU, leucovorin, and oxaliplatin (FOLFOX) $N = 350$ | 1. Capecitabine and oxaliplatin (XELOX) $N = 350$ 2. 5-FU, leucovorin, and oxaliplatin (FOLFOX) $N = 351$ | *Overall survival* Treatment arm: 21.3 months Comparison arm: 19.9 months $P = 0.077$ *Progression-free survival* Treatment arm: 9.4 months Comparison arm: 8 months $P = 0.0023$ |

**Table 16-1 Pivotal Trials Evaluating Bevacizumab in the Treatment of Advanced Colorectal Cancer (*continued*)**

| Trial Name | Study Design | Treatment Arm | Comparison Arm | Primary End Point |
|---|---|---|---|---|
| Bevacizumab regimens' investigation of treatment effects (BRITE) | Observational registry | Bevacizumab after disease progression $N = 642$ | 1. Cytotoxic chemotherapy without bevacizumab after disease progression $N = 531$<br>2. No therapy after disease progression $N = 253$ | *Overall survival*<br>Treatment arm: 31.8 months<br>Comparison arm 1: 19.9 months<br>Comparison arm 2: 12.6 months<br>$P < 0.001$, bevacizumab vs. no bevacizumab after disease progression |
| Treatment across multiple lines (TML) | Second line Metastatic colorectal cancer | Bevacizumab with cytotoxic chemotherapy $N = 409$ | Cytotoxic chemotherapy $N = 411$ | *Overall survival*<br>Treatment arm: 11.2 months<br>Comparison arm: 9.8 months<br>$P = 0.0062$<br>*Progression-free survival*<br>Treatment arm: 5.7 months<br>Comparison arm: 4.1 months<br>$P < 0.0001$ |
| ECOG 3200 | Second line Metastatic colorectal cancer | 1. Bevacizumab with 5-FU, leucovorin, and oxaliplatin (FOLFOX) $N = 286$<br>2. Bevacizumab alone $N = 243$ | 5-FU, leucovorin, and oxaliplatin (FOLFOX) $N = 291$ | *Overall survival*<br>Treatment arm 1: 12.9 months<br>Comparison arm: 10.8 months<br>$P = 0.0011$<br>Treatment arm 2: 10.2 months |

median overall survival and progression-free survival is somewhat limited compared to cytotoxic chemotherapy alone as a second-line agent (11.2 months and 5.7 months, respectively, vs. 9.8 months and 4.1 months, respectively).[28] These data suggest that once started, anti-VEGF treatment may lead to a survival advantage.

## Ziv-Aflibercept

Ziv-aflibercept is an antiangiogenic agent similar to bevacizumab. It is a protein comprising the extracellular domains of VEGFR-1 and VEGFR-2 and the constant region (Fc) of human IgG. It acts as a soluble decoy receptor to bind intravascular and extravascular VEGF. Sequestration of VEGF prevents binding and activation of VEGFR, thereby decreasing tumor angiogenesis.

Ziv-aflibercept inhibits cell signaling mediated by VEGF-A, VEGF-B, and platelet-like growth factor. Both ziv-aflibercept and bevacizumab are associated with a number of toxicities, although they tend to be greater when ziv-aflibercept is used. Typical antiangiogenic treatment toxicities include hypertension, proteinuria, gastrointestinal toxicity, and, rarely, venous and arterial thromboses. Bevacizumab may also be associated with gastrointestinal perforation.

Ziv-aflibercept prolongs overall survival among patients with stage IV colorectal cancer when used in combination with FOLFIRI as a second-line treatment.[32] Patients who received ziv-aflibercept have a 19.8% response rate compared to 11.1% among patients treated with FOLFIRI and a placebo. Improved progression-free survival is also associated with addition of ziv-aflibercept (6.9 months vs. 4.7 months for patients receiving FOLFIRI and placebo).[32] As a result, the Food and Drug Administration recently approved ziv-aflibercept for use in combination with FOLFIRI for treatment of patients with stage IV colorectal cancer that is either resistant to treatment or progresses following treatment with an oxaliplatin-containing regimen.

## MULTITARGETED KINASE INHIBITION

### Regorafenib

Regorafenib is a multitargeted kinase inhibitor that affects growth of both the tumor and its vasculature. It binds to and inhibits VEGFR-2 and VEGFR-3, as well as tumor cell signaling kinases (e.g., RET, KIT, PDGFR, and Raf). These actions effectively inhibit tumor angiogenesis and tumor cell proliferation. Regorafenib improves survival by 29% among patients with stage IV colorectal cancer who fail other lines of therapy, extending median overall survival to 6.4 months and progression-free survival to 1.7 months compared to 5.0 months and 1.7 months, respectively, for patients receiving a placebo.[33,34] Regorafenib was approved by the Food and Drug Administration for treatment of patients with stage IV colorectal cancer in October 2012. This agent is associated with several toxicities, including severe hand–foot skin reactions, fatigue, hypertension, diarrhea, and rashes.

## EPIDERMAL GROWTH FACTOR RECEPTOR

The epidermal growth factor receptor (EGFR) is expressed in many solid tumors, including colorectal cancer. This molecule is a member of the HER family of receptor tyrosine kinases that includes not only EGFR (ErbB/HER1) but also ErbB2 (HER2), ErbB3 (HER3), and ErbB4 (HER4). Activation of these proteins is ligand dependent, and they are specifically activated by epidermal growth factor and transforming growth factor–alpha. Ligand binding to the EGFR results in receptor phosphorylation and activation of several cell signaling mechanisms, including the Ras-Raf-MAPK, PI3K-AKT, protein kinase C, STAT, and Src kinase pathways. All of these signaling cascades play important roles in tumor cell proliferation, invasion, migration, and inhibition of apoptosis. Given the pivotal role of EGFR in the activation of multiple pathways and its relevance to tumor growth, this receptor is a target of several therapies, including monoclonal antibodies that recognize EGFR and small molecule inhibitors of EGFR tyrosine kinase activity, such as cetuximab and panitumumab (Figure 16.2).

### Cetuximab

Cetuximab is a mouse/human chimeric monoclonal antibody that binds to the EGFR and competitively inhibits ligand binding such that receptor dimerization and internalization do not occur. Cetuximab was approved for use in stage IV colorectal cancer by the Food and Drug Administration in 2004. It may be used as a single agent or in combination with irinotecan to treat EGFR-expressing, irinotecan-refractory tumors. Unfortunately, tumors that harbor alterations in cell signaling pathways downstream from EGFR may not respond well to anti-EGFR therapy, particularly if those changes include *KRAS* mutations (Figure 16.2). There is a positive

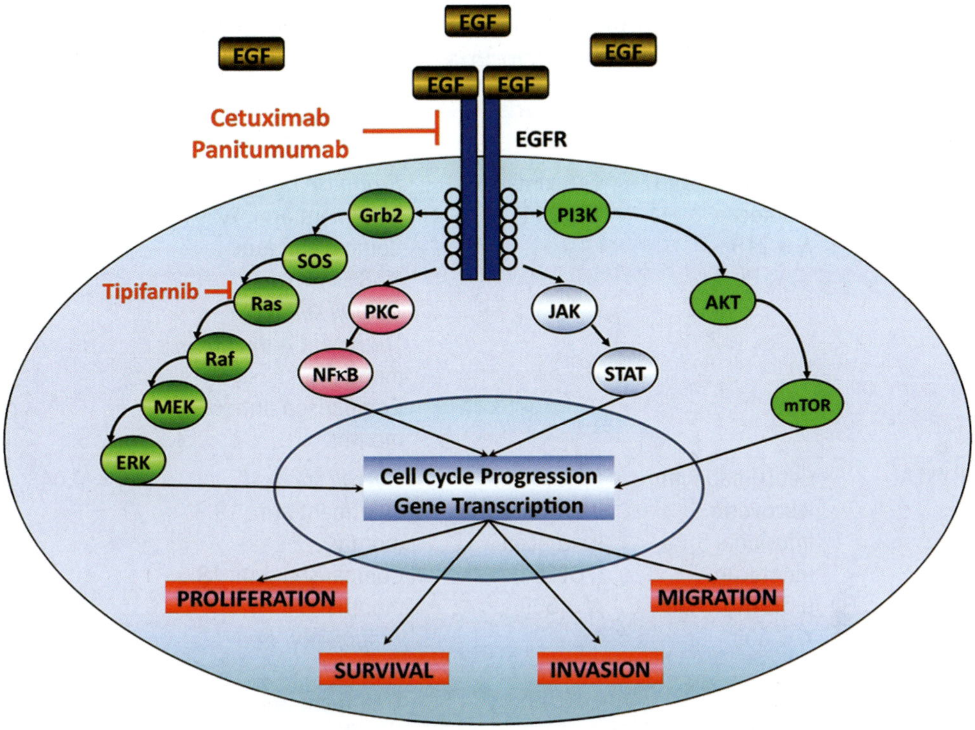


FIGURE 16.2: Binding of epidermal growth factor to its receptor results in dimerization and phosphorylation of intracellular domains that subsequently stimulates several cell signaling pathways that drive cell proliferation, prolonged survival, and cell migration. Targeted therapies, such as cetuximab and panitumumab, competitively inhibit binding of epidermal growth factor, whereas others target specific steps in signaling pathways. Inhibition of cell signaling is associated with diminished cell survival, proliferation, and migration.

relationship between treatment benefits of cetuximab in advanced colorectal cancers and wild-type *KRAS*. The Provisional Clinical Opinion issued by the American Society of Clinical Oncology recommends that all patients being considered for anti-EGFR therapy undergo *KRAS* mutation testing of their tumors and that such treatment be restricted to those with wild-type *KRAS*.[35]

Available data clearly support the role of cetuximab in the management of stage IV colorectal cancer (Table 16.2). The open-label phase II BOND trial showed that the combination of cetuximab and irinotecan was superior to cetuximab alone for treatment of irinotecan-refractory stage IV colorectal cancer. Response rates and interval to progression for the former were 22.9% and 4.1 months, compared to 10.8% and 1.5 months, respectively, for cetuximab alone.[36] The phase III Cetuximab Combined with Irinotecan in First-Line Therapy for Metastatic Colorectal Cancer (CRYSTAL) study evaluated the benefits of combining FOLFIRI and cetuximab. Response rates (46.9% vs. 38.7%) and progression-free survival (8.9 months vs. 8 months) were significantly higher among patients who received FOLFIRI and cetuximab compared to FOLFIRI alone.[37,38] Data from the study indicate that the addition of cetuximab to FOLFIRI reduces the risk of progression by 15%, although patients with *KRAS*-mutated tumors do not substantially benefit from cetuximab.[38]

## Panitumumab

Panitumumab is an anti-EGFR agent that binds EGFR and blocks its ligand. Unlike cetuximab, panitumumab is a fully humanized monoclonal antibody and, as such, has a lower rate of hypersensitivity reactions. It was approved by the Food and Drug Administration in 2006

**Table 16.2 Clinical Trials Evaluating the Role of Cetuximab in the Treatment of Stage IV Colorectal Carcinoma**

| Trial Name | Treatment Arm | Comparison Arm | Primary End Point | Significance |
|---|---|---|---|---|
| BOND | Cetuximab with irinotecan<br>*N* = 218 | Cetuximab<br>*N* = 111 | *Response rate*<br>Treatment arm: 22.9%<br>Comparison arm: 10.8%<br>*Overall survival*<br>Treatment arm: 8.6 months<br>Comparison arm: 6.9 months | *P* = 0.007 |
| CRYSTAL | Cetuximab with leucovorin<br>Infusional 5-FU<br>Irinotecan<br>(FOLFIRI)<br>*N* = 608 | Leucovorin<br>Infusional 5-FU<br>Irinotecan<br>(FOLFIRI)<br>*N* = 609 | *Overall survival*<br>Treatment arm: 19.9 months<br>Comparison arm: 18.6 months<br>*Progression free survival*<br>Treatment arm: 8.9 months<br>Comparison arm: 8.0 months | *P* = 0.048 |
| OPUS | Cetuximab with leucovorin<br>Infusional 5-FU<br>Oxaliplatin<br>(FOLFOX)<br>*N* = 169 | Leucovorin<br>Infusional 5-FU<br>Oxaliplatin<br>(FOLFOX)<br>*N* = 168 | *Response rate*<br>Treatment arm: 46%<br>Comparison arm: 36%<br>*Overall survival*: Not reported | *P* = 0.64 |
| Jonker et al. | Cetuximab with best supportive care<br>*N* = 287 | Best supportive care<br>*N* = 285 | *Overall survival*<br>Treatment arm: 6.1 months<br>Comparison arm: 4.6 months | *P* < 0.001 |

following a phase III clinical trial enrolling patients with EGFR-expressing stage IV colorectal carcinoma who failed fluoropyrimidine-, oxaliplatin-, and irinotecan-containing chemotherapy regimens. That study showed panitumumab monotherapy plus best supportive care improved survival compared to supportive care alone and decreased the rate of disease progression by 46%.[10] Importantly, panitumumab has a significantly greater effect on progression-free survival among patients with wild-type *KRAS* tumors (12.3 weeks) than mutant *KRAS* (7.4 weeks).[10] A current US clinical trial that addresses the use of EGFR antibody therapies in *KRAS* mutant tumors recently completed enrollment, and results are anticipated in 2014 (NCT00077233 www.clinicaltrials.gov).

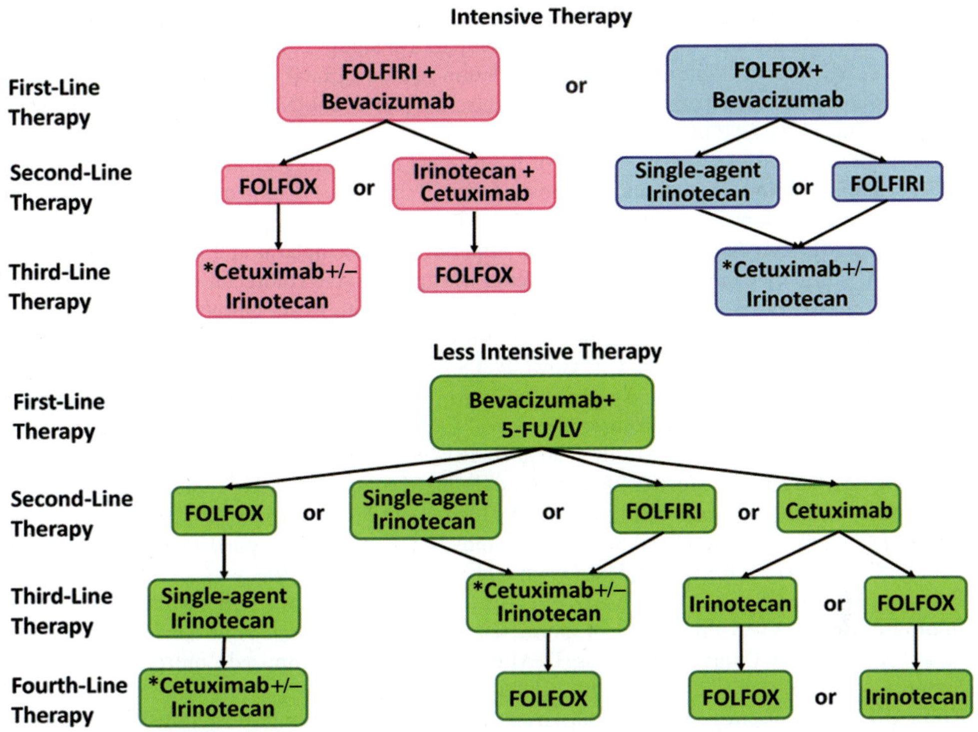


FIGURE 16.3: Treatment algorithms for advanced colorectal cancer include several agent combinations of variable intensity. Use of cetuximab and panitumumab is limited to *KRAS* wild-type tumors.

## SUMMARY AND CONCLUSIONS

Although surgery is the mainstay of therapy for early colorectal cancers, targeted therapeutics increasingly offer hope for improving the poor outcomes associated with advanced colorectal cancer. Seven new drugs have been approved for treatment of colorectal cancer since 1998, including all five new biologic agents. As a result of these advances, treatment algorithms for colorectal carcinoma have become increasingly complex. The challenge is to manage the entire course of treatment from initial first-line therapy through multiple additional lines of treatment, since patients who are able to receive multiple lines of cytotoxic and targeted therapy have the best overall survivals. These chemotherapeutic regimens may be used in conjunction with local–regional therapies, including resection of metastatic tumor deposits (Figure 16.3). Future refinement of treatment strategies will likely include targeted therapeutics, anti-inflammatory biologic agents, and cancer stem cell targeting to augment patient survival.

# References

1. Siegel R, Naishadham D, Jemal A. Cancer statistics, 2012. *CA Cancer J Clin* [Comparative Study] 2012;62(1):10–29.
2. Altekruse SF, K.C, Krapcho M, et al., eds. *SEER cancer statistics review, 1975–2007*. Bethesda, MD: National Cancer Institute, 2010. http://seer.cancer.gov/csr/1975_2007/

3. Gunderson LL, Jessup JM, Sargent DJ, et al. Revised TN categorization for colon cancer based on national survival outcomes data. *J Clin Oncol* [Comparative Study] 2010;28(2):264–271.
4. Thirion P, Michiels S, Pignon JP, et al. Modulation of fluorouracil by leucovorin in patients with advanced colorectal cancer: an updated meta-analysis. *J Clin Oncol* [Meta-Analysis Research Support, Non-U.S. Gov't] 2004;22(18):3766–3775.
5. Meta-Analysis Group In Cancer. Toxicity of fluorouracil in patients with advanced colorectal cancer: effect of administration schedule and prognostic factors. *J Clin Oncol* [Comparative Study Meta-Analysis Research Support, Non-U.S. Gov't] 1998;16(11):3537–3541.
6. Rothenberg ML, Oza AM, Bigelow RH, et al. Superiority of oxaliplatin and fluorouracil-leucovorin compared with either therapy alone in patients with progressive colorectal cancer after irinotecan and fluorouracil-leucovorin: interim results of a phase III trial. *J Clin Oncol* [Clinical Trial Clinical Trial, Phase III Comparative Study Multicenter Study Randomized Controlled Trial Research Support, Non-U.S. Gov't Research Support, U.S. Gov't, P.H.S.] 2003;21(11):2059–2069.
7. de Gramont A, Figer A, Seymour M, et al. Leucovorin and fluorouracil with or without oxaliplatin as first-line treatment in advanced colorectal cancer. *J Clin Oncol* [Clinical Trial Randomized Controlled Trial Research Support, Non-U.S. Gov't] 2000;18(16):2938–2947.
8. Goldberg RM, Sargent DJ, Morton RF, et al. A randomized controlled trial of fluorouracil plus leucovorin, irinotecan, and oxaliplatin combinations in patients with previously untreated metastatic colorectal cancer. *J Clin Oncol* [Clinical Trial Multicenter Study Randomized Controlled Trial Research Support, Non-U.S. Gov't Research Support, U.S. Gov't, P.H.S.] 2004;22(1):23–30.
9. Douillard JY, Cunningham D, Roth AD, et al. Irinotecan combined with fluorouracil compared with fluorouracil alone as first-line treatment for metastatic colorectal cancer: a multicentre randomised trial. *Lancet* [Clinical Trial Clinical Trial, Phase III Multicenter Study Randomized Controlled Trial Research Support, Non-U.S. Gov't] 2000;355(9209):1041–1047.
10. Kohne CH, van Cutsem E, Wils J, et al. Phase III study of weekly high-dose infusional fluorouracil plus folinic acid with or without irinotecan in patients with metastatic colorectal cancer: European Organisation for Research and Treatment of Cancer Gastrointestinal Group Study 40986. *J Clin Oncol* [Clinical Trial Clinical Trial, Phase III Comparative Study Multicenter Study Randomized Controlled Trial Research Support, Non-U.S. Gov't] 2005;23(22):4856–4865.
11. Saltz LB, Cox JV, Blanke C, et al. Irinotecan plus fluorouracil and leucovorin for metastatic colorectal cancer. Irinotecan Study Group. *N Engl J Med* [Clinical Trial Comparative Study Multicenter Study Randomized Controlled Trial Research Support, Non-U.S. Gov't] 2000;343(13):905–914.
12. Fuchs CS, Moore MR, Harker G, et al. Phase III comparison of two irinotecan dosing regimens in second-line therapy of metastatic colorectal cancer. *J Clin Oncol* [Clinical Trial Clinical Trial, Phase III Comparative Study Multicenter Study Randomized Controlled Trial Research Support, Non-U.S. Gov't] 2003;21(5):807–814.
13. Schuller J, Cassidy J, Dumont E, et al. Preferential activation of capecitabine in tumor following oral administration to colorectal cancer patients. *Cancer Chemother Pharmacol* [Clinical Trial Multicenter Study] 2000;45(4):291–297.
14. Hoff PM, Ansari R, Batist G, et al. Comparison of oral capecitabine versus intravenous fluorouracil plus leucovorin as first-line treatment in 605 patients with metastatic colorectal cancer: results of a randomized phase III study. *J Clin Oncol* [Clinical Trial Clinical Trial, Phase III Comparative Study Randomized Controlled Trial Research Support, Non-U.S. Gov't] 2001;19(8):2282–2292.
15. Van Cutsem E, Twelves C, Cassidy J, et al. Oral capecitabine compared with intravenous fluorouracil plus leucovorin in patients with metastatic colorectal cancer: results of a large phase III study. *J Clin Oncol* [Clinical Trial Clinical Trial, Phase III Multicenter Study Randomized Controlled Trial Research Support, Non-U.S. Gov't] 2001;19(21):4097–4106.
16. Arkenau HT, Arnold D, Cassidy J, et al. Efficacy of oxaliplatin plus capecitabine or infusional fluorouracil/leucovorin in patients with metastatic colorectal cancer: a pooled analysis of randomized trials. *J Clin Oncol* [Comparative Study Meta-Analysis] 2008;26(36):5910–5917.
17. Diaz-Rubio E, Tabernero J, Gomez-Espana A, et al. Phase III study of capecitabine plus oxaliplatin compared with continuous-infusion fluorouracil plus oxaliplatin as first-line therapy in metastatic colorectal cancer: final report of the Spanish Cooperative Group for the treatment of digestive tumors trial. *J Clin Oncol* [Clinical Trial, Phase III Multicenter Study Randomized Controlled Trial Research Support, Non-U.S. Gov't] 2007;25(27):4224–4230.

18. Cassidy J, Clarke S, Diaz-Rubio E, et al. Randomized phase III study of capecitabine plus oxaliplatin compared with fluorouracil/folinic acid plus oxaliplatin as first-line therapy for metastatic colorectal cancer. *J Clin Oncol* [Clinical Trial, Phase III Comparative Study Multicenter Study Randomized Controlled Trial] 2008;26(12):2006–2012.
19. Borgstrom P, Hillan KJ, Sriramarao P, et al. Complete inhibition of angiogenesis and growth of microtumors by anti-vascular endothelial growth factor neutralizing antibody: novel concepts of angiostatic therapy from intravital videomicroscopy. *Cancer Res* 1996;56(17):4032–4039.
20. El Zouhairi M, Charabaty A, Pishvaian MJ. Molecularly targeted therapy for metastatic colon cancer: proven treatments and promising new agents. *Gastrointest Cancer Res* 2011;4(1):15–21.
21. Wilhelm SM, Dumas J, Adnane L, et al. Regorafenib (BAY 73–4506): a new oral multikinase inhibitor of angiogenic, stromal and oncogenic receptor tyrosine kinases with potent preclinical antitumor activity. *Int J Cancer* 2011;129(1):245–255.
22. Kohne CH, Lenz HJ. Chemotherapy with targeted agents for the treatment of metastatic colorectal cancer. *Oncologist* [Review] 2009;14(5):478–488.
23. Cascinu S, Graziano F, Valentini M, et al. Vascular endothelial growth factor expression, S-phase fraction and thymidylate synthase quantitation in node-positive colon cancer: relationships with tumor recurrence and resistance to adjuvant chemotherapy. *Ann Oncol* 2001;12(2):239–244.
24. Folkman J. Tumor angiogenesis. *Adv Cancer Res* [Review] 1974;19(0):331–358.
25. Ferrara N, Gerber HP, LeCouter J. The biology of VEGF and its receptors. *Nat Med* [Review] 2003;9(6):669–676.
26. Grothey A, Sugrue MM, Purdie DM, et al. Bevacizumab beyond first progression is associated with prolonged overall survival in metastatic colorectal cancer: results from a large observational cohort study (BRiTE). *J Clin Oncol* [Multicenter Study Research Support, Non-U.S. Gov't] 2008;26(33): 5326–5334.
27. Cassidy J, Clarke S, Diaz-Rubio E, et al. XELOX vs FOLFOX-4 as first-line therapy for metastatic colorectal cancer: NO16966 updated results. *Br J Cancer* [Clinical Trial, Phase III Comparative Study Randomized Controlled Trial Research Support, Non-U.S. Gov't] 2011;105(1):58–64.
28. Bennouna J, Sastre J, Arnold D, et al. Continuation of bevacizumab after first progression in metastatic colorectal cancer (ML18147): a randomised phase 3 trial. *Lancet Oncol* 2013;14(1):29–37.
29. Giantonio BJ, Catalano PJ, Meropol NJ, et al. Bevacizumab in combination with oxaliplatin, fluorouracil, and leucovorin (FOLFOX4) for previously treated metastatic colorectal cancer: results from the Eastern Cooperative Oncology Group Study E3200. *J Clin Oncol* [Clinical Trial, Phase III Multicenter Study Randomized Controlled Trial Research Support, N.I.H., Extramural] 2007;25(12):1539–1544.
30. Hurwitz H, Fehrenbacher L, Novotny W, et al. Bevacizumab plus irinotecan, fluorouracil, and leucovorin for metastatic colorectal cancer. *N Engl J Med* [Clinical Trial Clinical Trial, Phase III Multicenter Study Randomized Controlled Trial Research Support, U.S. Gov't, P.H.S.] 2004;350(23):2335–2342.
31. Saltz LB, Clarke S, Diaz-Rubio E, et al. Bevacizumab in combination with oxaliplatin-based chemotherapy as first-line therapy in metastatic colorectal cancer: a randomized phase III study. *J Clin Oncol* [Clinical Trial, Phase III Multicenter Study Randomized Controlled Trial] 2008;26(12):2013–2019.
32. Van Cutsem E, Tabernero J, Lakomy R, et al. Addition of aflibercept to fluorouracil, leucovorin, and irinotecan improves survival in a phase III randomized trial in patients with metastatic colorectal cancer previously treated with an oxaliplatin-based regimen. *J Clin Oncol* [Clinical Trial, Phase III Randomized Controlled Trial Research Support, Non-U.S. Gov't] 2012;30(28):3499–3506.
33. Grothey A. Regorafenib in metastatic colorectal cancer. *Clin Adv Hematol Oncol* 2012;10(5):324–325.
34. Grothey A, Cutsem EV, Sobrero A, et al. Regorafenib monotherapy for previously treated metastatic colorectal cancer (CORRECT): an international, multicentre, randomised, placebo-controlled, phase 3 trial. *Lancet* 2013;381(9863):303–312.
35. Allegra CJ, Jessup JM, Somerfield MR, et al. American Society of Clinical Oncology provisional clinical opinion: testing for KRAS gene mutations in patients with metastatic colorectal carcinoma to predict response to anti-epidermal growth factor receptor monoclonal antibody therapy. *J Clin Oncol* [Review] 2009;27(12):2091–2096.
36. Cunningham D, Humblet Y, Siena S, et al. Cetuximab monotherapy and cetuximab plus irinotecan in irinotecan-refractory metastatic colorectal cancer. *N Engl J Med* [Clinical Trial Comparative Study Multicenter Study Randomized Controlled Trial Research Support, Non-U.S. Gov't] 2004;351(4): 337–345.

37. Van Cutsem E, Kohne CH, Hitre E, et al. Cetuximab and chemotherapy as initial treatment for metastatic colorectal cancer. *N Engl J Med* [Comparative Study Multicenter Study Randomized Controlled Trial Research Support, Non-U.S. Gov't] 2009;360(14):1408–1417.
38. Van Cutsem E, Kohne CH, Lang I, et al. Cetuximab plus irinotecan, fluorouracil, and leucovorin as first-line treatment for metastatic colorectal cancer: updated analysis of overall survival according to tumor KRAS and BRAF mutation status. *J Clin Oncol* [Clinical Trial, Phase III Multicenter Study Randomized Controlled Trial Research Support, Non-U.S. Gov't] 2011;29(15):2011–2019.

# Surgical Management of Stage IV Colorectal Cancer

# 17

▶ Michael D. Kluger
▶ Ser Yee Lee
▶ Daniel Cherqui

Colorectal cancer is a leading cause of cancer-related death worldwide, and successful long-term management generally requires surgical intervention with, or without, other treatment modalities. Unfortunately, a substantial number of patients have distant extracolonic disease at the time of diagnosis, or they develop metastases at some point following initial presentation. Up to 25% of colorectal cancer patients have synchronous liver metastases, and 50% will develop them over their lives, followed in frequency by disseminated disease within the peritoneal cavity and extra-abdominal metastases.[1] Although stage IV colorectal cancer was historically treated in a palliative manner, the increased use of targeted chemotherapeutic and biologic agents, improved operative safety, and a better understanding of anatomy and physiology have facilitated surgical management of distant metastatic disease. Indeed, it is now possible to achieve long-term survival in patients with stage IV colorectal cancer who are managed with a combination of chemotherapy and surgery. Five-year survival rates as high as 58% and 68% have been reported among patients with extracolonic disease limited to the liver and lung, respectively.[2–5]

Pathologists play an increasingly important role in management decisions of patients with stage IV colorectal cancer, particularly as biologic therapies and interventional technologies advance. Accurate assessment of pathologic stage and adequacy of resection are required to determine prognosis and make informed decisions regarding subsequent chemotherapeutic options. Pathologic evaluation for the presence and extent of underlying liver disease also facilitates planning of surgical treatment when patients have potentially resectable hepatic metastases. The purpose of this chapter is to discuss the necessity of multidisciplinary interactions in management of patients with stage IV colorectal cancer, clinical and pathologic risk factors that impact surgical decisions, and operative and interventional strategies in the modern era of chemotherapy.

## MULTIDISCIPLINARY MANAGEMENT OF PATIENTS WITH STAGE IV COLORECTAL CANCER

Colorectal cancer patients who present with obstructive symptoms or substantial bleeding may require emergent surgical intervention. However, treatment decisions for most other patients are best arrived upon following discussion with a multidisciplinary team comprising diagnostic and interventional radiologists, oncologists, colorectal and hepatobiliary surgeons, gastroenterologists, radiation oncologists, and pathologists (Figure 17.1). Expertise of other individuals, such as thoracic surgeons and genetic counselors, should be called upon, as necessary. The European Colorectal Metastases Treatment Group, the American Hepato-Pancreato-Biliary Association (AHPBA), the Society of Surgical Oncology (SSO), and the Society for Surgery of Alimentary Tract (SSAT) all emphasize a multidisciplinary approach to managing cancer patients, which improves efficiency and efficacy of patient care and generally results in better outcomes.[6–8]

Multidisciplinary management improves comprehensive preoperative evaluation (i.e., computerized tomography imaging, serology testing for carcinoembryonic antigen [CEA] levels, transrectal ultrasound for local staging of rectal cancer), and better adherence to the

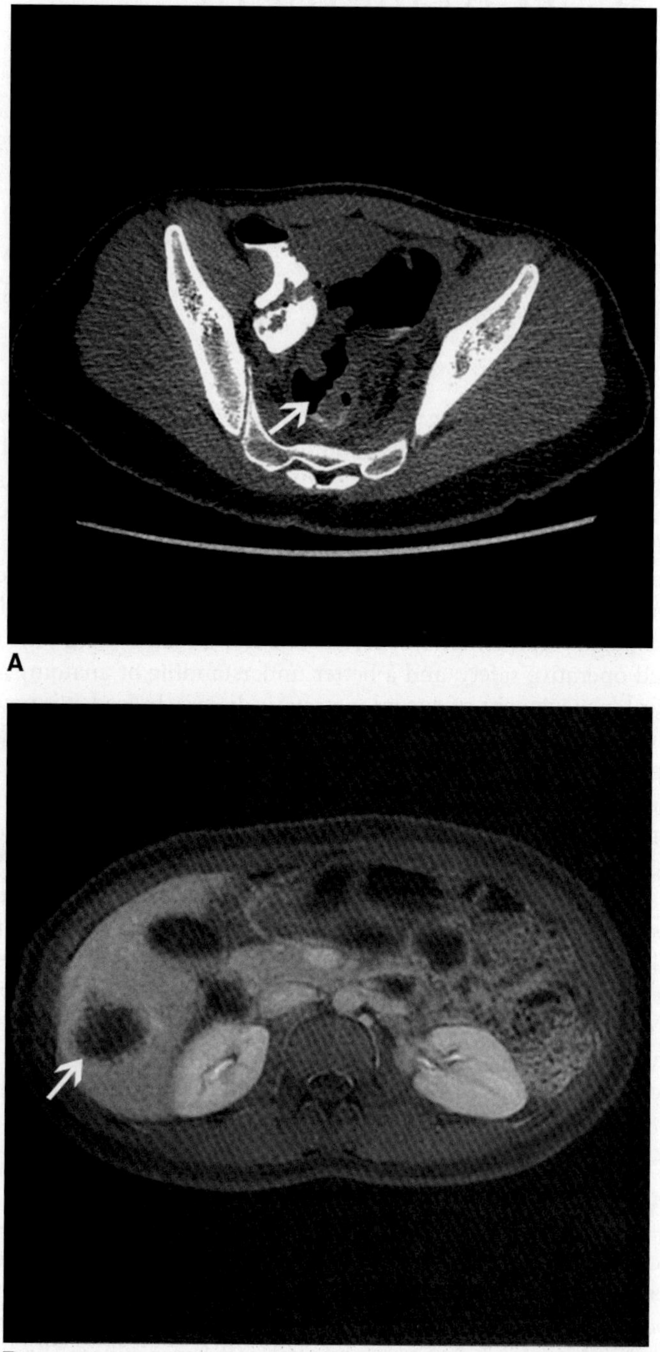

A

B

FIGURE 17.1: A 21-year-old woman with Gardner syndrome and stage IV colon cancer underwent evaluation by a multidisciplinary team. Virtual colonoscopy and imaging demonstrated a nearly obstructing mass (*arrow*) in the recto-sigmoid colon (**A**). Magnetic resonance imaging revealed a metastasis (*arrow*) in segments 5 and 6 (**B**).

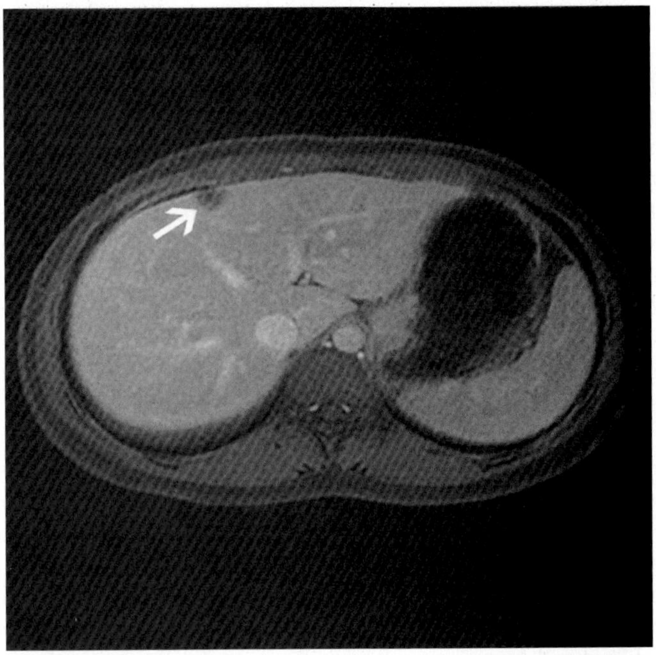

C

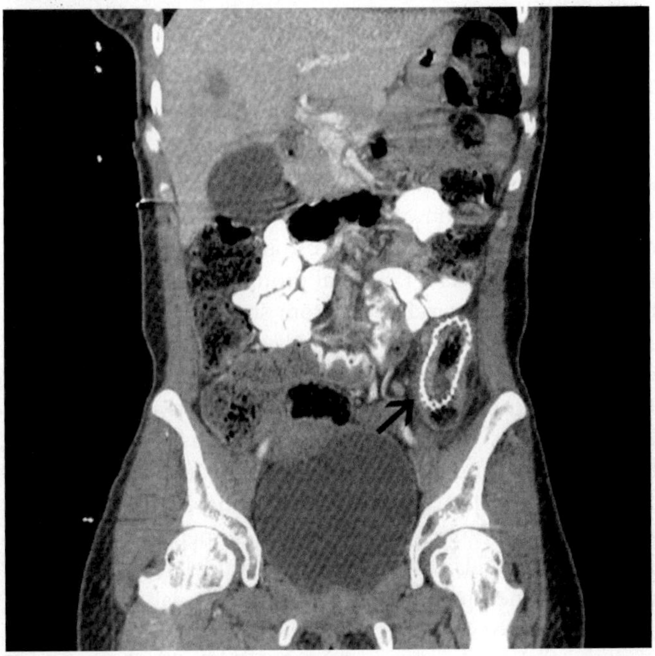

D

FIGURE 17.1: (*Continued*) A second tumor deposit (*arrow*) was present in segment 4 (**C**). Discussion at a multidisciplinary conference led to placement of a colonic stent (*arrow*) through the tumor and rapid initiation of neoadjuvant chemotherapy (**D**). The primary cancer and segment 4 lesion were removed simultaneously, and the tumor in segments 5 and 6 was treated with a subsequent right hepatectomy. The patients received a complete course of adjuvant chemotherapy and remains disease-free more than 1 year later.

National Comprehensive Cancer Network guidelines. Patients initially treated in specialized centers enjoy enhanced access to multimodal therapy and more frequent oncology consultation (99% vs. 62%) with higher rates of neoadjuvant therapy implementation (76% vs. 20%) as compared to institutions that utilize a more general surgical approach to colorectal cancer.[9] Primary surgeries for colorectal cancers performed at specialized care centers are often of higher quality than those from institutions in which cancer patients are managed by general surgeons and pathologists. For example, longitudinal data from institutions transitioning to a subspecialized cancer management model show improvement in quality assurance measures after implementation of a multidisciplinary approach. They report higher numbers of harvested lymph nodes ($16 \pm 1$ vs. $9 \pm 1$), more frequent negative surgical resection margins (95% vs. 78%), and a decline in the frequency of grossly positive resection margins (15% to 2.5%) among primary colorectal cancer resection specimens.[10] Pathologic evaluation of colorectal cancers also improves when performed in the multidisciplinary setting and more commonly includes ancillary testing that may be clinically important, such as evaluation for microsatellite instability (30% vs. 11%).[9]

Finally, access to specialists affords colorectal cancer patients with more surgical options, particularly when they present with, or develop, advanced disease. Only a minority of patients with liver metastases treated in specialized centers receive palliative therapy alone, and nearly two-thirds of patients with hepatic metastases deemed unresectable by nonliver surgeons are considered potentially resectable by those with expertise in hepatobiliary surgery.[11] Most data demonstrate the value of collaboration and centralized specialty care in affecting treatment decisions, decreasing the number of interventions, shortening delays in care, reducing the number of chemotherapy cycles, and decreasing postoperative morbidity.

## PROGNOSTIC FACTORS

Many clinical and tumor-related factors are considered when patients with stage IV colorectal cancer contemplate surgical management of extracolonic disease. Clinical features that are commonly assessed in the preoperative evaluation of these individuals include patient age, gender, Eastern Cooperative Oncology Group performance status, and American Society of Anesthesiologists physical status classification (Table 17.1). Several groups have proposed prognostic scoring systems to identify individuals unlikely to benefit from surgical management of advanced disease. Of these, seven tumor-related features have emerged as independent factors associated with poor prognosis: the presence of extrahepatic distant disease, positive surgical margins, lymph node metastases from the primary tumor, fewer than 12 months between treatment of primary tumor and detection of liver metastases, size of largest tumor deposit in the liver (>5 cm), number of metastatic deposits in liver (>1), and CEA level in excess of 200 ng/mL.[2,12]

Some molecular alterations also correlate with prognosis among colorectal cancer patients with advanced disease. Increased expression of human telomerase reverse transcriptase (hTERT), glucose transporter-1 protein (GLUT-1), p27, and thymidylate synthase (TS) promote tumor growth, and tritiated thymidine uptake, high Ki-67 immunolabeling, and *TP53* mutations are adverse prognostic factors among colorectal cancer patients.[13–15] Alterations that affect cell signaling pathways, such as those involving COX-2, KRAS, BRAF, iNOS, HMG-CoA, RXR-$\alpha$, $\beta$-catenin, and STAT3, impact response to targeted chemotherapeutic agents and, thus, affect overall prognosis. Some of these molecular markers help identify patients who may respond to specific chemotherapy regimens. For example, *KRAS* mutational status directly affects the efficacy of epidermal growth factor receptor (EGFR) inhibitors, such as cetuximab, as discussed in Chapter 16.[16] The American Society of Clinical Oncology and National Comprehensive Cancer Network now recommend that all patients with stage IV colorectal cancer who are candidates for anti-EGFR therapy undergo *KRAS* mutational testing of their tumors prior to initiation of treatment.[17]

**Table 17.1** Performance Status Scales Used in Preoperative Evaluation of Patients with Stage IV Colorectal Cancer

| | American Society of Anesthesiologists Physical Status Classification | Eastern Cooperative Oncology Group Performance Status Scale |
|---|---|---|
| **Status Grade 0** | | Fully active without restrictions |
| **Status Grade 1** | A normal healthy patient | Restricted strenuous activity; able to carry out light work of sedentary nature |
| **Status Grade 2** | Mild systemic disease | Ambulatory and capable of self-care, unable to carry out work activities Up and about >50% of waking hours |
| **Status Grade 3** | Severe systemic disease | Capable of limited self-care<br>Confined to bed or chair >50% of waking hours |
| **Status Grade 4** | Severe life-threatening systemic disease | Completely disabled; incapable of any self-care<br>Totally confined to bed or chair |
| **Status Grade 5** | Moribund patient not expected to survive without intervention | Dead |
| **Status Grade 6** | Brain-dead patient whose organs are being harvested | |

## INTERVENTIONAL STRATEGIES IN THE ERA OF MODERN CHEMOTHERAPEUTICS

Patients with stage IV colorectal cancer and extraintestinal disease at multiple sites may be considered for staged resection, provided that the managing team has a reasonable expectation of achieving complete surgical resection. Potential candidates must have excellent functional status and be in good health with family support and psychosocial stability. They must be able to tolerate systemic chemotherapy and show no disease progression during chemotherapy. Metastatic deposits that are least amenable to complete eradication are approached first, as patients should not be subjected to multiple procedures and cycles of chemotherapy before undergoing the least feasible operation.

Colorectal cancer patients presenting with colorectal disease and synchronous resectable liver metastases should be considered for curative therapy *via* simultaneous, or staged, resections of the primary tumor and hepatic metastases with integration of neoadjuvant and adjuvant therapy (Figure 17.2). Treatment strategies and their timing are individualized according to patient needs and, thus, are best determined in a multidisciplinary setting. All patients with synchronous or metachronous distant metastases deserve consideration by physicians with expertise in the management of advanced colorectal cancer, particularly if they are initially deemed unresectable. Key elements of current management strategies are discussed below.

### Defining Resectability

Decisions regarding potential resection of colorectal cancer liver metastases were historically based on algorithms that utilized various prognostic factors as previously mentioned.[2,3,18,19] More

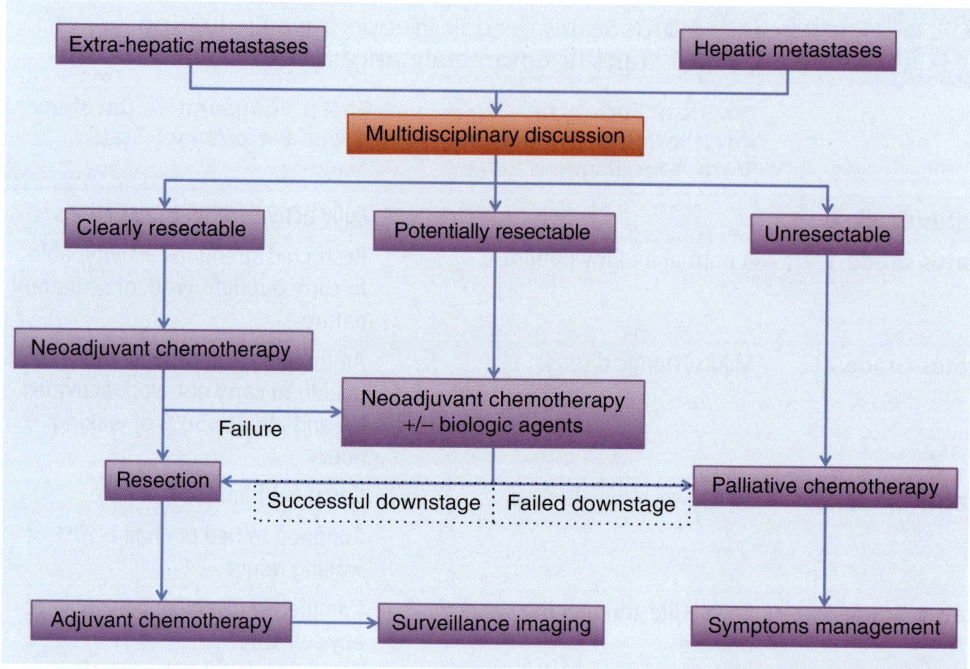


**FIGURE 17.2:** Multimodal treatment plans are not static, and comprehensive management requires reevaluation at several time points. Failure to initially respond to chemotherapy requires modification of agents to achieve maximal success. Extracolonic cancer resection may occur prior to removal of the primary tumor, at the time of colorectal surgery, or following management of colorectal disease. Hepatic metastases are often managed with a combination of interventional strategies, such as portal vein embolization and tumor ablation, as well as surgical resection.

recent guidelines suggest that tumor resections may be considered if it is possible to preserve a liver remnant volume representing at least 20% of the healthy liver and consisting of at least two contiguous hepatic segments with adequate vascular inflow, vascular outflow, and biliary drainage, as well as a reasonable expectation of achieving complete surgical resection.[8] The presence of extrahepatic disease is not considered an absolute contraindication to liver resection, provided the patient is medically fit to tolerate the procedure and complete resection of intra- and extrahepatic disease is feasible. Thus, decisions regarding potential resectability require input from a multidisciplinary team. Patients with pulmonary metastases require assessment by a pulmonologist and thoracic surgeon. Input from radiologists with a firm understanding of liver anatomy and experience using imaging software to assess underlying liver disease (e.g., cirrhosis, hepatosteatosis, hemosiderosis) and measure liver volumes is essential. Although preoperative liver biopsies are infrequently obtained, patients who undergo tumor biopsy should also be assessed for underlying disease and chemotherapy effects in the nonlesional liver, since the presence of abnormalities may impact operative strategies.

## Chemotherapy

Perioperative chemotherapy reduces risk of colorectal cancer recurrence among patients with resectable liver metastases and improves recurrence-free survival, although prospective data justifying the use of chemotherapy prior to surgical management of patients with stage IV colorectal cancer are lacking.[20,21] Chemotherapy may be used to indirectly assess tumor aggressiveness and biology prior to surgery, or to decrease the size and number of metastatic deposits to the point that surgical resection is possible.[20] Overall, patients with initially unresectable liver metastases show an objective response rate of 64% (range 43% to 79%) to neoadjuvant chemotherapy. Complete tumor resection is achieved in most (87%) patients who show an acceptable response to neoadjuvant chemotherapy and undergo surgical removal of liver metastases.[22,23] However, potential disadvantages to neoadjuvant chemotherapy in this setting include increased perioperative morbidity and unclear long-term survival benefits.[24–27]

Use of neoadjuvant chemotherapy among patients with stage IV disease can cause hepatotoxicity and result in postoperative complications. Thus, colorectal cancer patients with advanced disease generally receive no more than three cycles of neoadjuvant chemotherapy before they undergo additional radiographic evaluation to assess for a response to treatment. Chemotherapeutic regimens and overall treatment plans may be reconsidered, or altered, when patients respond poorly in order to maximize the potential utility of chemotherapy while minimizing its negative effects.[28,29] Importantly, only 17% to 69% of colorectal cancer metastases in the liver that show a complete radiographic response to chemotherapy are entirely nonviable upon pathologic examination, so these lesions should ultimately be resected if possible.[30–33] Operative management is generally postponed for 4 to 5 weeks after completion of chemotherapy such that risks for liver-specific morbidity and mortality are decreased.

## Resection Strategies

Surgical approaches to management of advanced colorectal cancers are influenced by location of extracolonic disease as well as its immediate and long-term threat to patient well-being. Some patients who present with synchronous liver metastases undergo hepatectomy prior to surgical management of the primary tumor. This approach is suitable for patients with large but resectable liver metastases who may lose the window of opportunity for curative surgery if hepatectomy is delayed, but is generally applied only to patients who have asymptomatic primary tumors.[34–36] Other hepatic metastases may be managed during a one-stage operation that also involves removal of the primary tumor or a two-stage operation.[37] The latter strategy is commonly applied to patients with bilobar hepatic metastases who undergo simultaneous resection of the primary tumor and limited liver metastases followed by a second-stage major hepatic resection (Figure 17.3). A single-stage procedure generally results in shorter hospital stays, faster recovery from surgical therapy, and earlier initiation of adjuvant therapy with comparable morbidity to that of a two-stage approach.[8] However, patients who require complex procedures to remove the primary colorectal tumor as well as substantial liver surgery are probably best managed with a staged approach.

Intervals between surgical procedures are variable, but are timed to allow for maximal hypertrophy of the remnant liver. Patients may also undergo interventions to increase remnant mass, including portal vein embolization, parenchyma preserving techniques, and combination therapy with ablation (Figure 17.4). Preoperative portal vein embolization produces ipsilateral atrophy and contralateral hypertrophy of the liver remnant, thereby minimizing risk of postoperative liver failure, particularly among patients with underlying liver disease.[38] This technique is also useful when applied to patients with bilobar liver metastases in whom a two-stage liver resection is required to achieve complete surgical removal. Parenchymal preserving techniques, such as removal of posterior or anterior segments rather than formal right hepatectomy, achieve clear margins for many tumors while maximally preserving normal parenchyma. Parenchyma-sparing procedures are particularly useful in anticipation of repetitive operative needs.

## Interventional Procedures

Interventional endoscopists and radiologists facilitate care patients with stage IV disease. They perform a number of procedures that circumvent complications associated with invasive operations, such as stenting of partially obstructing lesions rather than operative colostomy, and prepare the patient for future, complex operative procedures. Radiofrequency ablation is used in combination with surgical resection as well as to treat unresectable lesions, provided all sites of disease are amenable to ablation or resection.[39] This technique utilizes high-frequency alternating current delivered *via* electrodes to increase tissue temperature, thereby promoting protein denaturation, tissue coagulation, and desiccation. Microwave ablation affects a larger tissue zone, is faster than radiofrequency ablation, and is associated with less blood vessel deflection and

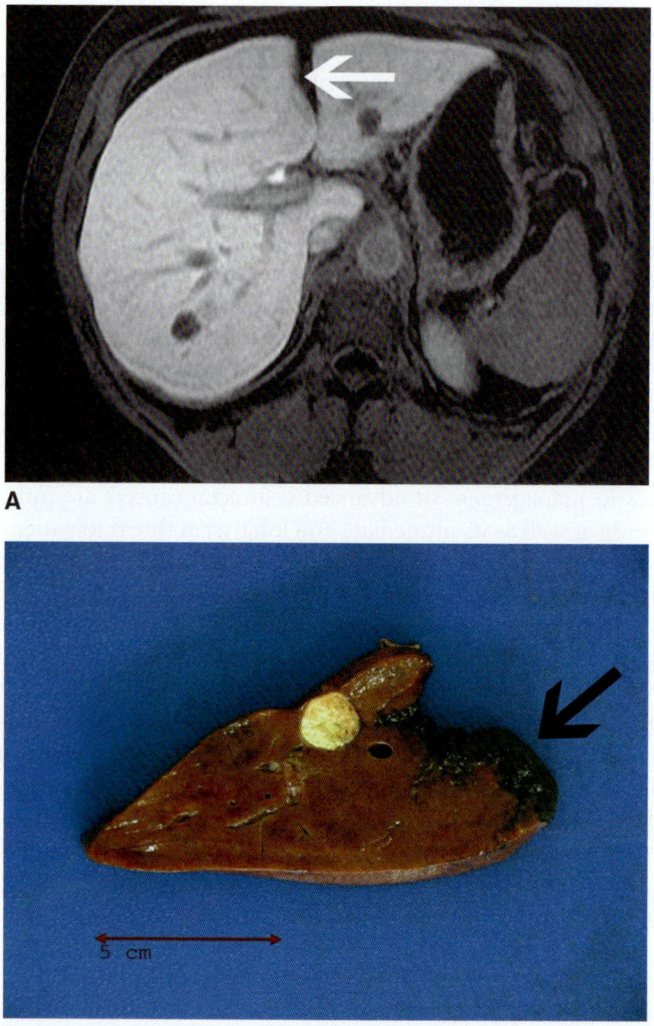


FIGURE 17.3: A patient with bilobar hepatic metastases may be successfully managed with multiple surgical procedures. First, a left-lateral sectionectomy removes a lesion in segment 2 with an adequate resection margin (*arrow*), yet deposits in the right lobe are not resected (**A**). The corresponding resection specimen contains the tumor, which is distant from the inked resection margin (*arrow*) (**B**).

heat-sink effect.[40] Ablative techniques are used to treat patients with bilobar hepatic metastases who require preservation of hepatic parenchyma, in which case they are applied to tumors in one lobe in combination with resection of tumors in another area. Repetitive ablation can be applied to tumor recurrences with reduced morbidity and affords progression-free survival benefit compared to chemotherapy alone for patients with inoperable disease.[41,42]

Arterial therapies, such as transarterial chemoembolization, hepatic arterial infusion chemotherapy, and selective internal radiation therapy, represent options for patients who are not surgical candidates and display a suboptimal response to systemic chemotherapy. Transarterial chemoembolization is a relatively selective method for targeting tumors, since they derive most of their blood supply from arteries rather than the portal venous system, which supplies the nonneoplastic hepatic parenchyma.[43–46] Hepatic arterial infusion chemotherapy can be used in combination with modern systemic chemotherapy in the neoadjuvant, second-line, and adjuvant treatment settings and is associated with higher response rates (22% to 62%) than systemic chemotherapy (9% to 25%).[45,47] Yttrium-90 microspheres delivered by selective internal radiation

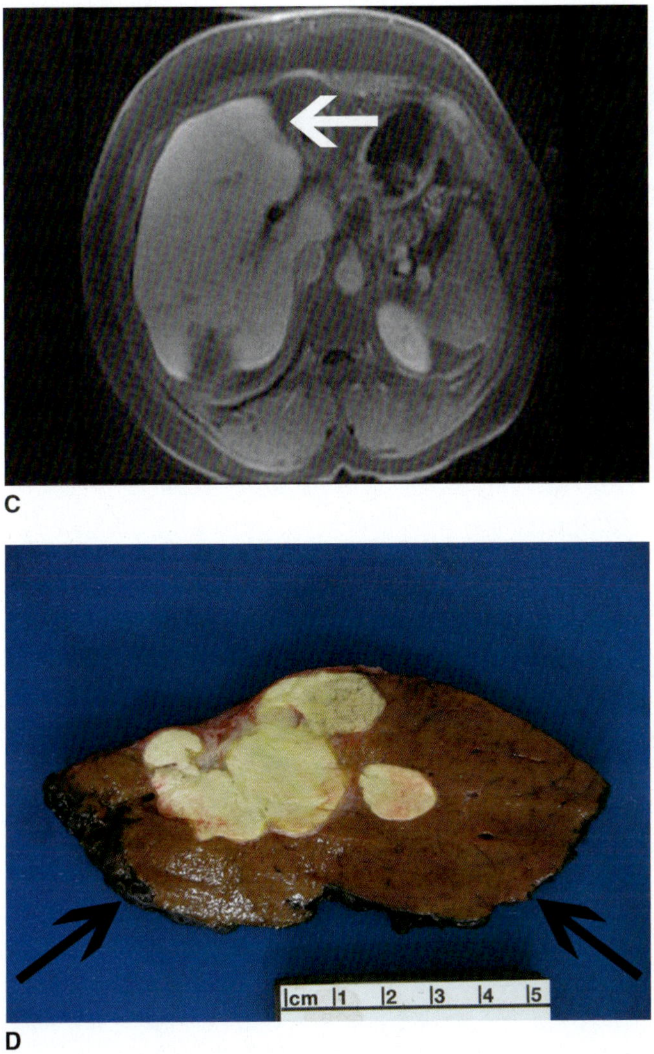


FIGURE 17.3: (*Continued*) Postoperative imagine demonstrates the resection margin (*arrow*) as well as a second larger mass in segment 7 (**C**). The subsequent resection specimen contains a large metastatic deposit with a clearly negative resection margin (*arrow*) (**D**).

therapy provide higher local doses than can be achieved by conventional radiation therapy because the microspheres are too large (mean diameter 20 to 40 μm) to pass through the arteriole–capillary plexus. Thus, a high radiation dose (>100 Gy) is delivered selectively to metastatic sites while sparing normal liver parenchyma.

## Treatment of Extrahepatic Metastases

The incidence of synchronous lung metastases among patients with colorectal cancer has increased over time, particularly among patients with rectal cancer in whom they are more common.[48] Many patients with pulmonary metastases also have hepatic tumor deposits, and, thus, successful surgical intervention requires that tumors in both sites be amenable to resection. Individuals with pulmonary and hepatic metastases treated by surgical removal may enjoy 5-year survival rates in excess of 50%, which are superior to those of patients who undergo treatment of hepatic metastases alone.[49,50] Thus, extrahepatic disease is no longer a contraindication to hepatectomy among patients with stage IV colorectal cancer, although surgical candidates require careful selection.[51]

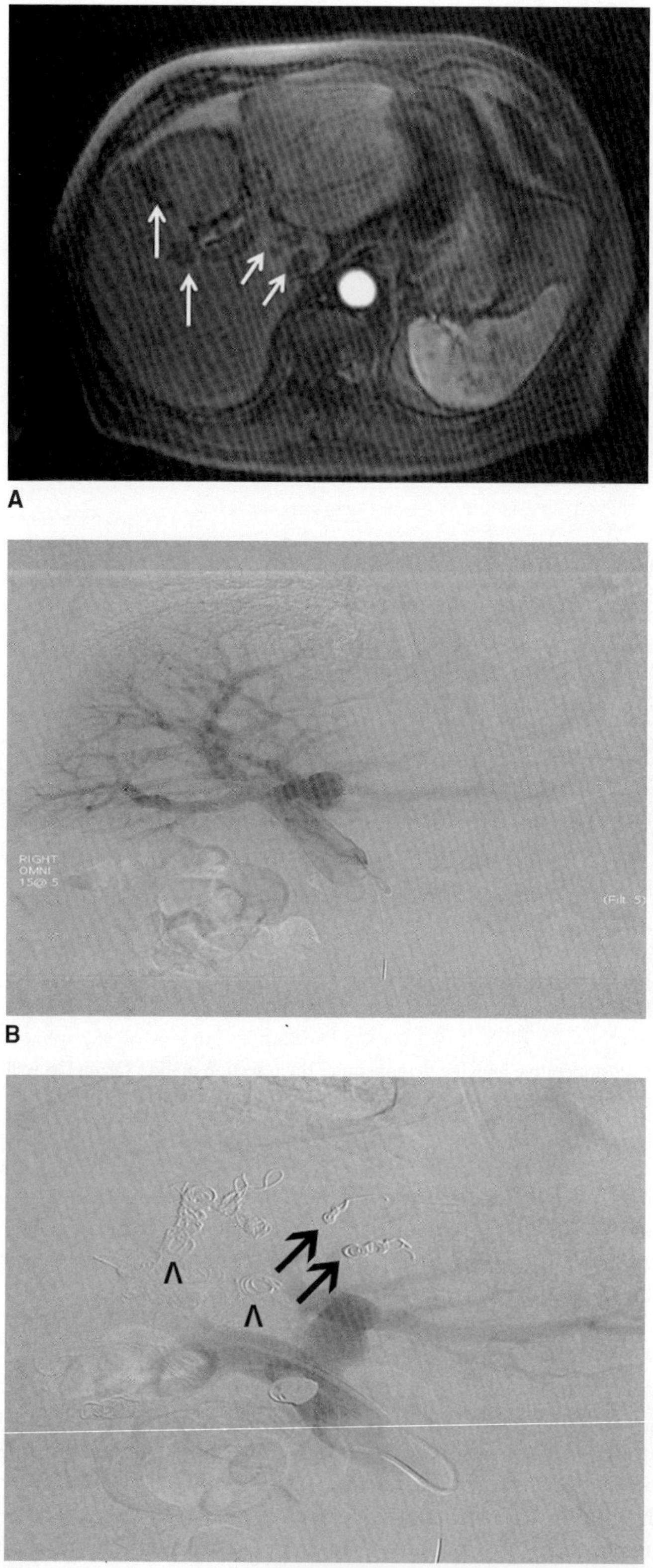


FIGURE 17.4: Colorectal cancer metastases (*arrows*) are present in segments 1, 4, and 5 (**A**). The right portal venous system is illustrated (**B**). Imaging of the portal venous system shows markedly diminished flow in the right portal vein branches (*arrowheads*) and segment 4 branches from the left portal vein (*arrows*) after successful embolization (**C**).

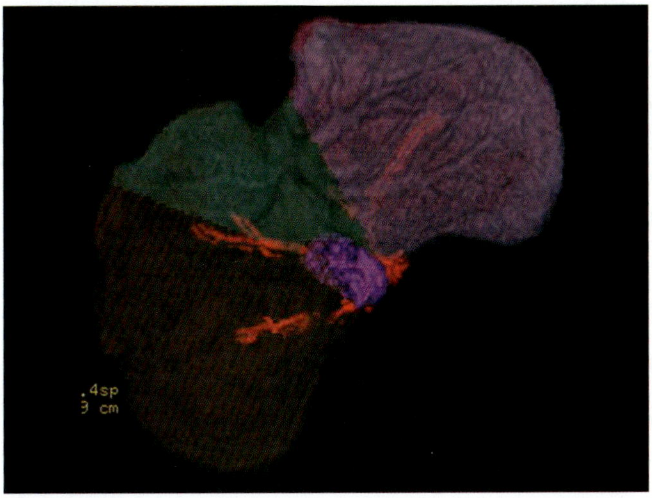


**D**

FIGURE 17.4: (*Continued*) Volume imaging 4 weeks after portal vein embolization demonstrates hypertrophy of segments 2 and 3 (s3), which are now similar in size to atrophic segments 5, 6, 7, and 8 (s5–8). The volumes of remnant segments 2 and 3 increased from less than 20% of total liver volume to 29% following embolization (**D**).

Management of multiorgan metastases, including peritoneal dissemination, is more challenging.[52] Peritoneal carcinomatosis develops in up to 44% of patients with recurrent colorectal cancer who undergo laparotomy and nearly 80% of patients who eventually succumb to cancer, so it is generally regarded as a terminal condition. Emerging techniques involving cytoreductive surgery with hyperthermic perioperative intraperitoneal chemotherapy provide a survival benefit in selected patients with this condition, especially when used in conjunction with systemic chemotherapy.[53–55] Initial aggressive surgical removal of all macroscopic peritoneal disease is followed by heated chemotherapy that presumably treats residual microscopic (i.e., nonvisible) peritoneal disease. Highly selected patients who complete cytoreductive surgery with hyperthermic perioperative intraperitoneal chemotherapy have prolonged survival (mean, 63 months) compared to patients treated with modern systemic chemotherapy (mean, 24 months).[56] Survivals are generally better among patients with low tumor burden in the peritoneal cavity who are treated at specialized centers.[53]

## SUMMARY AND CONCLUSIONS

Nearly half of colorectal cancer patients present with, or develop, distant metastases during the course of their lives, the presence of which powerfully impacts long-term survival. Multidisciplinary management of advanced disease is essential to providing state-of-the-art care and improving both survival and quality of life among these individuals. Application of aggressive surgical techniques, advanced endoscopic approaches, and interventional radiology procedures are increasingly used to control systemic disease, often in combination with modern chemotherapy and targeted biologic agents. Pathologists play an important role in assessing the efficacies of these modalities and facilitate planning of care for patients with stage IV colorectal cancer.

# References

1. Manfredi S, Lepage C, Hatem C, et al. Epidemiology and management of liver metastases from colorectal cancer. *Ann Surg* 2006;244(2):254–259.
2. Fong Y, Fortner J, Sun RL, et al. Clinical score for predicting recurrence after hepatic resection for metastatic colorectal cancer: analysis of 1001 consecutive cases. *Ann Surg* [Research Support, U.S. Gov't, P.H.S.] 1999;230(3):309–318; discussion 18–21.

3. Rees M, Tekkis PP, Welsh FK, et al. Evaluation of long-term survival after hepatic resection for metastatic colorectal cancer: a multifactorial model of 929 patients. *Ann Surg* 2008;247(1):125–135.
4. Watanabe K, Nagai K, Kobayashi A, et al. Factors influencing survival after complete resection of pulmonary metastases from colorectal cancer. *Br J Surg* 2009;96(9):1058–1065.
5. Pfannschmidt J, Dienemann H, Hoffmann H. Surgical resection of pulmonary metastases from colorectal cancer: a systematic review of published series. *Ann Thorac Surg* [Review] 2007;84(1):324–338.
6. Brown G. Specialist multidisciplinary team working in the treatment of cancer. *BMJ* [Editorial] 2012;344:e2780.
7. Van Cutsem E, Nordlinger B, Adam R, et al. Towards a pan-European consensus on the treatment of patients with colorectal liver metastases. *Eur J Cancer* [Review] 2006;42(14):2212–2221.
8. Charnsangavej C, Clary B, Fong Y, et al. Selection of patients for resection of hepatic colorectal metastases: expert consensus statement. *Ann Surg Oncol* 2006;13(10):1261–1268.
9. Levine RA, Chawla B, Bergeron S, et al. Multidisciplinary management of colorectal cancer enhances access to multimodal therapy and compliance with National Comprehensive Cancer Network (NCCN) guidelines. *Int J Colorectal Dis* 2012;27(11):1531–1538.
10. Wilks JA, Liebig C, Tasleem SH, et al. Rectal cancer patients benefit from implementation of a dedicated colorectal cancer center in a Veterans Affairs Medical Center. *Am J Surg* [Comparative Study] 2009;198(1):100–104.
11. Jones RP, Vauthey JN, Adam R, et al. Effect of specialist decision-making on treatment strategies for colorectal liver metastases. *Br J Surg* 2012;99(9):1263–1269.
12. Mala T, Bohler G, Mathisen O, et al. Hepatic resection for colorectal metastases: can preoperative scoring predict patient outcome? *World J Surg* 2002;26(11):1348–1353.
13. Chen YT, Henk MJ, Carney KJ, et al. Prognostic significance of tumor markers in colorectal cancer patients: DNA index, S-phase fraction, p53 expression, and Ki-67 index. *J Gastrointest Surg* 1997;1(3):266–272; discussion 73.
14. Domont J, Pawlik TM, Boige V, et al. Catalytic subunit of human telomerase reverse transcriptase is an independent predictor of survival in patients undergoing curative resection of hepatic colorectal metastases: a multicenter analysis. *J Clin Oncol* [Research Support, Non-U.S. Gov't] 2005;23(13):3086–3093.
15. Lee JK, Chan AT. Molecular prognostic and predictive markers in colorectal cancer: current status. *Curr Colorectal Cancer Rep* 2011;7(2):136–144.
16. Karapetis CS, Khambata-Ford S, Jonker DJ, et al. K-ras mutations and benefit from cetuximab in advanced colorectal cancer. *N Engl J Med* [Clinical Trial, Phase III Multicenter Study Randomized Controlled Trial Research Support, Non-U.S. Gov't] 2008;359(17):1757–1765.
17. Allegra CJ, Jessup JM, Somerfield MR, et al. American Society of Clinical Oncology provisional clinical opinion: testing for KRAS gene mutations in patients with metastatic colorectal carcinoma to predict response to anti-epidermal growth factor receptor monoclonal antibody therapy. *J Clin Oncol* [Review] 2009;27(12):2091–2096.
18. Abdel-Misih SR, Schmidt CR, Bloomston PM. Update and review of the multidisciplinary management of stage IV colorectal cancer with liver metastases. *World J Surg Oncol* [Review] 2009;7:72.
19. Gomez D, Cameron IC. Prognostic scores for colorectal liver metastasis: clinically important or an academic exercise? *HPB (Oxford)* [Review] 2010;12(4):227–238.
20. Juez I, Rubio C, Figueras J. Multidisciplinary approach of colorectal liver metastases. *Clin Transl Oncol* [Review] 2011;13(10):721–727.
21. Wieser M, Sauerland S, Arnold D, et al. Peri-operative chemotherapy for the treatment of resectable liver metastases from colorectal cancer: a systematic review and meta-analysis of randomized trials. *BMC Cancer* [Research Support, Non-U.S. Gov't Review] 2010;10:309.
22. Folprecht G, Grothey A, Alberts S, et al. Neoadjuvant treatment of unresectable colorectal liver metastases: correlation between tumour response and resection rates. *Ann Oncol* [Meta-Analysis] 2005;16(8):1311–1319.
23. Lam VW, Spiro C, Laurence JM, et al. A systematic review of clinical response and survival outcomes of downsizing systemic chemotherapy and rescue liver surgery in patients with initially unresectable colorectal liver metastases. *Ann Surg Oncol* [Review] 2012;19(4):1292–1301.
24. Goyer P, Karoui M, Vigano L, et al. Single-center multidisciplinary management of patients with colorectal cancer and resectable synchronous liver metastases improves outcomes. *Clin Res Hepatol Gastroenterol* 2013;37(1):47–55.

25. Karoui M, Soprani A, Charachon A, et al. Primary chemotherapy with or without colonic stent for management of irresectable stage IV colorectal cancer. *Eur J Surg Oncol* 2010;36(1):58–64.
26. Nordlinger B, Van Cutsem E, Gruenberger T, et al. Combination of surgery and chemotherapy and the role of targeted agents in the treatment of patients with colorectal liver metastases: recommendations from an expert panel. *Ann Oncol* [Consensus Development Conference Research Support, Non-U.S. Gov't] 2009;20(6):985–992.
27. Pinto Marques H, Barroso E, de Jong MC, et al. Peri-operative chemotherapy for resectable colorectal liver metastasis: does timing of systemic therapy matter? *J Surg Oncol* 2012;105(6):511–519.
28. Zorzi D, Laurent A, Pawlik TM, et al. Chemotherapy-associated hepatotoxicity and surgery for colorectal liver metastases. *Br J Surg* [Review] 2007;94(3):274–286.
29. Karoui M, Penna C, Amin-Hashem M, et al. Influence of preoperative chemotherapy on the risk of major hepatectomy for colorectal liver metastases. *Ann Surg* 2006;243(1):1–7.
30. Auer RC, White RR, Kemeny NE, et al. Predictors of a true complete response among disappearing liver metastases from colorectal cancer after chemotherapy. *Cancer* 2010;116(6):1502–1509.
31. Benoist S, Brouquet A, Penna C, et al. Complete response of colorectal liver metastases after chemotherapy: does it mean cure? *J Clin Oncol* [Clinical Trial Research Support, Non-U.S. Gov't] 2006;24(24):3939–3945.
32. van Vledder MG, de Jong MC, Pawlik TM, et al. Disappearing colorectal liver metastases after chemotherapy: should we be concerned? *J Gastrointest Surg* 2010;14(11):1691–1700.
33. Tanaka K, Takakura H, Takeda K, et al. Importance of complete pathologic response to prehepatectomy chemotherapy in treating colorectal cancer metastases. *Ann Surg* [Comparative Study] 2009;250(6): 935–942.
34. Aloia TA, Fahy BN. A decision analysis model predicts the optimal treatment pathway for patients with colorectal cancer and resectable synchronous liver metastases. *Clin Colorectal Cancer* 2008;7(3):197–201.
35. Cai GX, Cai SJ. Multi-modality treatment of colorectal liver metastases. *World J Gastroenterol*[Review] 2012;18(1):16–24.
36. Mentha G, Roth AD, Terraz S, et al. 'Liver first' approach in the treatment of colorectal cancer with synchronous liver metastases. *Dig Surg* 2008;25(6):430–435.
37. Karoui M, Vigano L, Goyer P, et al. Combined first-stage hepatectomy and colorectal resection in a two-stage hepatectomy strategy for bilobar synchronous liver metastases. *Br J Surg* [Evaluation Studies Multicenter Study] 2010;97(9):1354–1362.
38. Vauthey JN, Chaoui A, Do KA, et al. Standardized measurement of the future liver remnant prior to extended liver resection: methodology and clinical associations. *Surgery* 2000;127(5):512–519.
39. Wong SL, Mangu PB, Choti MA, et al. American Society of Clinical Oncology 2009 clinical evidence review on radiofrequency ablation of hepatic metastases from colorectal cancer. *J Clin Oncol*[Review] 2010;28(3):493–508.
40. Alberts SR. Update on the optimal management of patients with colorectal liver metastases. *Crit Rev Oncol Hematol* 2012;84(1):59–70.
41. Ruers T, Punt C, Van Coevorden F, et al. Radiofrequency ablation combined with systemic treatment versus systemic treatment alone in patients with non-resectable colorectal liver metastases: a randomized EORTC Intergroup phase II study (EORTC 40004). *Ann Oncol* 2012;23(10):2619–2626.
42. Kingham TP, Tanoue M, Eaton A, et al. Patterns of recurrence after ablation of colorectal cancer liver metastases. *Ann Surg Oncol* 2012;19(3):834–841.
43. Thng CH, Koh TS, Collins DJ, et al. Perfusion magnetic resonance imaging of the liver. *World J Gastroenterol* [Research Support, Non-U.S. Gov't Review] 2010;16(13):1598–1609.
44. de Baere T, Deschamps F. Arterial therapies of colorectal cancer metastases to the liver. *Abdom Imaging* [Review] 2011;36(6):661–670.
45. Kanat O, Gewirtz A, Kemeny N. What is the potential role of hepatic arterial infusion chemo-therapy in the current armamentarium against colorectal cancer. *J Gastrointest Oncol* 2012;3(2):130–138.
46. Abdullah SS, Pialat JB, Wiart M, et al. Characterization of hepatocellular carcinoma and colorectal liver metastasis by means of perfusion MRI. *J Magn Reson Imaging* 2008;28(2):390–395.
47. Kemeny NE, Niedzwiecki D, Hollis DR, et al. Hepatic arterial infusion versus systemic therapy for hepatic metastases from colorectal cancer: a randomized trial of efficacy, quality of life, and molecular markers (CALGB 9481). *J Clin Oncol* [Multicenter Study Randomized Controlled Trial Research Support, N.I.H., Extramural] 2006;24(9):1395–1403.

48. Mitry E, Guiu B, Cosconea S, et al. Epidemiology, management and prognosis of colorectal cancer with lung metastases: a 30-year population-based study. *Gut* [Multicenter Study] 2010;59(10):1383–1388.
49. Brouquet A, Vauthey JN, Contreras CM, et al. Improved survival after resection of liver and lung colorectal metastases compared with liver-only metastases: a study of 112 patients with limited lung metastatic disease. *J Am Coll Surg* [Research Support, N.I.H., Extramural] 2011;213(1):62–69; discussion 69–71.
50. Schule S, Dittmar Y, Knosel T, et al. Long-term results and prognostic factors after resection of hepatic and pulmonary metastases of colorectal cancer. *Int J Colorectal Dis* 2012;28(4):537–545.
51. Elias D, Liberale G, Vernerey D, et al. Hepatic and extrahepatic colorectal metastases: when resectable, their localization does not matter, but their total number has a prognostic effect. *Ann Surg Oncol* [Comparative Study] 2005;12(11):900–909.
52. Croner RS, Merkel S, Papadopoulos T, et al. Multivisceral resection for colon carcinoma. *Dis Colon Rectum* [Comparative Study] 2009;52(8):1381–1386.
53. Sugarbaker PH. Cytoreductive surgery plus hyperthermic perioperative chemotherapy for selected patients with peritoneal metastases from colorectal cancer: a new standard of care or an experimental approach? *Gastroenterol Res Pract* 2012;2012:309417.
54. Koppe MJ, Boerman OC, Oyen WJ, et al. Peritoneal carcinomatosis of colorectal origin: incidence and current treatment strategies. *Ann Surg* [Research Support, Non-U.S. Gov't Review] 2006;243(2):212–222.
55. Macri A, Saladino E, Bartolo V, et al. Peritoneal carcinomatosis of colorectal origin. *World J Gastrointest Oncol* 2010;2(2):98–101.
56. Elias D, Lefevre JH, Chevalier J, et al. Complete cytoreductive surgery plus intraperitoneal chemohyperthermia with oxaliplatin for peritoneal carcinomatosis of colorectal origin. *J Clin Oncol* [Research Support, Non-U.S. Gov't] 2009;27(5):681–685.

SECTION

# VI

# Neoplasms of the Vermiform Appendix

# 18 Endocrine Cell (Carcinoid) Tumors of the Vermiform Appendix

Rhonda K. Yantiss

A variety of neoplasms develop in the appendix, many of which are incidentally discovered tumors encountered in appendectomy specimens obtained for other reasons. Of these, endocrine (carcinoid) tumors are, by far, most common. Endocrine neoplasms are recognized by their histologic patterns, cytoplasmic argentaffinity or argyrophilia, and immunohistochemical staining for cytosolic markers (e.g., neuron-specific enolase and CD56), vesicles (e.g., synaptophysin), or secretory granules (e.g., chromogranin). Most endocrine tumors of the appendix are composed of enterochromaffin cells similar to those of tumors involving the distal small intestine and have been termed "classic" carcinoid tumors. These lesions should be distinguished from goblet cell carcinoid tumors, as discussed in Chapter 20.

## CLINICAL FEATURES OF ENDOCRINE (CARCINOID) TUMORS

Endocrine tumors account for slightly more than 50% of all appendiceal neoplasms and nearly 20% of all gastrointestinal endocrine tumors. They are identified in less than 1% of patients undergoing appendectomy.[1] Most tumors are identified in appendices obtained from adults but tend to occur in a slightly younger age group than endocrine tumors elsewhere in the gastrointestinal tract. Females are affected more often than males, although some of the difference may reflect the greater number of incidental appendectomies performed on women undergoing gynecologic surgery.[2] Appendiceal endocrine tumors are usually located in the distal appendix and, thus, are asymptomatic. Some tumors that develop in the mid or proximal appendix are associated with appendicitis, presumably due to obstruction of the lumen.

## PATHOLOGIC FEATURES OF ENDOCRINE TUMORS

### Enterochromaffin Cell Endocrine Tumors (Classic Carcinoid Tumors)

Appendiceal endocrine tumors appear as yellow, or white, firm nodules in the appendiceal tip, and most are composed of enterochromaffin cells (Figure 18.1). These serotonin-producing tumors are usually low grade and contain cells that are argentaffin and argyrophil positive. The tumors are well circumscribed, but unencapsulated, and consist of tightly packed nests and acini containing neoplastic cells that fill the mucosa and variably extend into the appendiceal wall (Figure 18.2). Acinar structures may harbor luminal material that is positive for periodic acid–Schiff stain but lack mucin production. The tumor cells contain abundant amphophilic or eosinophilic granular cytoplasm with round, smooth nuclei and coarse "salt and pepper" chromatin and rare mitoses (Figure 18.3). Some may contain spindle cells, whereas others show nuclear pleomorphism and multinucleation. Enterochromaffin cells show strong immunohistochemical staining for

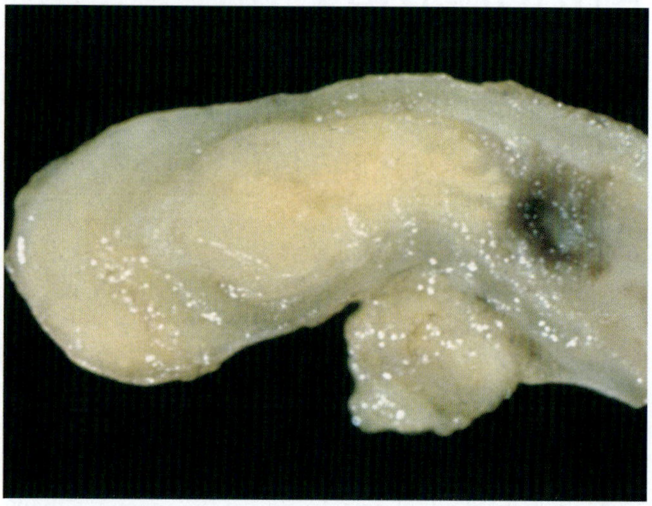

FIGURE 18.1: An endocrine tumor forms an unencapsulated yellow nodule in the distal tip of the appendix. The lesion fills the submucosa and extends into the muscularis propria. (Reprinted from Panarelli N, Yantiss R. *Frozen Section Laboratory: Appendix, Colon, and Anus*. New York, NY: Springer; 2010, with permission.)

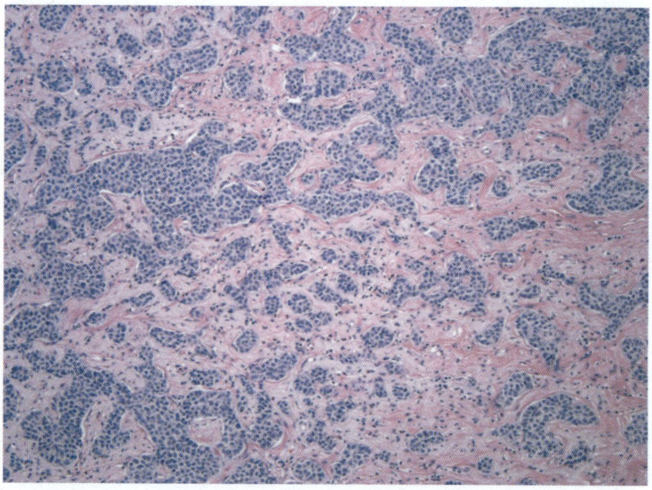

FIGURE 18.2: Enterochromaffin cell endocrine tumors resemble lesions of the distal jejunum and ileum. They contain solid cell nests and trabeculae enmeshed in a collagenous stroma.

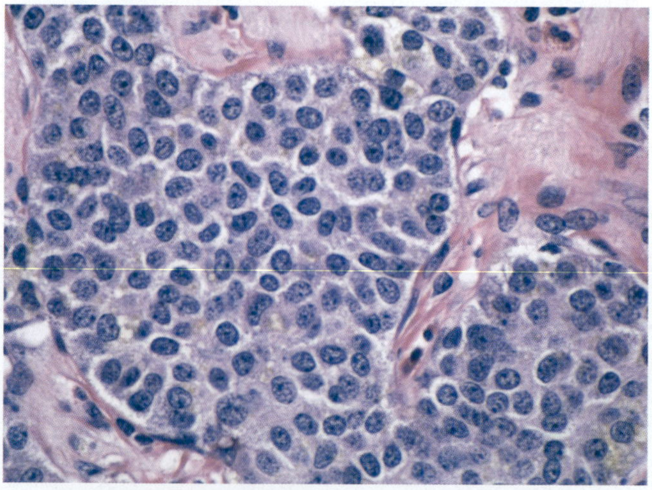

FIGURE 18.3: Lesional cells of an enterochromaffin cell tumor contain abundant faintly eosinophilic cytoplasm and ovoid nuclei with smooth membranes. The nuclei are small with inconspicuous nucleoli and stippled chromatin.

chromogranin A, synaptophysin, serotonin, and substance P. Tumor cell nests are surrounded by sustentacular cells that are immunopositive for S-100 protein. More than 70% of serotonin-producing endocrine tumors of the appendix span less than 1 cm in diameter and show very low proliferation indices by Ki-67 immunolabeling.[3]

## Enteroglucagon (L) Cell Endocrine Tumors

Enteroglucagon cell endocrine tumors composed of L cells are much less common. They contain cells arranged in a trabecular pattern that harbor enteroglucagons (glicentin and oxyntomodulin), glucagon-like peptides (GLP1 and GLP2), pancreatic polypeptide, or peptide YY. These lesions are small, often spanning only 2 to 3 mm in diameter, and consist of tumor cells arranged in anastomosing trabeculae and cords (Figure 18.4). The tumor cells are argyrophilic and show immunopositivity for chromogranin B and carcinoembryonic antigen (CEA) but are often negative for chromogranin A.[4] Immunolabeling indices for Ki-67 are quite low, and most tumors behave in an indolent fashion.

## Tubular Endocrine Tumors

Tubular endocrine tumors may represent a variant of enteroglucagon (L) cell endocrine tumor with a predominantly acinar growth pattern. They generally behave in a benign fashion and show a predilection for the distal appendix of young adults (Figure 18.5).[5] Tubular endocrine tumors

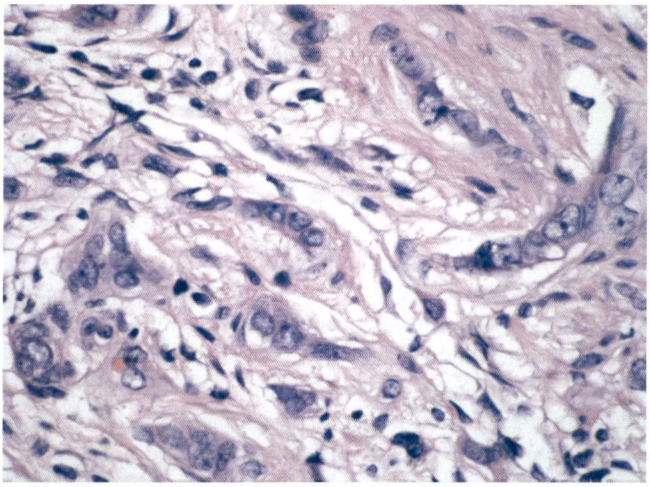

FIGURE 18.4: An enteroglucagon (L) cell tumor contains cords and clusters of lesional cells associated with cellular stroma.

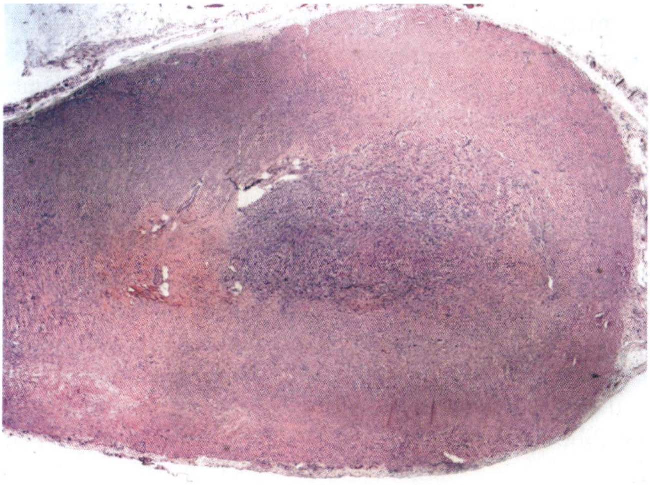

FIGURE 18.5: A tubular endocrine tumor in the tip of the appendix is associated with obliteration of the lumen.

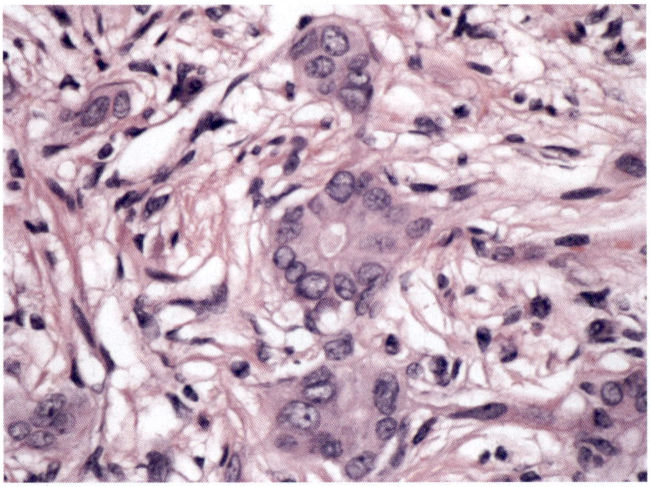

FIGURE 18.6: A tubular endocrine tumor contains bland cells arranged in small tubules and acini that do not contain mucin.

are composed of small tubules, some of which harbor inspissated mucin. They contain cytologically bland tumor cells without substantial mitotic activity (Figure 18.6). These tumors are usually positive for chromogranin B and glucagon similar to L cell tumors but are negative for chromogranin A and S-100 protein.[5] They may show focal or diffuse immunopositivity for cytokeratins 7 and 20, and thus, these markers may not be of value when distinguishing these lesions from appendiceal carcinomas.[6]

## PATHOLOGIC REPORTING OF APPENDICEAL ENDOCRINE TUMORS

The WHO has moved away from the "carcinoid" terminology throughout the gastrointestinal tract and recommends three general categories to describe a spectrum of neoplasms, well-differentiated (neuro)endocrine tumors, poorly differentiated (neuro)endocrine carcinomas, and mixed adeno(neuro)endocrine carcinomas, based on mitotic activity, Ki-67 immunohistochemical labeling, and morphologic features (Table 18.1).[7] Virtually all endocrine neoplasms of the appendix are well-differentiated tumors, whereas poorly differentiated carcinomas are distinctly uncommon. Mixed adeno(neuro)endocrine carcinomas are derived from goblet cell carcinoid tumors, as discussed in Chapter 20. The most recent version of the American Joint Commission on *Cancer Staging Manual* incorporated appendiceal carcinoid tumors into the TNM staging system.[8] Other key information included in pathology reports includes margin status, proliferation indices, and the presence of any aggressive features, such as lymphovascular invasion and involvement of mesoappendiceal soft tissues. Perineural invasion is commonly observed among appendiceal endocrine neoplasms, but this feature is not an independent prognostic factor.

## BIOLOGIC BEHAVIOR AND MANAGEMENT

Most appendiceal endocrine tumors behave in a clinically benign fashion, but those that metastasize spread first to regional lymph nodes followed by the liver, at which point they may produce the carcinoid syndrome. Less than 1% of tumors smaller than 2 cm in diameter metastasize. For this reason, small (≤1 cm) appendiceal endocrine tumors are adequately treated with appendectomy alone. Tumors larger than 2 cm are treated with right colectomy and lymph node dissection owing to the greater likelihood of regional lymph node metastases and vascular

**Table 18.1 World Health Organization Classification of Appendiceal Endocrine Tumors**

| Tumor Differentiation and Subtypes | Characteristics | Immunohistochemistry Positivity |
|---|---|---|
| **Well-Differentiated Endocrine Neoplasm** | | |
| Enterochromaffin cell endocrine tumor | Most common<br>Variable size, most <1 cm<br>Nests and acini<br>Up to 40% show deep mural invasion | Serotonin<br>Substance P<br>S-100<br>Chromogranin A |
| Enteroglucagon L cell endocrine tumor | Uncommon<br>Small (2–3 mm)<br>Tubular and trabecular pattern | Glucagon-like peptides<br>Pancreatic polypeptide<br>Peptide YY |
| Tubular endocrine tumor | Least common<br>Small tubules with mucin in lumina | Glucagons<br>Serotonin |
| **Poorly Differentiated Endocrine Carcinoma** | | |
| Small cell carcinoma | Rare | Chromogranin A |
| Large cell carcinoma | Usually associated with adenocarcinoma | Synaptophysin |
| **Mixed Adenoendocrine Carcinoma** | | |
| Usually derived from goblet cell carcinoid | Older patients<br>Submucosal concentric growth<br>Mucin production<br>Often overt carcinomatous component | Chromogranin A<br>Serotonin<br>Somatostatin<br>Carcinoembryonic antigen (CEA) |

invasion. Tumors that span 1 to 2 cm may be treated with additional surgery depending on the presence, or absence, of other features suggestive of aggressive behavior, such as invasion of the mesoappendix, vascular invasion, mitotic activity, and high proliferation rates.[9] Most studies have failed to show a survival benefit to extensive surgery among patients with larger tumors.[10]

## SUMMARY AND CONCLUSIONS

Appendiceal endocrine tumors display a variety of growth patterns and immunohistochemical expression profiles depending on the peptides they elaborate. Most of these lesions are small, incidentally discovered tumors detected in appendectomy specimens obtained for other indications, and thus, they tend to be small and asymptomatic. Tumors more frequently occur in the distal appendix distant from the resection margin. Small lesions are adequately managed by appendectomy alone, whereas larger tumors (i.e., more than 2 cm in diameter) are at increased risk for aggressive biologic behavior and generally require more extensive surgery with lymph node dissection. New guidelines recommend use of Ki-67 immunohistochemistry for pathologic grade assessment, whereas staging criteria are enumerated in the AJCC *Cancer Staging Manual*, seventh Edition.[8]

# References


1. In't Hof KH, van der Wal HC, Kazemier G, et al. Carcinoid tumour of the appendix: an analysis of 1,485 consecutive emergency appendectomies. *J Gastrointest Surg* [Comparative Study Multicenter Study]. 2008;12(8):1436–1438.
2. Hemminki K, Li X. Incidence trends and risk factors of carcinoid tumors: a nationwide epidemiologic study from Sweden. *Cancer* [Research Support, Non-U.S. Gov't] 2001;92(8):2204–2210.
3. Deans GT, Spence RA. Neoplastic lesions of the appendix. *Br J Surg* [Review] 1995;82(3):299–306.
4. Williams GT. Endocrine tumours of the gastrointestinal tract-selected topics. *Histopathology* [Review] 2007;50(1):30–41.
5. Burke AP, Sobin LH, Federspiel BH, et al. Goblet cell carcinoids and related tumors of the vermiform appendix. *Am J Clin Pathol* 1990;94(1):27–35.
6. Matsukuma KE, Montgomery EA. Tubular carcinoids of the appendix: the CK7/CK20 immunophenotype can be a diagnostic pitfall. *J Clin Pathol* 2012;65(7):666–668.
7. Komminoth P, Arnold R, Capella C, et al. Neuroendocrine neoplasms of the appendix. In: Bosman FT, Carneiro F, Hruban RH, et al., eds. *WHO Classification of Tumours of the Digestive System*. 4th ed. Lyon, France: International Agency for Research on Cancer; 2010:126–128.
8. Appendix. In: Edge SB, Byrd DR, Compton CC, et al., eds. *AJCC Cancer Staging Manual*. 7th ed. New York, NY: Springer; 2009:133–141.
9. Stinner B, Rothmund M. Neuroendocrine tumours (carcinoids) of the appendix. *Best Pract Res Clin Gastroenterol* [Comparative Study Review] 2005;19(5):729–738.
10. Plockinger U, Couvelard A, Falconi M, et al. Consensus guidelines for the management of patients with digestive neuroendocrine tumours: well-differentiated tumour/carcinoma of the appendix and goblet cell carcinoma. *Neuroendocrinology* 2008;87(1):20–30.

# Appendiceal Mucinous Neoplasms and Pseudomyxoma Peritonei

# 19

Joseph Misdraji

Most epithelial neoplasms of the appendix are of mucinous type and characteristically cause cystic dilatation of the appendix with accumulation of copious gelatinous material. Their importance lies in the fact that they can disseminate in the peritoneal cavity and coat serosal surfaces with mucinous tumor deposits, a finding that has been called "pseudomyxoma peritonei." The appendiceal mucinous neoplasm has been the subject of numerous debates since its recognition as the source of pseudomyxoma peritonei. Philosophical differences regarding the nature of pseudomyxoma peritonei have generated a number of classification systems for appendiceal mucinous neoplasms. The inconsistent diagnostic terminology has resulted in considerable confusion with respect to the pathologic classification of appendiceal mucinous neoplasms and pseudomyxoma peritonei, with ramifications on patient management and research in this area. The purpose of this chapter is to discuss the pathologic and clinical features of these lesions, as well as their biologic behavior and clinical management. Other epithelial tumors of the appendix are discussed in Chapter 20.

## CLASSIFICATION OF MUCINOUS NEOPLASMS OF THE APPENDIX AND PERITONEUM

There is considerable controversy regarding the most appropriate terminology for appendiceal mucinous tumors and pseudomyxoma peritonei because tumors that resemble appendiceal adenomas can disseminate to the peritoneum and cause the death of the patient. Most of the debate is due to philosophical differences regarding the nature of pseudomyxoma peritonei. One viewpoint is that pseudomyxoma peritonei results from rupture of an adenoma of the appendix, with seeding of the peritoneum by low-grade neoplastic, but noninvasive mucinous epithelium. Investigators with this viewpoint classify pseudomyxoma peritonei as disseminated peritoneal adenomucinosis.[1] The opposing view is that peritoneal dissemination is equivalent to carcinoma and that the source appendiceal tumors are actually adenocarcinomas.[2,3] However, the criteria for invasion in appendiceal tumors are poorly defined, and their proposed classifications reflect the difficulty of assigning them into benign or malignant categories (Table 19.1).[1–5] The Armed Forces Institute of Pathology proposed that appendiceal mucinous neoplasms be classified as adenomas, tumors of uncertain malignant potential, and invasive mucinous carcinoma, based on tumor stage.[2] That scheme defines adenomas as mucinous neoplasms confined to the mucosa with intact muscularis mucosae, whereas tumors with infiltrative mural invasion or proliferation of neoplastic epithelium outside the appendix (pseudomyxoma peritonei) are considered to be carcinomas. More problematic tumors that show "pushing" invasion with tongues of epithelium dissecting outward in a "diverticulum-like" fashion or acellular mucin outside the appendix associated with loss of the muscularis mucosae are classified as mucinous tumor of uncertain

Table 19.1 Classification Schemes for Mucinous Neoplasms of the Appendix

| Pathologic Features | Carr and Sobin[2] | Misdraji et al.[4] | Pai and Longacre[5] | World Health Organization[7] |
|---|---|---|---|---|
| Tumors without invasion (intact muscularis mucosae) | Adenoma | LAMN | Adenoma | Adenoma |
| Tumors with Pushing Invasion | | | | |
| • Tumor confined to the appendix | Mucinous tumor of uncertain malignant potential | LAMN | Adenoma | LAMN |
| • Tumor with acellular mucin outside the appendix | Mucinous tumor of uncertain malignant potential | LAMN | Low-grade mucinous neoplasm with low risk of recurrence | LAMN |
| • Tumor with extraappendiceal tumor | Mucinous adenocarcinoma | LAMN | Low-grade mucinous neoplasm with high risk of recurrence | LAMN |
| Tumors with Infiltrative Invasion | | | | |
| Infiltrative invasion of wall, with or without desmoplasia, regardless of stage | Invasive mucinous adenocarcinoma | Invasive mucinous adenocarcinoma | Invasive mucinous adenocarcinoma | Invasive mucinous adenocarcinoma |

malignant potential. Others define the uncertain malignant potential category as tumors with involvement of the proximal margin, tumors with mucin or epithelium in the appendiceal wall that is not clearly invasive, and cases in which the possibility of extraappendiceal epithelium cannot be excluded.[5,6] Some have suggested that, to avoid nomenclature confusion, the entire spectrum of mucinous tumors, from adenomas to mucinous tumors with presumed pushing invasion and pseudomyxoma peritonei, be classified using a single-term, low-grade appendiceal mucinous neoplasms (LAMN) and that the pathology report describes the stage of disease.[4] In its most recent classification of gastrointestinal tumors, the World Health Organization adopted this terminology to describe low-grade carcinomas but maintained the term adenoma for tumors confined to the mucosa.[7]

## APPENDICEAL ADENOMA AND CYSTADENOMA

Adenomas are benign tumors of the appendix that are often incidental lesions detected in appendectomy specimens obtained for other reasons, but they can present with right lower quadrant pain and infrequently a palpable right lower quadrant mass. They might not produce any gross abnormalities or can cause cystic dilatation due to accumulation of tenacious mucin, but they do not display mucin on the external surface. Adenomas are confined to the appendiceal mucosa and surrounded by intact muscularis mucosae, although the lymphoid tissue of the lamina propria is often atrophic (Figure 19.1).[2,4,8] Tumors are composed of a villous or flat proliferation of mucinous epithelial cells with abundant intracytoplasmic mucin (Figure 19.2). Deeper glands typically have straight luminal edges, although serrated architecture may also be present, mimicking the appearance of a serrated polyp, as discussed in Chapter 20.[1,2] Mucin accumulation frequently produces cystic dilatation of the appendix, in which case the term cystadenoma may be applied. Cystadenomas mostly contain a flat, undulating epithelial cell lining with infrequent villous areas that distinguish these lesions from retention cysts (Figure 19.3).[2,4,8,9]

Appendiceal mucinous adenomas display a spectrum of cytologic atypia, which is classified as low- or high-grade dysplasia in the same manner as in other parts of the gastrointestinal tract. Most tumors are low grade with nuclear hyperchromasia, pseudostratification, rare mitoses, and apoptotic nuclear debris.[4,9,10] High-grade tumors show a greater degree of nuclear pleomorphism with stratification and loss of cell polarity equivalent to intraepithelial carcinoma (Figure 19.4). However, appendiceal mucinous adenomas have no potential for aggressive clinical behavior and are cured by appendectomy. Mucinous neoplasms associated with mural changes, such as disruption of the muscularis mucosae or replacement of the muscularis mucosae by fibrous tissue, or with extraappendiceal mucin are better classified as LAMN to convey some degree of uncertainty regarding the biologic potential of the lesion.

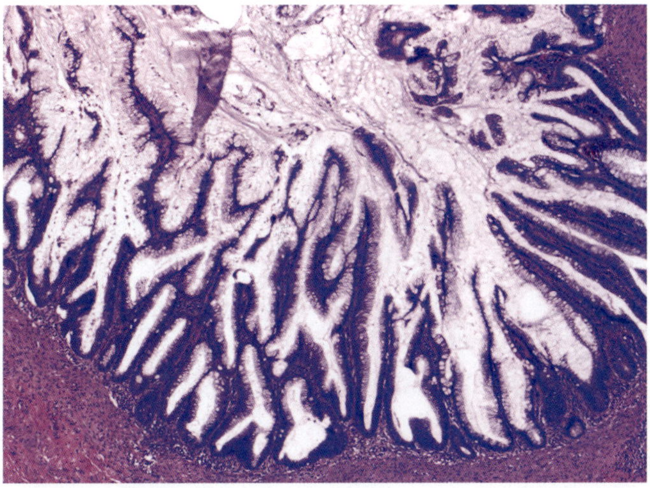

**FIGURE 19.1:** An appendiceal villous adenoma is composed of slender villi lined by mucinous epithelial cells with an intact muscularis mucosae. The appendiceal lymphoid tissue is atrophic.

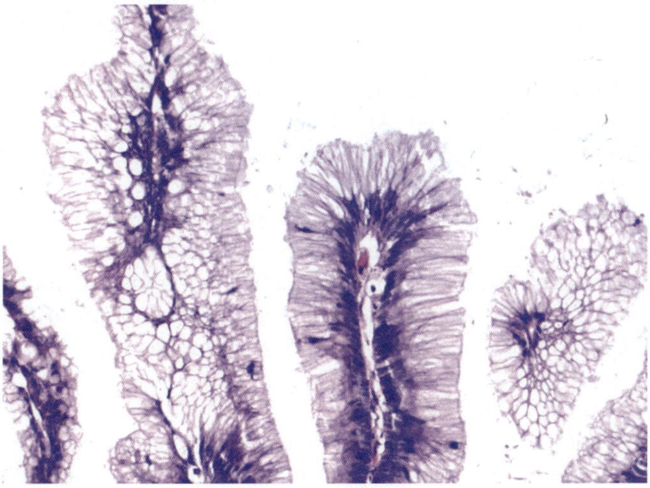

**FIGURE 19.2:** The villi of an appendiceal mucinous adenoma are lined by columnar mucinous epithelial cells containing tall mucin vacuoles. The nuclei show mild hyperchromasia and nuclear pseudostratification, similar to low-grade dysplasia in other parts of the gastrointestinal tract.

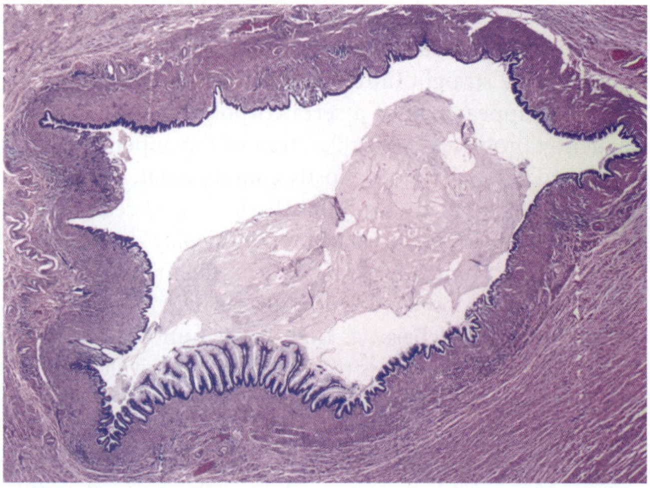

FIGURE 19.3: An appendiceal mucinous cystadenoma contains an undulating, flat lining of mucinous epithelial cells with only a small area of villous projections (**lower left**). The muscularis mucosae is intact.

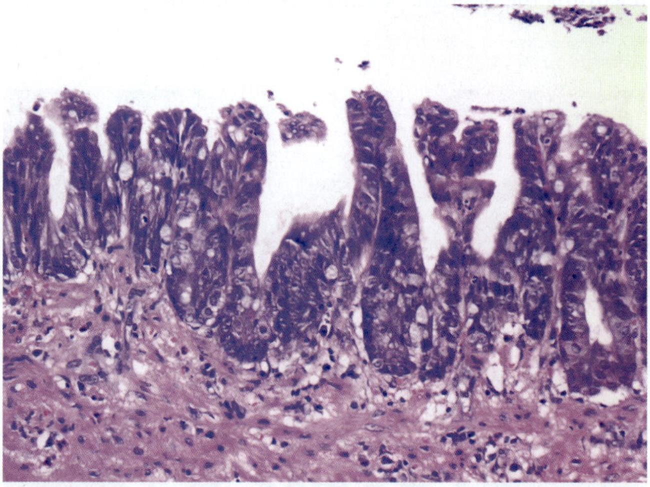

FIGURE 19.4: A mucinous adenoma with high-grade dysplasia is confined to the mucosa but shows nuclear hyperchromasia, nuclear disarray, and full-thickness nuclear stratification.

# LOW-GRADE APPENDICEAL MUCINOUS NEOPLASM

LAMN resemble appendiceal adenomas but have the propensity to spread to the peritoneum, recur, and result in the death of the patient. They contain mucinous epithelium and display a villous architecture or undulating, flat luminal surface. Unlike adenomas, LAMN show pushing invasion through the muscularis mucosae, hyalinizing fibrosis of the muscularis mucosae, or frank rupture of the appendix with extruded mucin. Unfortunately, criteria for mural invasion in appendiceal mucinous neoplasms are not well defined. As a result, they have been variably classified as ruptured adenomas, tumors of uncertain malignant potential, and adenocarcinomas reflecting the difficulty of classifying them as benign or malignant (Table 19.1).[1–3,5,7–9,11,12] The most recent World Health Organization classification scheme denotes low-grade mucinous tumors with pushing invasion as LAMN, whereas the term mucinous adenocarcinoma is reserved for high-grade tumors or those with conventional invasion.[7] Both low- and high-grade mucinous neoplasms that extend beyond the muscularis mucosae are staged as adenocarcinomas in the seventh edition of the American Joint Committee on *Cancer (AJCC) Staging Manual.*[13]

## Clinical Features

LAMN typically occur in the sixth decade of life.[2] Abdominal pain that mimics acute appendicitis and an abdominal mass are the most common presentations, but many lesions are discovered incidentally, particularly in women undergoing gynecologic surgery.[4,9]

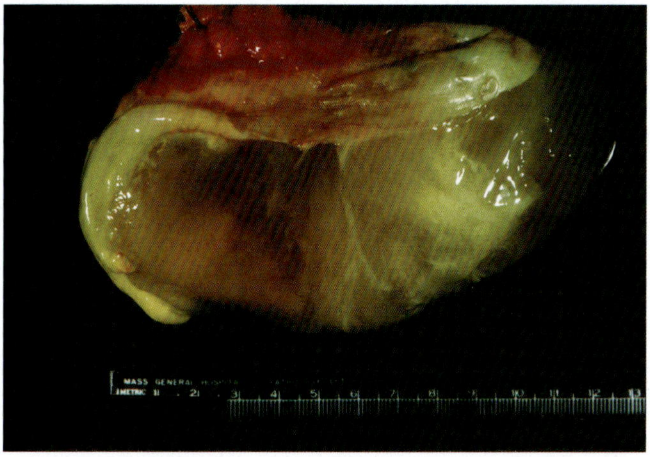


FIGURE 19.5: A ruptured low-grade mucinous neoplasm produces appendiceal dilatation. The rupture exposes copious mucin in the lumen.

## Pathologic Features

LAMN may appear grossly unremarkable or produce a cystically dilated appendix filled with tenacious mucin. The wall is variably fibrotic and calcified. Mucin extruding onto the serosal surface is important to note at the time of gross examination (Figure 19.5). The appendix may even be encased in, or replaced by, mucinous tumor.

LAMN resemble mucinous adenomas; they are villous or flat, composed of tall mucinous epithelial cells, and show atrophy of lamina propria lymphoid tissue.[2,4,8] The villi are typically slender with scant lamina propria and have straight luminal edges. Mucin accumulation and cystic dilatation of the appendix produce attenuation or denudation of the lining epithelium.[8] Some tumors may show denudation of virtually the entire appendiceal mucosa that simulates a retention cyst, and thus, extensive sampling to uncover a focus of neoplastic mucinous epithelium should be performed in such cases.[9,11] The mucinous epithelial cells are columnar with abundant mucin and display low-grade cytologic atypia.[4,9,10]

LAMN are cytologically indistinguishable from appendiceal adenomas but show a distinct manner of invasion of the underlying appendiceal wall. They do not invade in the conventional manner with desmoplastic stroma and a destructive proliferation of irregularly infiltrative glands. Rather, these lesions are associated with pushing invasion and effacement of the muscularis mucosae, mural fibrosis, hyalinization, and dystrophic calcification.[4,8,14] LAMN may dissect into or through the wall and create diverticula-like herniations or grow directly on fibrotic or hyalinized tissue rather than on muscularis mucosae (Figure 19.6). Some tumors overtly perforate the appendix and have been historically classified as "ruptured adenomas." However, designation of these tumors as adenomas should be avoided because such terminology does not adequately describe the risk of developing pseudomyxoma peritonei.[7]

## Natural History

The prognosis of LAMN is dependent on their stage.[6,13] Tumors confined to the appendix that are unassociated with extraappendiceal mucin are almost always cured by appendectomy. Tumors associated with acellular mucin in the peritoneal cavity or mucinous neoplasia confined to the right lower quadrant ("localized pseudomyxoma peritonei") are associated with an extremely low risk of progression to widespread pseudomyxoma peritonei, particularly if the entire appendix and all the periappendiceal mucin are histologically evaluated to exclude the presence of extraappendiceal neoplastic epithelium.[15] However, up to 33% of patients with any neoplastic epithelium outside the appendix, yet limited to the right lower quadrant, may develop disseminated peritoneal disease that can result in the eventual death of the patient.[6,15] Extensive peritoneal dissemination (pseudomyxoma peritonea) has a progressive clinical course with a high risk of death of disease as described below.

FIGURE 19.6: LAMN herniate through the muscularis propria (**upper left**) and are bound only by fibrous tissue along the bottom of the image (**A**). Another tumor irregularly dissects into the muscularis propria resembling a diverticulum (**B**).

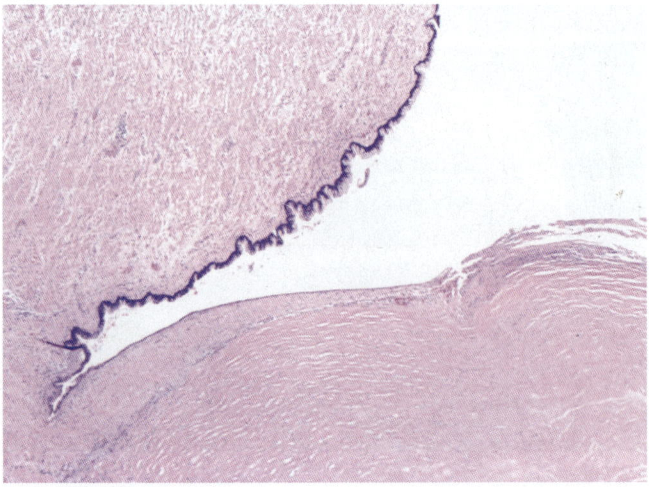

A

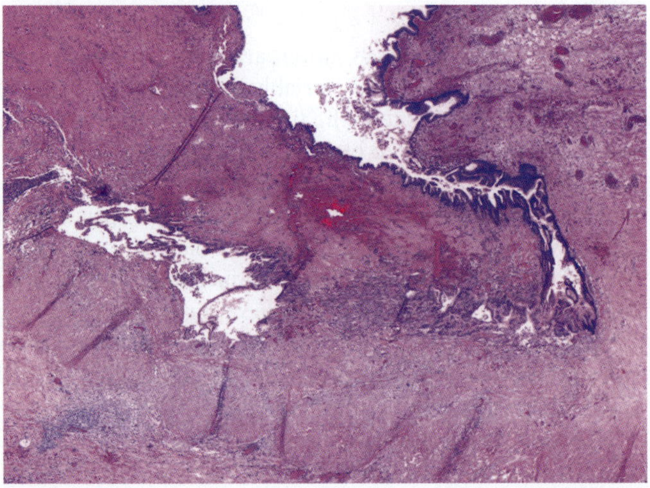

B

## Treatment

Simple appendectomy is sufficient treatment for LAMN confined to the appendix. Patients with acellular mucin on the appendiceal serosa should undergo radiographic surveillance to ensure that mucinous ascites does not develop. Tumors that have spread to the right lower quadrant have a somewhat higher risk of recurrence, but appropriate management for these patients is not standardized. Right hemicolectomy offers no benefit over appendectomy for patients with LAMN, even in the event of rupture.[16,17] Tumors that have disseminated widely throughout the peritoneal cavity are treated by either debulking or complete peritonectomy with heated intraperitoneal chemotherapy as discussed in the next section.

# PSEUDOMYXOMA PERITONEI AND PERITONEAL MUCINOUS ADENOCARCINOMA

## Clinical Features

Pseudomyxoma peritonei is a descriptive term used to denote accumulation of mucin in the peritoneal cavity secondary to dissemination of a mucinous neoplasm (Figure 19.7). Most cases develop secondary to spread of a LAMN or, less commonly, mucinous adenocarcinoma. Patients

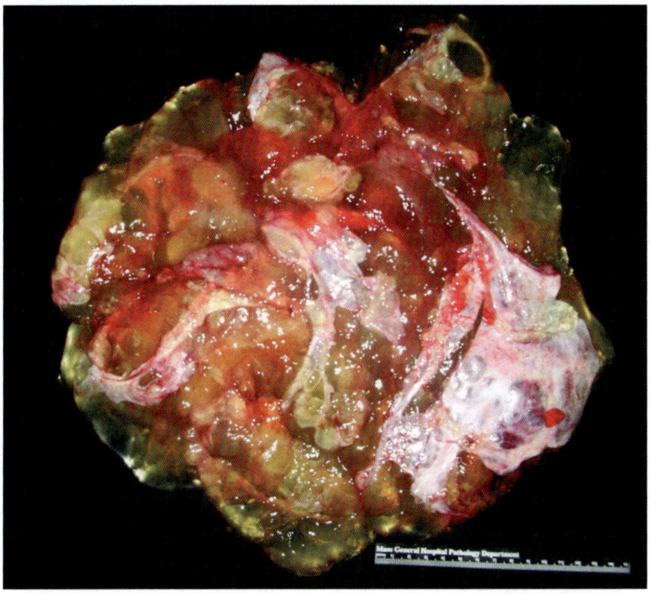

FIGURE 19.7: Classic pseudomyxoma peritonei shows bulky peritoneal tumors composed of abundant tenacious mucin.

are typically in the seventh decade of life, and women are affected more often than men.[18] Mucin accumulates in those areas from which ascitic fluid is resorbed or in dependent areas.[11] These areas include the greater omentum, undersurface of the right hemidiaphragm, pelvis, right retrohepatic space, left abdominal gutter, and ligament of Treitz.[19]

## Pathologic Features

The morphology and grade of peritoneal tumor deposits generally correlates with the appearance of the appendiceal tumor.[1] Peritoneal tumors associated with LAMN are composed of abundant mucin pools that contain scant strips of simple or focally proliferative epithelium with minimal to moderate cytologic atypia and no significant mitotic activity (Figure 19.8). Tumor cells and mucin pools dissect through hyalinized, fibrotic stroma unassociated with destructive invasion of underlying tissues. Peritoneal mucinous tumors with high-grade cytologic atypia usually arise from an appendiceal or intestinal mucinous adenocarcinoma. They display complex epithelial proliferations arranged as glands, nests, or individual cells and often show parenchymal organ invasion and lymph node metastases (Figure 19.9).[1,4,20] Some tumors show discordant histologic features in the appendiceal tumor compared to that of the peritoneum, and progression from low-grade to high-grade histology has been described in patients who fail treatment.[21,22]

## Prognosis

Long-term survival is significantly better for patients with low-grade peritoneal disease compared to those with overtly malignant cells in peritoneal mucin. Five- and ten-year survival rates are 75% and 68% for patients with low-grade epithelium in the peritoneal cavity but are substantially worse among patients with high-grade mucinous carcinoma in the peritoneal cavity (14% and 3%, respectively).[1] The biologic potential of low-grade tumors with foci of overtly malignant epithelium in the peritoneum is somewhat ambiguous. Some data suggest that tumors with these features are associated with a poor clinical outcome, whereas other reports describe a natural history comparable to that of low-grade tumors in the peritoneum.[3,20]

## Treatment

Surgical debulking was the mainstay of therapy for pseudomyxoma peritonei for decades, but this approach is limited by complications related to the procedure. Most patients with peritoneal

**FIGURE 19.8:** Pseudomyxoma peritonei associated with a low-grade peritoneal mucinous neoplasm shows abundant mucin dissecting through fibrotic or hyalinized tissue with relatively scant epithelium (**A**). Scant strips of cohesive low-grade mucinous epithelium are present in the peritoneal tumor (**B**).

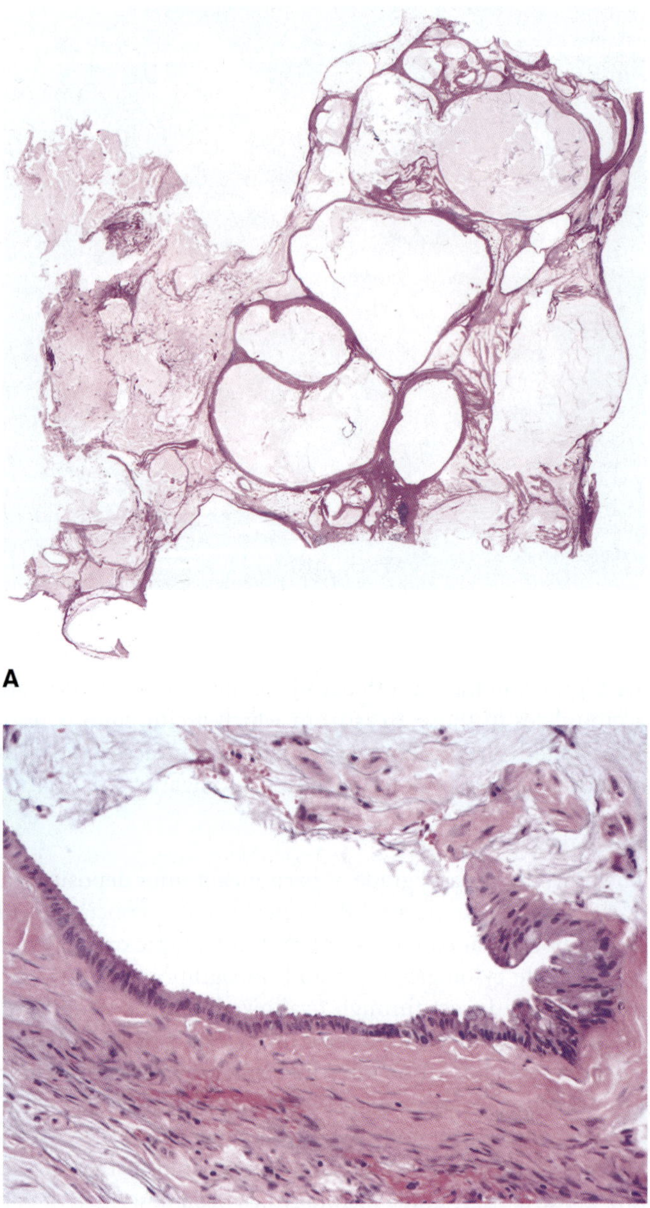

A

B

disease develop multiple tumor recurrences necessitating repetitive interventions that ultimately produce adhesions and complications that prohibit further surgical therapy.[23,24] Two-, five-, and ten-year survival rates for patients treated with serial debulking are approximately 86%, 60%, and 32%.[23–25] More aggressive approaches include a combination of peritonectomy with resection of multiple organs to achieve complete tumor cytoreduction with hyperthermic intraoperative intraperitoneal chemotherapy (HIPEC) supplemented by additional cycles of early postoperative intraperitoneal chemotherapy.[26–29] Potentially resectable organs include part or all of the stomach and/or colon, gallbladder, omentum, spleen, and affected small intestine. Women are also treated with hysterectomy and bilateral salpingo-oophorectomy. This aggressive approach achieves 5- and 10-year survival rates of 72% and 55%.[16] Patients with low-grade peritoneal tumors have improved survival following this aggressive approach relative to patients with

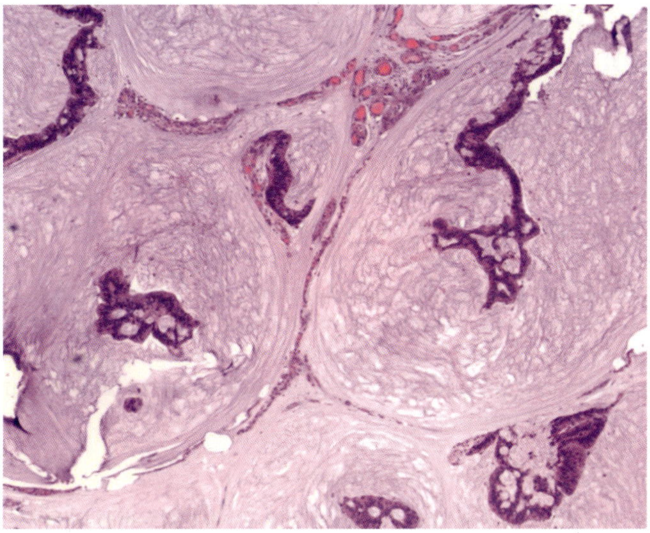

A

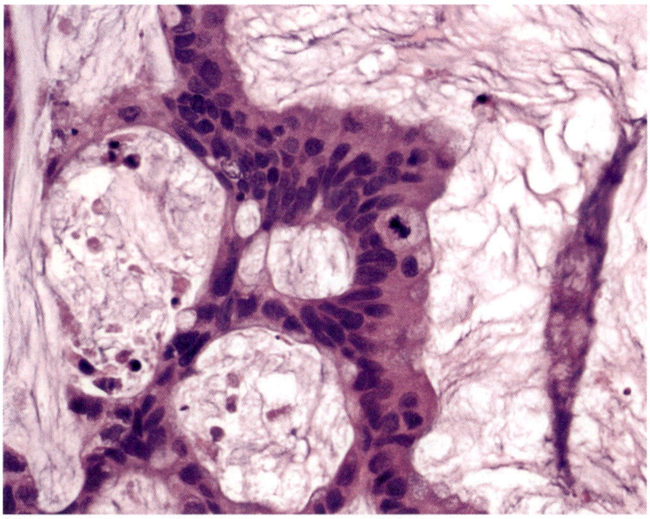

B

FIGURE 19.9: Peritoneal tumor deposits with high-grade cytologic features show abundant mucin similar to classic pseudomyxoma peritonei but contain more numerous groups of epithelial cells arranged in architecturally complex groups (**A**). The tumor cells display malignant cytologic features with enlarged hyperchromatic nuclei, mitotic figures, and cribriform architecture (**B**).

high-grade peritoneal disease. Low-grade tumors that are treated with cytoreductive surgery and chemotherapy are associated with 5-year survival rates of 86% compared to 50% for high-grade tumors, although emerging data suggest better outcomes among patients with high-grade disease.[27,30–32]

Although aggressive approaches show promise in the management of patients with pseudomyxoma peritonei, they are associated with high morbidity and mortality rates and are of questionable benefit in some situations, particularly since short-term survival rates are similar to those following less aggressive surgical debulking.[25,26,33] One critical factor that determines outcome following peritonectomy and HIPEC is whether complete cytoreduction is achieved.[26,32] Five- and ten-year survival rates of 87% and 74% are associated with complete cytoreduction but drop to 34% and 23% among patients in whom complete cytoreduction cannot be achieved.[32] Extensive involvement of the small bowel or its mesentery predicts a high likelihood of incomplete cytoreduction. Low-grade histology and experience of both the surgeon and surgical center are other factors that affect outcome.[27,31]

## ANCILLARY TESTING OF APPENDICEAL MUCINOUS NEOPLASMS AND PSEUDOMYXOMA PERITONEI

### Immunohistochemistry

Appendiceal mucinous neoplasms and pseudomyxoma peritonei usually express cytokeratin 20, and up to 40% coexpress cytokeratin 7.[34,35] Immunohistochemical staining for CDX2 and MUC2 are universal in appendiceal mucinous tumors and pseudomyxoma peritonei.[34–37] Most appendiceal adenomas are negative for MUC1, but adenocarcinomas may be positive and staining for MUC5AC and MUC6 is variable.[35] Immunohistochemical staining for p53 in adenomas is uncommon and limited to areas of severe atypia; however, up to 67% of cells in carcinomas stain for this marker, reflecting the presence of underlying mutations.[35] N-cadherin staining is increased in appendiceal mucinous tumors and pseudomyxoma peritonei, whereas E-cadherin staining is reduced in tumors relative to normal mucosa.[34]

### Molecular Alterations in Appendiceal Mucinous Neoplasms

Appendiceal adenomas and LAMN show frequent *KRAS* mutations and infrequent loss of chromosome 5q, but no loss of heterozygosity of *APC* or *DCC*.[38–41] Adenomas and LAMN do not show microsatellite instability or *BRAF* mutations.[40,42]

Appendiceal carcinomas commonly show allelic loss of chromosome 18q and less frequent mutations of *DPC4,* suggesting that tumor suppressor genes located on 18q play a role in their pathogenesis.[43] Approximately 50% of tumors harbor *KRAS* mutations.[44] These tumors lack *β-catenin* mutations and are microsatellite stable without immunohistochemical evidence of DNA mismatch repair protein deficiency.[43–45]

## SUMMARY AND CONCLUSIONS

Despite apparent controversies, appendiceal mucinous neoplasms pursue a predictable clinical course based on grade and stage. Tumors confined to the appendiceal mucosa are cured by excision and, thus, are appropriately classified as adenomas regardless of the degree of dysplasia present in the lesion. Mucinous neoplasms with acellular mucin in the appendiceal wall or limited to periappendiceal soft tissue are associated with an excellent prognosis. These cases can be managed similarly to appendiceal adenomas, provided the possibility of extraappendiceal epithelium is excluded and patients are clinically followed. Appendiceal mucinous tumors associated with neoplastic epithelium beyond the muscularis mucosae are potentially biologically aggressive and may be associated with progressive mucinous ascites. Once the presence of extraappendiceal epithelium is confirmed, pathologists must assign a histologic grade to the neoplastic cells, since surgical and chemotherapeutic management decisions may depend on the grade of peritoneal tumor deposits.

# References

1. Ronnett BM, Zahn CM, Kurman RJ, et al. Disseminated peritoneal adenomucinosis and peritoneal mucinous carcinomatosis. A clinicopathologic analysis of 109 cases with emphasis on distinguishing pathologic features, site of origin, prognosis, and relationship to "pseudomyxoma peritonei." *Am J Surg Pathol* 1995;19(12):1390–1408.
2. Carr NJ, McCarthy WF, Sobin LH. Epithelial noncarcinoid tumors and tumor-like lesions of the appendix. A clinicopathologic study of 184 patients with a multivariate analysis of prognostic factors. *Cancer* 1995;75(3):757–768.
3. Bradley RF, Stewart JHT, Russell GB, et al. Pseudomyxoma peritonei of appendiceal origin: a clinicopathologic analysis of 101 patients uniformly treated at a single institution, with literature review. *Am J Surg Pathol* 2006;30(5):551–559.

4. Misdraji J, Yantiss RK, Graeme-Cook FM, et al. Appendiceal mucinous neoplasms: a clinicopathologic analysis of 107 cases. *Am J Surg Pathol* 2003;27(8):1089–1103.
5. Pai RK, Longacre TA. Appendiceal mucinous tumors and pseudomyxoma peritonei: histologic features, diagnostic problems, and proposed classification. *Adv Anat Pathol* 2005;12(6):291–311.
6. Pai RK, Beck AH, Norton JA, et al. Appendiceal mucinous neoplasms: clinicopathologic study of 116 cases with analysis of factors predicting recurrence. *Am J Surg Pathol* 2009;33(10):1425–1439.
7. Carr NJ, Sobin LH. Tumors of the appendix. In: Bosman FT, Carneir F, Hruban RH, et al., eds. *WHO Classification of Tumours of the Digestive System*. 4th ed. Lyon, France: International Agency for Research on Cancer (IARC); 2010:122–125.
8. Qizilbash AH. Mucoceles of the appendix. Their relationship to hyperplastic polyps, mucinous cystadenomas, and cystadenocarcinomas. *Arch Pathol* 1975;99(10):548–555.
9. Higa E, Rosai J, Pizzimbono CA, et al. Mucosal hyperplasia, mucinous cystadenoma, and mucinous cystadenocarcinoma of the appendix. A re-evaluation of appendiceal "mucocele." *Cancer* 1973;32(6):1525–1541.
10. Appelman HD. Epithelial neoplasia of the appendix. In: Norris HT, ed. *Pathology of the Colon, Small Intestine, and Anus*. New York, NY: Churchill Livingstone; 1991:263–303.
11. Carr NJ, Sobin LH. Unusual tumors of the appendix and pseudomyxoma peritonei. *Semin Diagn Pathol* 1996;13(4):314–325.
12. Parsons J, Gray GF, Thorbjarnarson B. Pseudomyxoma peritonei. *Arch Surg* 1970;101(5):545–549.
13. Appendix. In: Edge S, Byrd D, Compton CC, et al., eds. *AJCC Cancer Staging Manual*. 7th ed. New York, NY: Springer; 2009:133–141.
14. Prayson RA, Hart WR, Petras RE. Pseudomyxoma peritonei. A clinicopathologic study of 19 cases with emphasis on site of origin and nature of associated ovarian tumors. *Am J Surg Pathol* 1994;18(6):591–603.
15. Yantiss RK, Shia J, Klimstra DS, et al. Prognostic significance of localized extra-appendiceal mucin deposition in appendiceal mucinous neoplasms. *Am J Surg Pathol* 1009;33:248–255.
16. Gonzalez-Moreno S, Sugarbaker PH. Right hemicolectomy does not confer a survival advantage in patients with mucinous carcinoma of the appendix and peritoneal seeding. *Br J Surg* 2004;91(3): 304–311.
17. Foster JM, Gupta PK, Carreau JH, et al. Right hemicolectomy is not routinely indicated in pseudomyxoma peritonei. *Am Surg* [Comparative Study] 2012;78(2):171–177.
18. Smeenk RM, van Velthuysen ML, Verwaal VJ, et al. Appendiceal neoplasms and pseudomyxoma peritonei: a population based study. *Eur J Surg Oncol* 2008;34(2):196–201.
19. Sugarbaker PH. Pseudomyxoma peritonei. A cancer whose biology is characterized by a redistribution phenomenon. *Ann Surg* [Comment Editorial] 1994;219(2):109–111.
20. Ronnett BM, Yan H, Kurman RJ, et al. Patients with pseudomyxoma peritonei associated with disseminated peritoneal adenomucinosis have a significantly more favorable prognosis than patients with peritoneal mucinous carcinomatosis. *Cancer* 2001;92:85–91.
21. Yan H, Pestieau SR, Shmookler BM, et al. Histopathologic analysis in 46 patients with pseudomyxoma peritonei syndrome: failure versus success with a second-look operation [Evaluation Studies]. *Mod Pathol* 2001;14(3):164–171.
22. Chua TC, Al-Zahrani A, Saxena A, et al. Secondary cytoreduction and perioperative intraperitoneal chemotherapy after initial debulking of pseudomyxoma peritonei: a study of timing and the impact of malignant dedifferentiation. *J Am Coll Surg* 2010;211(4):526–535.
23. Gough DB, Donohue JH, Schutt AJ, et al. Pseudomyxoma peritonei. Long-term patient survival with an aggressive regional approach. *Ann Surg* 1994;219(2):112–119.
24. Miner TJ, Shia J, Jaques DP, et al. Long-term survival following treatment of pseudomyxoma peritonei: an analysis of surgical therapy. *Ann Surg* 2005;241(2):300–308.
25. Jarvinen P, Jarvinen HJ, Lepisto A. Survival of patients with pseudomyxoma peritonei treated by serial debulking. *Colorectal Dis* 2010;12(9):868–872.
26. Moran B, Baratti D, Yan TD, et al. Consensus statement on the loco-regional treatment of appendiceal mucinous neoplasms with peritoneal dissemination (pseudomyxoma peritonei). *J Surg Oncol* [Review] 2008;98(4):277–282.
27. Elias D, Gilly F, Quenet F, et al. Pseudomyxoma peritonei: a French multicentric study of 301 patients treated with cytoreductive surgery and intraperitoneal chemotherapy. *Eur J Surg Oncol* [Multicenter Study] 2010;36(5):456–462.
28. Sugarbaker PH, Jablonski KA. Prognostic features of 51 colorectal and 130 appendiceal cancer patients with peritoneal carcinomatosis treated by cytoreductive surgery and intraperitoneal chemotherapy. *Ann Surg* [Clinical Trial Clinical Trial, Phase II Comparative Study Multicenter Study] 1995;221(2):124–132.

29. Sugarbaker PH, Zhu BW, Sese GB, et al. Peritoneal carcinomatosis from appendiceal cancer: results in 69 patients treated by cytoreductive surgery and intraperitoneal chemotherapy. *Dis Colon Rectum* 1993;36(4):323–329.
30. Sugarbaker PH, Chang D. Results of treatment of 385 patients with peritoneal surface spread of appendiceal malignancy. *Ann Surg Oncol* 1999;6(8):727–731.
31. Smeenk RM, Verwaal VJ, Antonini N, et al. Survival analysis of pseudomyxoma peritonei patients treated by cytoreductive surgery and hyperthermic intraperitoneal chemotherapy. *Ann Surg* 2007;245(1): 104–109.
32. Youssef H, Newman C, Chandrakumaran K, et al. Operative findings, early complications, and long-term survival in 456 patients with pseudomyxoma peritonei syndrome of appendiceal origin. *Dis Colon Rectum* 2011;54(3):293–299.
33. Schomas DA, Miller RC, Donohue JH, et al. Intraperitoneal treatment for peritoneal mucinous carcinomatosis of appendiceal origin after operative management: long-term follow-up of the Mayo Clinic experience. *Ann Surg* 2009;249(4):588–595.
34. Bibi R, Pranesh N, Saunders MP, et al. A specific cadherin phenotype may characterise the disseminating yet non-metastatic behaviour of pseudomyxoma peritonei. *Br J Cancer* [Research Support, Non-U.S. Gov't] 2006;95(9):1258–1264.
35. Yajima N, Wada R, Yamagishi S, et al. Immunohistochemical expressions of cytokeratins, mucin core proteins, p53, and neuroendocrine cell markers in epithelial neoplasm of appendix. *Hum Pathol* [Historical Article] 2005;36(11):1217–1225.
36. O'Connell JT, Hacker CM, Barsky SH. MUC2 is a molecular marker for pseudomyxoma peritonei [Comparative Study Research Support, Non-U.S. Gov't]. *Mod Pathol* 2002;15(9):958–972.
37. Nonaka D, Kusamura S, Baratti D, et al. CDX-2 expression in pseudomyxoma peritonei: a clinicopathological study of 42 cases. *Histopathology* 2006;49(4):381–387.
38. Szych C, Staebler A, Connolly DC, et al. Molecular genetic evidence supporting the clonality and appendiceal origin of Pseudomyxoma peritonei in women. *Am J Pathol* 1999;154(6):1849–1855.
39. Cuatrecasas M, Matias-Guiu X, Prat J. Synchronous mucinous tumors of the appendix and the ovary associated with pseudomyxoma peritonei. A clinicopathologic study of six cases with comparative analysis of c-Ki-ras mutations. *Am J Surg Pathol* [Case Reports Comparative Study Research Support, Non-U.S. Gov't] 1996;20(6):739–746.
40. Zauber P, Berman E, Marotta S, et al. Ki-ras gene mutations are invariably present in low-grade mucinous tumors of the vermiform appendix. *Scand J Gastroenterol* [Research Support, Non-U.S. Gov't] 2011;46(7–8):869–874.
41. Chuaqui RF, Zhuang Z, Emmert-Buck MR, et al. Genetic analysis of synchronous mucinous tumors of the ovary and appendix. *Hum Pathol* 1996;27(2):165–171.
42. Yantiss RK, Panczykowski A, Misdraji J, et al. A comprehensive study of nondysplastic and dysplastic serrated polyps of the vermiform appendix. *Am J Surg Pathol* [Comparative Study] 2007;31(11): 1742–1753.
43. Maru D, Wu TT, Canada A, et al. Loss of chromosome 18q and DPC4 (Smad4) mutations in appendiceal adenocarcinomas. *Oncogene* 2004;23(3):859–864.
44. Kabbani W, Houlihan PS, Luthra R, et al. Mucinous and nonmucinous appendiceal adenocarcinomas: different clinicopathological features but similar genetic alterations. *Mod Pathol* 2002;15(6):599–605.
45. Misdraji J, Burgart LJ, Lauwers GY. Defective mismatch repair in the pathogenesis of low-grade appendiceal mucinous neoplasms and adenocarcinomas. *Mod Pathol* [Comparative Study] 2004;17(12):14471454.

# Nonmucinous Epithelial Tumors of the Appendix

# 20

Rhonda K. Yantiss

The vast majority of clinically important appendices epithelial neoplasms are mucinous tumors, as discussed in Chapter 19, whereas nonmucinous neoplasms are less frequent. These tumors generally simulate their colonic counterparts in that they display tubular, villous, or serrated crypt architecture. Most nonmucinous neoplasms are detected in appendectomy specimens obtained for presumed appendicitis or in appendices removed during procedures performed for other reasons. Invasive nonmucinous adenocarcinomas are even more rare, and their clinicopathologic features and biologic potential are not well described. Most arise in association with precursor lesions, such as goblet cell carcinoid tumors and serrated neoplasms. Their pathologic stage groupings essentially mirror those of colorectal neoplasms.

## COLONIC-TYPE ADENOMAS

### Clinical Features

Colonic-type adenomas are the least common type of epithelial neoplasm in the appendix. Appendiceal adenomatous polyps are typically asymptomatic. Virtually all of them are identified in prophylactic colectomy specimens from patients with familial polyposis, although rare sporadic lesions are occasionally encountered. Thus, they show an equal predilection for males and females and occur in pediatric patients as well as adults.[1] Cancer development occurs in less than 20% of appendiceal adenomas, probably reflecting the relatively small size of these lesions.[2,3]

### Pathologic Features

Colonic-type adenomas of the proximal appendix likely represent extension of sessile colonic polyps into the appendiceal orifice. Lesions that develop in the appendix appear as polypoid projections that protrude into the lumen (Figure 20.1). Unlike appendiceal mucinous neoplasms, they do not circumferentially involve the mucosa but are sharply demarcated from adjacent non-neoplastic mucosa. They resemble their colonic counterparts and contain crowded, tubular crypts lined by overtly dysplastic epithelial cells with elongated, hyperchromatic nuclei (Figure 20.2).

## SERRATED LESIONS OF THE APPENDIX

### Clinical Features

Serrated appendiceal polyps tend to develop in older adults and show an equal sex distribution.[4,5] *In situ* lesions are asymptomatic and incidentally detected in appendices removed for other reasons, including colon cancers, and thus, early evidence pointed toward a strong relationship between serrated appendiceal lesions and colon cancer. Indeed, retrospective data suggested that nearly 50% of serrated appendiceal neoplasms occurred in patients with proximal colonic carcinomas.[6] However, recent reports have shown that serrated appendiceal neoplasms are more commonly observed in resection specimens obtained for medical reasons, such as appendicitis, enterocolitis, or indications unrelated to the gastrointestinal tract.[4,5]

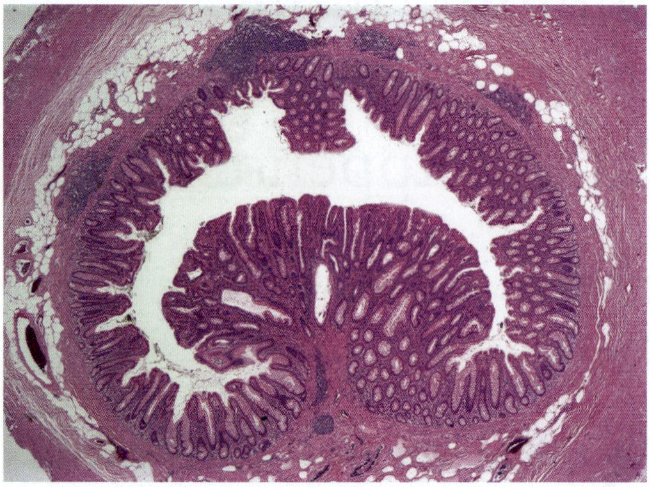

FIGURE 20.1: A sporadic colonic-type adenoma in the appendix has a polypoid appearance and is sharply demarcated from the adjacent nonneoplastic epithelium. (Photograph Courtesy of Dr. Henry Appelman, University of Michigan, Ann Arbor, MI.)

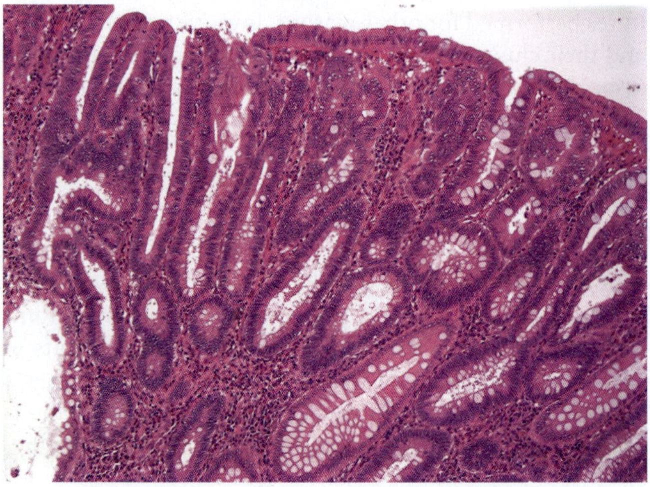

FIGURE 20.2: A sporadic colonic-type adenoma of the appendix contains crypts lined by neoplastic cells with elongated, hyperchromatic nuclei similar to its counterpart in the colorectum. (Photograph Courtesy of Dr. Henry Appelman, University of Michigan, Ann Arbor, MI.)

## Pathologic Features

Serrated appendiceal neoplasms show a spectrum of morphologic features similar to serrated colorectal polyps. Most lack dysplasia and resemble colonic hyperplastic polyps or sessile serrated polyps. Hyperplastic polyps typically protrude into the lumen and appear as plaque-like excrescences but do not involve the entire luminal circumference (Figure 20.3). They contain serrated crypts and mucinous epithelial cells similar to "microvesicular" hyperplastic polyps of the colorectum (Figure 20.4). Sessile serrated polyps circumferentially involve the appendiceal mucosa (Figure 20.5). These lesions contain elongated, somewhat dilated, serrated crypts with lateral branching, dystrophic goblet cells, and mild cytologic atypia (Figure 20.6).

Dysplastic serrated polyps of the appendix are classified as either serrated adenomas or sessile serrated polyps with dysplasia. Serrated adenomas contain serrated crypts lined by cells with abundant eosinophilic cytoplasm and pencillate nuclei (Figure 20.7). Sessile serrated polyps with dysplasia may harbor nondysplastic areas that resemble hyperplastic polyp or sessile serrated polyp intimately admixed with overtly dysplastic crypts that display a tubular, villous, or serrated appearance. Less frequently, sessile serrated polyps with dysplasia contain dilated, laterally branched crypts lined by dysplastic epithelium (Figure 20.8).

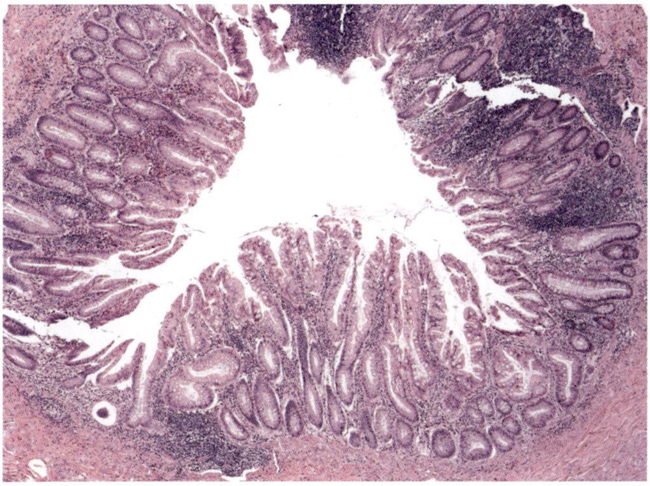

FIGURE 20.3: A hyperplastic polyp protrudes into the lumen of the appendix.

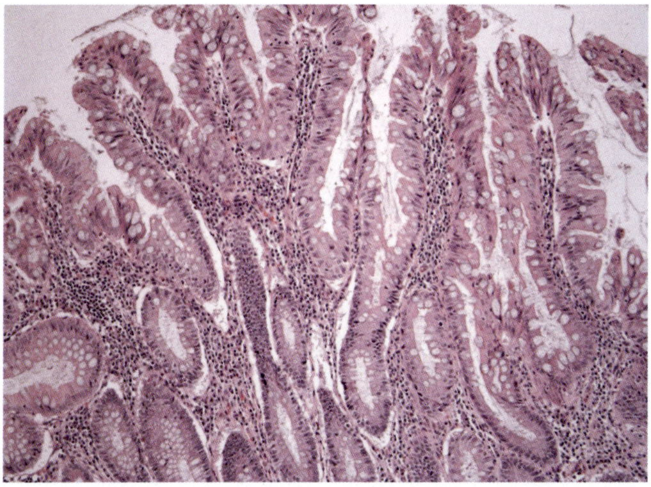

FIGURE 20.4: Hyperplastic appendiceal polyps contain serrated crypts lined by goblet and nongoblet mucinous epithelial cells, similar to colonic microvesicular polyps.

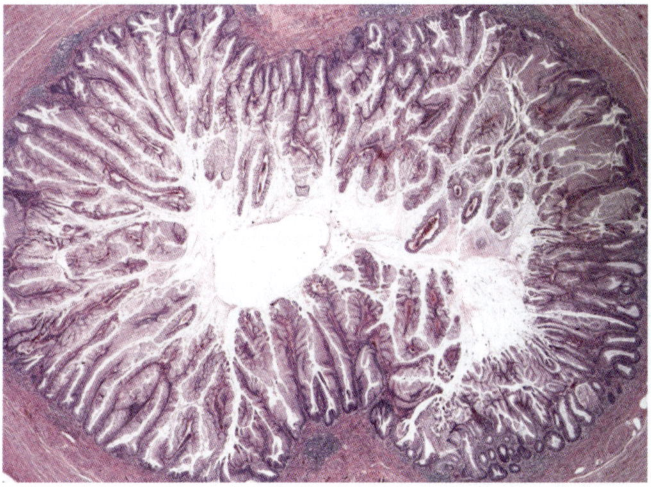

FIGURE 20.5: Sessile serrated polyps circumferentially involve the mucosa of the appendix. Dilated, elongated crypts expand the mucosa.

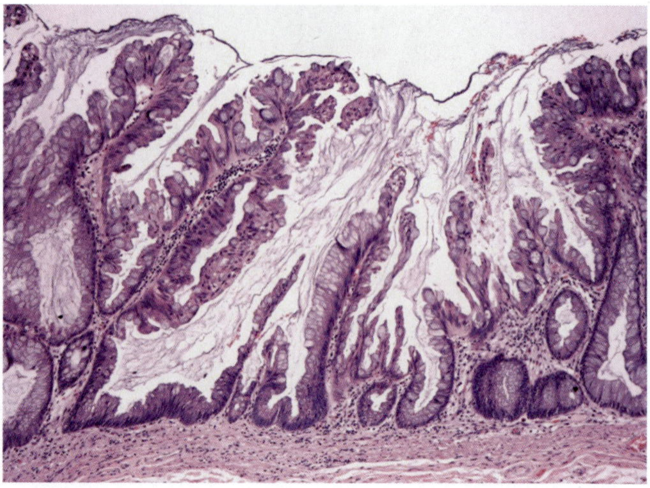

FIGURE 20.6: This sessile serrated polyp of the appendix contains distended crypts, some of which show branching above the muscularis mucosae.

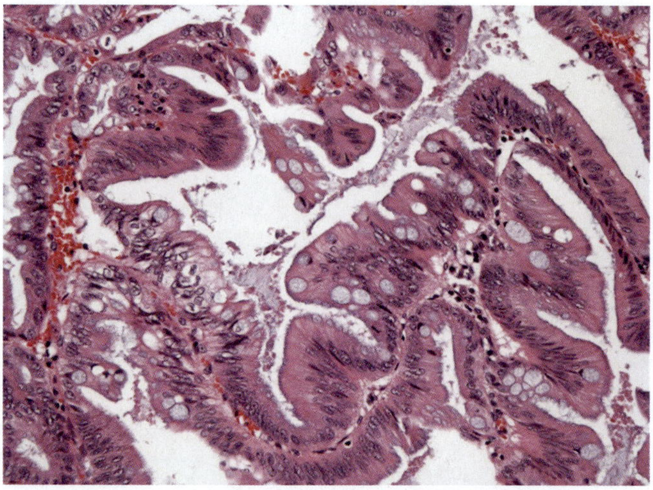

FIGURE 20.7: Serrated adenomas of the appendix contain serrated crypts lined by cells with abundant eosinophilic cytoplasm and pencillate nuclei.

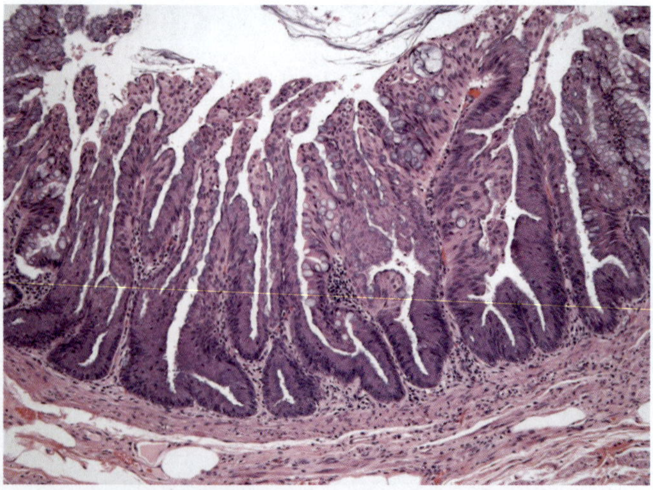

FIGURE 20.8: Sessile serrated polyps with dysplasia contain elongated, dilated crypts that show budding and branching in the deep mucosa. The cells lining the crypts are overtly dysplastic with enlarged, hyperchromatic nuclei.

## Immunohistochemical and Molecular Features

Sessile serrated polyps of the appendix are positive for MUC6 and display asymmetric Ki-67 labeling of crypt epithelial cells.[7] Similar to nondysplastic serrated polyps of the colon, appendiceal lesions may show partial loss of DNA repair protein expression, including MGMT and MLH1, but this finding reflects the nonproliferative nature of superficial serrated epithelium and does not correlate with detectable MSI.[5] Mutually exclusive *BRAF* and *KRAS* mutations occur in the majority of cases. Approximately one-half of appendiceal sessile serrated polyps harbor *BRAF* mutations and one-fifth have *KRAS* mutations, whereas *BRAF* mutations are far more common (>80%) among nondysplastic serrated polyps of the colon.

## Natural History

Invasive adenocarcinomas that develop in association with serrated neoplasms typically produce symptoms only when they penetrate the visceral peritoneum, thereby simulating symptoms of acute appendicitis.[8] As a result, most appendiceal carcinomas are locally advanced at the time of diagnosis. They show a destructive growth pattern and overtly malignant cytologic features characteristic of cancers of the lower gastrointestinal tract (Figure 20.9). These cancers may contain abundant extracellular mucin, but peritoneal disease is in the form of solid tumor nodules, or carcinomatosis, and pursues a uniformly aggressive course (Figure 20.10).

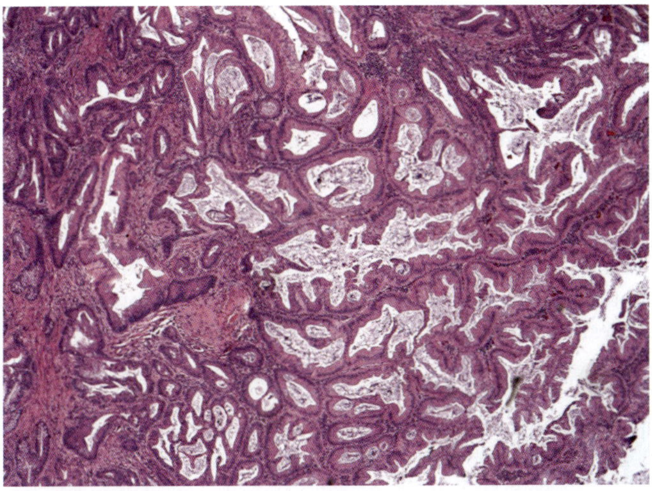

**FIGURE 20.9:** Invasive appendiceal adenocarcinoma derived from a serrated adenoma of the appendix consists of glands with a serrated architecture juxtaposed to single cells enmeshed in desmoplastic stroma.

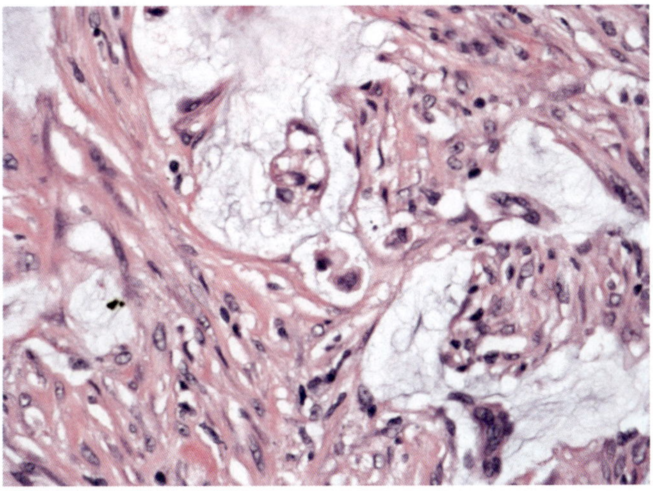

**FIGURE 20.10:** Appendiceal carcinomas are often locally advanced at the time of diagnosis and may spread to the peritoneal surfaces in the form of tumor implants. Although the tumor cells are associated with extracellular mucinous material, the cells are overtly malignant with high-grade cytologic features and poor gland formation. This growth pattern is associated with a poor prognosis.

# GOBLET CELL CARCINOID TUMOR (CRYPT CELL CARCINOMA)

## Clinical Features

Goblet cell carcinoid tumors occur in middle-aged adults and demonstrate a near equal sex distribution. Most tumors are discovered in appendices removed for indications of acute appendicitis, and the diagnosis is rarely suspected at the time of surgery. However, goblet cell carcinomas have a propensity to give rise to overtly malignant invasive adenocarcinomas, nearly half of which cause symptoms related to an abdominal or pelvic mass.[9] Female patients typically come to clinical attention owing to the presence of ovarian metastases.[10]

## Pathologic Features

Goblet cell carcinoid tumors are unique to the vermiform appendix. These uncommon neoplasms display features of both endocrine and epithelial differentiation and show a propensity to dedifferentiate to overtly malignant invasive adenocarcinomas with successive recurrences.[11] They occur in any region of the appendix, typically resulting in ill-defined mural thickening that is difficult to appreciate prior to histologic examination of the appendix.[12] Similar to classic carcinoid tumors, they may involve the deep mucosa but are not associated with dysplasia of the surface epithelium. Tumor cells in the mucosa are arranged in round solid cell clusters that resemble colonic crypts (Figure 20.11). These neoplasms grow as nests, cords, and clusters circumferentially arranged in the appendiceal wall, where they induce a densely collagenous stroma, but do not form a discreet mass or elicit a desmoplastic tissue reaction (Figure 20.12). Goblet cell carcinoid tumors display mild cytologic atypia and contain numerous cells distended with cytoplasmic mucin. The lesional cells contain small, crescentic nuclei with inconspicuous nucleoli and monotonous nuclear features (Figure 20.13).

More than half of goblet cell carcinoid tumors contain carcinomatous elements, and thus, the entire appendix should be submitted for evaluation if only goblet cell carcinoid tumor is identified in initial sections. Overtly malignant areas are usually of signet ring cell type, although mucinous, intestinal, and poorly differentiated areas may also be observed (Figure 20.14). Single infiltrating cells, loss of mucin production, or detection of overt adenocarcinomatous elements should prompt concern for a more aggressive lesion.

## Pathologic Reporting of Goblet Cell Carcinoid Tumors

Goblet cell carcinoid tumors are classified as well-differentiated, low-grade malignancies with potential to metastasize to the peritoneum, similar to other types of appendiceal carcinoma.[13] However,

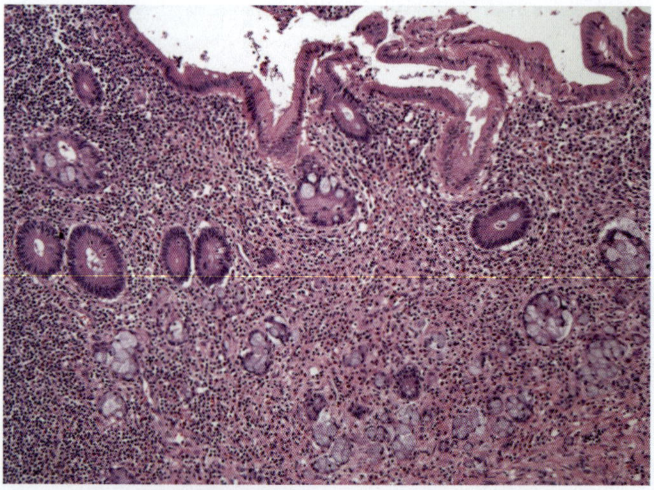

**FIGURE 20.11:** Goblet cell carcinoid tumors consist of round tumor cell nests that simulate the appearance of colonic crypts. These lesions are unassociated with surface dysplasia.

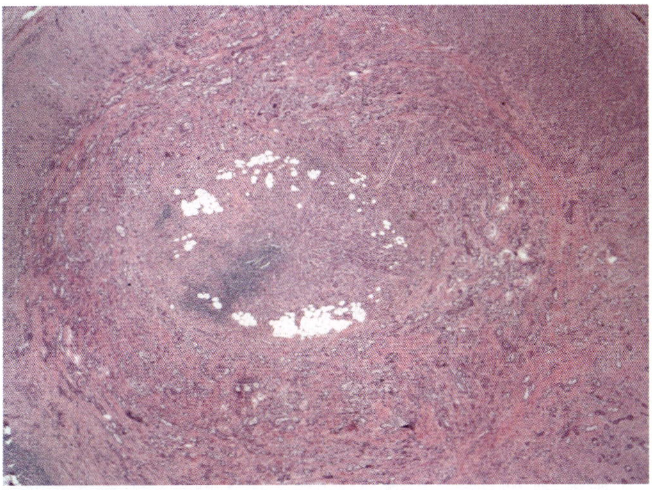

FIGURE 20.12: Goblet cell carcinoid tumors grow in a circumferential fashion within the appendiceal wall. The tumor cells are associated with densely collagenous stroma, but desmoplasia is lacking.

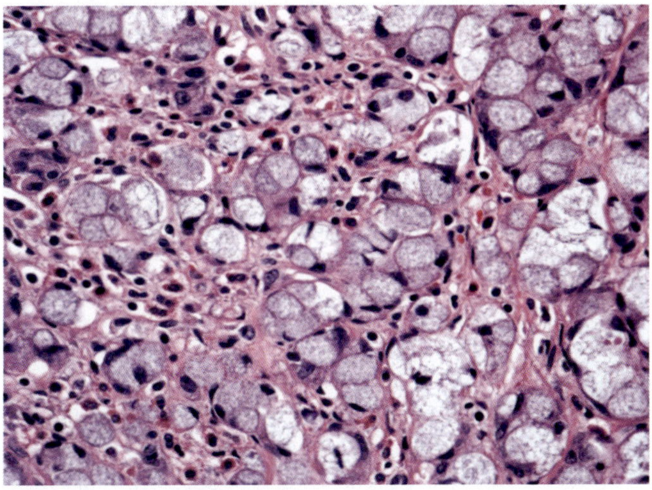

FIGURE 20.13: Goblet cell carcinoid tumors contain rounded nests of tumor cells that harbor large cytoplasmic mucin vacuoles and eccentrically placed bland nuclei.

more than half of these lesions are associated with foci of overtly malignant invasive carcinomas that are frequently associated with disseminated disease and pursue an aggressive clinical course.[14] Both the World Health Organization and American Joint Committee on Cancer classify and stage goblet cell carcinoid tumors as adenocarcinomas, regardless of the presence or absence of high-grade elements.[15,16] Criteria for staging of (neuro)endocrine neoplasms should not be applied to these lesions.

Additional features to note in the surgical pathology report include tumor size and extent of invasion, status of the resection margin, and presence of lymphovascular invasion. Goblet cell carcinoid tumors commonly show neurotropism, but this feature does not appear to be clinically important. Notably the entire appendix should be submitted for histologic evaluation if initial sections demonstrate only the presence of a goblet cell carcinoid tumor, in order to exclude the presence of an overtly malignant component. One may also consider including a comment in pathology reports indicating to clinicians that, despite the terminology, goblet cell carcinoid tumors are more aggressive than classic carcinoid tumors.

## Immunohistochemical, Histochemical, and Molecular Features

Goblet cell carcinoid tumors show divergent differentiation with patchy immunopositivity for endocrine markers as well as evidence of secretory cell differentiation with strong mucicarmine positivity (Figure 20.15). They also express CK20 and CEA similar to colonic adenocarcinomas

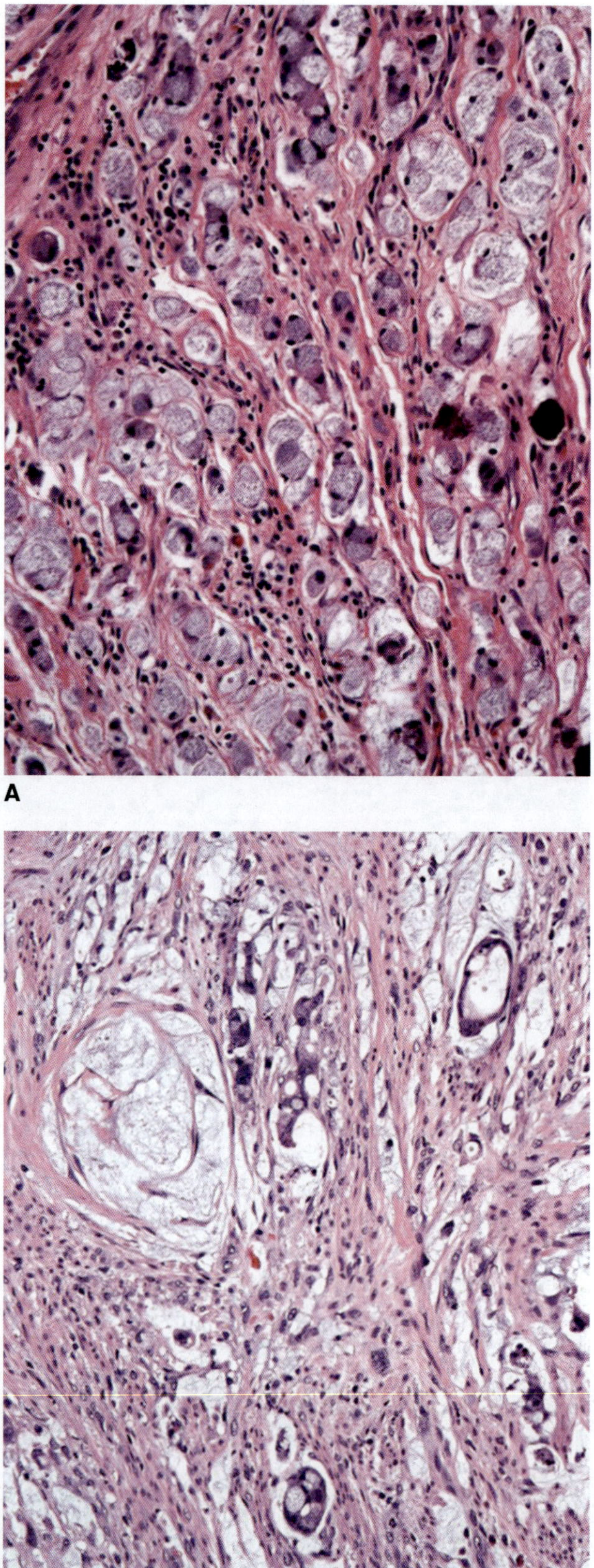

A

B

**FIGURE 20.14:** Goblet cell carcinoid tumors frequently contain foci of invasive carcinoma. Single infiltrating signet ring cells are most commonly encountered (**A**). A mucinous growth pattern with clusters of cells in extracellular mucin pools is not uncommon (**B**).

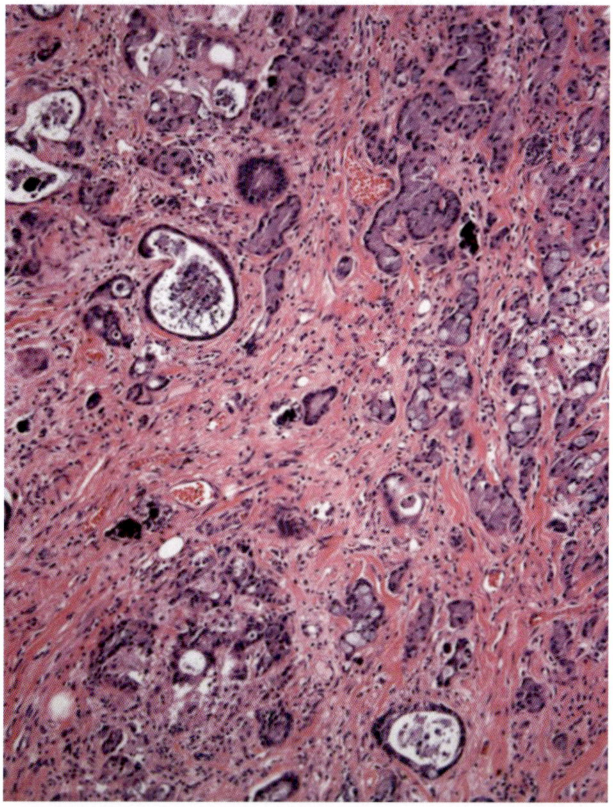

**C**

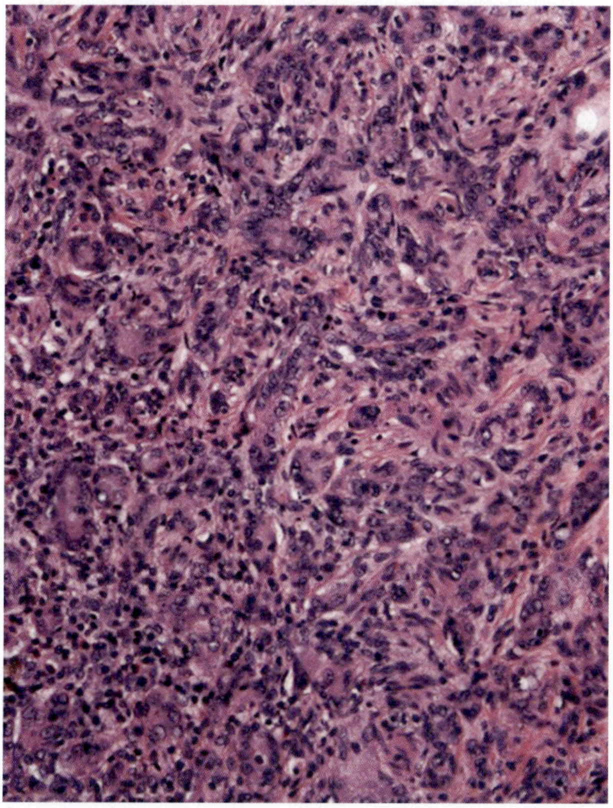

**D**

FIGURE 20.14: (*Continued*) Goblet cell carcinoid infrequently contain intestinal-type glands (**C**) and poorly differentiated areas may be encountered (**D**).

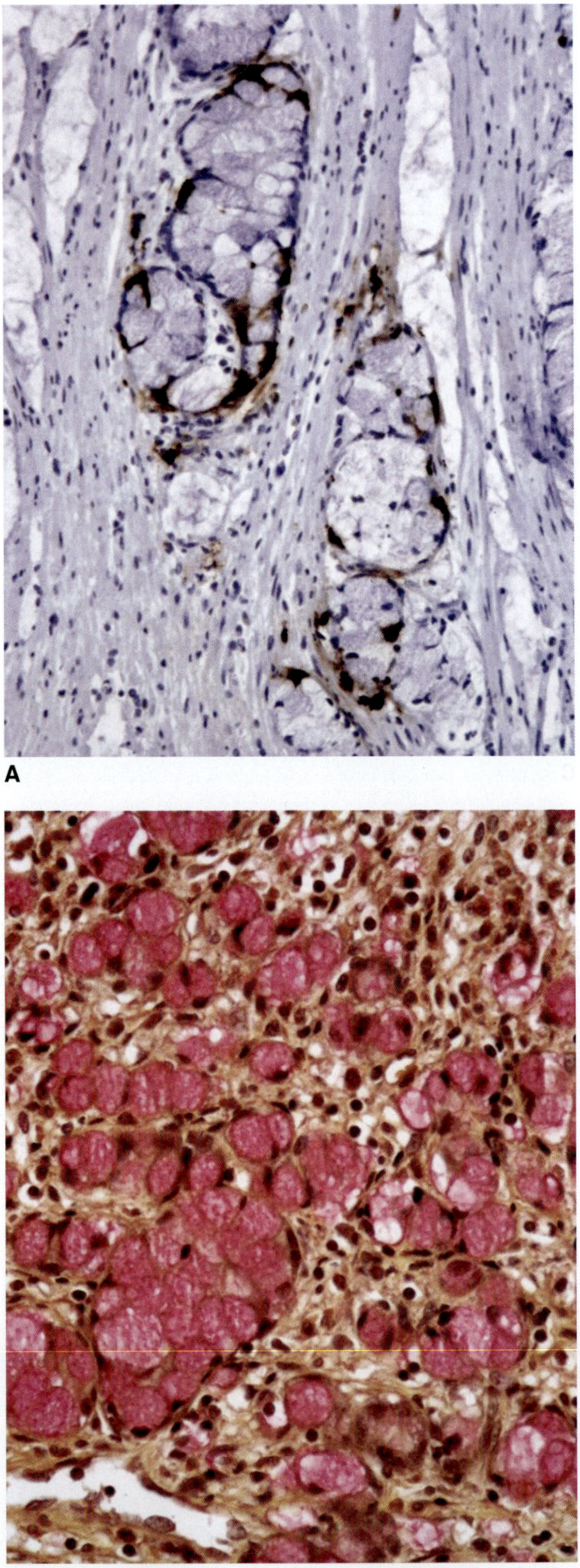


**FIGURE 20.15:** Immunohistochemical stains demonstrate patchy chromogranin positivity among tumor cells (**A**). The tumor shows strong, diffuse mucicarmine staining (**B**).

but display a relatively low Ki-67 proliferation index.[17] Carcinomas derived from goblet cell carcinoid tumors lack molecular alterations typical of malignancies of the lower gastrointestinal tract in that they do not show *KRAS* or *DPC4* mutations, abnormalities in β-catenin, or alterations affecting TP53.[18]

### Natural History

Early evidence suggested that goblet cell carcinoid tumors may pursue a benign clinical course, although more recent data suggest they are more aggressive than other (neuro)endocrine tumors of the appendix.[12] Most invade deeply into the wall and penetrate the serosa, and a substantial number of cases are associated with regional lymph node metastases as well as peritoneal and/or ovarian deposits. Tumors that spread beyond the appendix often contain overtly carcinomatous elements, in which case the natural history is dictated by the tumor grade and stage, similar to carcinomas of other organs. These overtly malignant tumors are commonly associated with regional lymph node and distant metastases, as well as decreased survival. For these reasons, goblet cell carcinoid has been labeled with a variety of terms, including adenocarcinoid tumor, mucinous carcinoid tumor, crypt cell carcinoma, microglandular carcinoma, and mixed adenocarcinoma–carcinoid tumor of the appendix.[19]

Goblet cell carcinoid tumors are commonly detected in appendectomy specimens obtained for other indications, in which case appropriate subsequent management strategies are somewhat controversial. Most investigators consider appendectomy alone to be inadequate therapy because of their relatively high propensity to metastasize.[20,21] Surgical management generally consists of right colectomy with lymph node staging.

## SUMMARY AND CONCLUSIONS

Most nonmucinous carcinomas of the appendix are derived from serrated appendiceal neoplasms and goblet cell carcinoid tumors. Serrated appendiceal polyps resemble their colonic counterparts and may be nondysplastic (hyperplastic polyp and sessile serrated polyp) or dysplastic (serrated adenoma and sessile serrated polyp with dysplasia). They show either *BRAF* or *KRAS* mutations, and some cancers derived from them display MSI, indicating that appendiceal serrated lesions share some elements of the serrated neoplastic pathway of colorectal carcinogenesis. Goblet cell carcinoid tumors have been increasingly recognized as a distinct clinicopathologic entity with secretory and endocrine differentiation. These lesions are now recognized and classified as adenocarcinomas, rather than endocrine tumors, because they behave in a more aggressive fashion than classic endocrine (carcinoid) tumors of the appendix. They frequently give rise to overtly malignant carcinomas that behave in a grade- and stage-dependent fashion.

# References

1. Carr NJ, McCarthy WF, Sobin LH. Epithelial noncarcinoid tumors and tumor-like lesions of the appendix. A clinicopathologic study of 184 patients with a multivariate analysis of prognostic factors. *Cancer* 1995;75(3):757–768.
2. Maisel B, Foot NC. Multiple polyposis of the colon with malignant change involving colon and appendix: case report. *Ann Surg* 1947;126(3):262–269.
3. Collins DC. 71,000 human appendix specimens. A final report, summarizing forty years' study. *Am J Proctol* 1963;14:265–281.
4. Renshaw AA, Kish R, Gould EW. Sessile serrated adenoma is associated with acute appendicitis in patients 30 years or older. *Am J Clin Pathol* 2006;126(6):875–877.
5. Yantiss RK, Panczykowski A, Misdraji J, et al. A comprehensive study of nondysplastic and dysplastic serrated polyps of the vermiform appendix. *Am J Surg Pathol* 2007;31(11):1742–1753.

6. Younes M, Katikaneni PR, Lechago J. Association between mucosal hyperplasia of the appendix and adenocarcinoma of the colon. *Histopathology* 1995;26(1):33–37.
7. Bellizzi AM, Rock J, Marsh WL, et al. Serrated lesions of the appendix: a morphologic and immunohistochemical appraisal. *Am J Clin Pathol* 2010;133(4):623–632.
8. Rubio CA. Serrated adenomas of the appendix. *J Clin Pathol* 2004;57(9):946–949.
9. Butler JA, Houshiar A, Lin F, et al. Goblet cell carcinoid of the appendix. *Am J Surg* 1994;168(6): 685–687.
10. Hristov AC, Young RH, Vang R, et al. Ovarian metastases of appendiceal tumors with goblet cell carcinoidlike and signet ring cell patterns: a report of 30 cases. *Am J Surg Pathol* 2007;31(10):1502–1511.
11. Carr NJ, Sobin LH. Neuroendocrine tumors of the appendix. *Semin Diagn Pathol* 2004;21(2):108–119.
12. Burke AP, Sobin LH, Federspiel BH, et al. Goblet cell carcinoids and related tumors of the vermiform appendix. *Am J Clin Pathol* 1990;94(1):27–35.
13. McCusker ME, Cote TR, Clegg LX, et al. Primary malignant neoplasms of the appendix: a population-based study from the surveillance, epidemiology and end-results program, 1973–1998. *Cancer* 2002;94(12):3307–3312.
14. Lin BT, Gown AM. Mixed carcinoid and adenocarcinoma of the appendix: report of 4 cases with immunohistochemical studies and a review of the literature. *Appl Immunohistochem Mol Morphol* 2004;12(3):271–276.
15. Appendix. In: Edge S, Byrd D, Compton CC, et al., eds. *AJCC Cancer Staging Manual.* 7th ed. New York, NY: Springer; 2009:133–141.
16. Komminoth P, Arnold R, Capella C, et al. Tumors of the appendix. In: Bosman FT, Carneir F, Hruban RH, et al., eds. *WHO Classification of Tumours of the Digestive System.* 4th ed. Lyon, France: International Agency for Research on Cancer (IARC); 2010:126–128.
17. Li CC, Hirowaka M, Qian ZR, et al. Expression of E-cadherin, b-catenin, and Ki-67 in goblet cell carcinoids of the appendix: an immunohistochemical study with clinical correlation. *Endocr Pathol* 2002;13(1):47–58.
18. Stancu M, Wu TT, Wallace C, et al. Genetic alterations in goblet cell carcinoids of the vermiform appendix and comparison with gastrointestinal carcinoid tumors. *Mod Pathol* 2003;16(12):1189–1198.
19. Tang LH, Shia J, Soslow RA, et al. Pathologic classification and clinical behavior of the spectrum of goblet cell carcinoid tumors of the appendix. *Am J Surg Pathol* 2008;32(10):1429–1443.
20. Maes M, Segers K, Cheyns P. Goblet cell carcinoid of the appendix: laparoscopic appendectomy or right hemicolectomy? *Acta Chir Belg* 2008;108(4):447–450.
21. Palanivelu C, Rangarajan M, Annapoorni S, et al. Laparoscopic right hemicolectomy for goblet-cell carcinoid of the appendix: report of a rare case and literature survey. *J Laparoendosc Adv Surg Tech* 2008;18(3):417–421.

# Index

Note: Page numbers followed by *f* indicate figures; those followed by *t* indicate tables.